Cardiac Anesthesia

Editor

COLLEEN G. KOCH

ANESTHESIOLOGY CLINICS

www.anesthesiology.theclinics.com

Consulting Editor
LEE A. FLEISHER

June 2013 • Volume 31 • Number 2

ELSEVIER

1600 John F. Kennedy Boulevard • Suite 1800 • Philadelphia, Pennsylvania, 19103-2899

http://www.theclinics.com

ANESTHESIOLOGY CLINICS Volume 31, Number 2
June 2013 ISSN 1932-2275, ISBN-13: 978-1-4557-7065-6

Editor: Pamela Hetherington

Anesthesiology Clinics (ISSN 1932-2275) is published quarterly by Elsevier Inc., 360 Park Avenue South, New York, NY 10010-1710. Months of issue are March, June, September, and December. Periodicals postage paid at New York, NY and at additional mailing offices. Subscription prices are $154.00 per year (US student/resident), $313.00 per year (US individuals), $383.00 per year (Canadian individuals), $516.00 per year (US institutions), $639.00 per year (Canadian institutions), $216.00 per year (Canadian and foreign student/resident), $434.00 per year (foreign individuals), and $639.00 per year (foreign institutions). To receive student and resident rate, orders must be accompanied by name of affiliated institution, date of term, and the *signature* of program/residency coordinator on institutions letterhead. Orders will be billed at individual rate until proof of status is received. Foreign air speed delivery is included in all *Clinics'* subscription prices. All prices are subject to change without notice. POSTMASTER: Send address changes to *Anesthesiology Clinics,* Elsevier Health Sciences Division, Subscription Customer Service, 3251 Riverport Lane, Maryland Heights, MO 63043. Customer Service (orders, claims, online, change of address): Elsevier Health Sciences Division, Subscription Customer Service, 3251 Riverport Lane, Maryland Heights, MO 63043. Tel:1-800-654-2452 (U.S. and Canada); 314-447-8871 (outside U.S. and Canada). Fax: 314-447-8029. E-mail: journalscustomerservice-usa@elsevier.com (for print support); journalsonlinesupport-usa@elsevier.com (for online support).

Reprints. For copies of 100 or more of articles in this publication, please contact the Commercial Reprints Department, Elsevier Inc., 360 Park Avenue South, New York, NY 10010-1710. Tel.: 212-633-3812; Fax: 212-462-1935; E-mail: reprints@elsevier.com.

Anesthesiology Clinics, is also published in Spanish by McGraw-Hill Inter-americana Editores S. A., P.O. Box 5-237, 06500 Mexico D. F., Mexico.

Anesthesiology Clinics, is covered in *MEDLINE/PubMed (Index Medicus), Current Contents/Clinical Medicine, Excerpta Medica, ISI/BIOMED,* and *Chemical Abstracts.*

Printed and bound by CPI Group (UK) Ltd, Croydon, CR0 4YY

Transferred to digital print 2013

Contributors

CONSULTING EDITOR

LEE A. FLEISHER, MD, FACC, FAHA
Robert D. Dripps Professor and Chair of Anesthesiology and Critical Care, Professor of Medicine, Perelman School of Medicine, University of Pennsylvania School of Medicine, Philadelphia, Pennsylvania

EDITOR

COLLEEN G. KOCH, MD, MS, MBA
Professor of Anesthesiology, Department of Cardiothoracic Anesthesia and The Quality and Patient Safety Institute, Cleveland Clinic Lerner College of Medicine of Case Western Reserve University, Cleveland Clinic, Cleveland, Ohio

AUTHORS

ANDREJ ALFIREVIC, MD
Staff, Cardiothoracic Anesthesiology, Assistant Professor of Anesthesiology, Cleveland Clinic Lerner College of Medicine of Case Western Reserve University, Cleveland Clinic, Cleveland, Ohio

RYAN ANDERSON, MD, PhD
Cardiothoracic Anesthesia Fellow, Division of Adult Cardiothoracic Anesthesia, Department of Anesthesiology and Perioperative Medicine, Oregon Health and Science University, Portland, Oregon

SOLOMON ARONSON, MD, MBA
Executive Vice Chair, Division of Cardiac Anesthesia, Department of Anesthesiology, Duke University Medical Center, Durham, North Carolina

PAVAN ATLURI, MD
Assistant Professor of Surgery, Division of Cardiovascular Surgery, Department of Surgery, University of Pennsylvania, Philadelphia, Pennsylvania

MOISES AURON, MD, FAAP, FACP, SFHM
Assistant Professor of Medicine and Pediatrics, Cleveland Clinic Lerner College of Medicine Staff, Department of Hospital Medicine and Department of Pediatric Hospital Medicine, Cleveland Clinic, Cleveland, Ohio

EUGENE H. BLACKSTONE, MD
Head, Clinical Investigations, Heart and Vascular Institute, Cleveland Clinic, Cleveland, Ohio

MICHELLE CAPDEVILLE, MD
Associate Professor, Department of Cardiothoracic Anesthesia, Cleveland Clinic, Cleveland, Ohio

FREDERICK Y. CHEN, MD, PhD
Division of Cardiac Surgery, Brigham and Women's Hospital, Harvard Medical School, Boston, Massachusetts

DAVY CHENG, MD, MSc, FRCPC, FCAHS
Department of Anesthesia and Perioperative Medicine, London Health Sciences Centre, Schulich School of Medicine and Dentistry, Western University, London, Ontario, Canada

ANNE CHERRY, MD
Duke University Medical Center, Durham, North Carolina

JOHN M. CONNELL, MD, MPH
Division of Cardiac Surgery, Brigham and Women's Hospital, Harvard Medical School, Boston, Massachusetts

MARK ERETH, MD, MA
Professor, Department of Anesthesiology, Mayo Clinic, Rochester, Minnesota

SOFIA FISCHER, MD
Assistant Professor, Department of Anesthesiology, Emory University School of Medicine, Atlanta, Georgia

KATHRYN E. GLAS, MD, FASE, MBA
Associate Professor, Department of Anesthesiology, Emory University School of Medicine, Atlanta, Georgia

IZUMI HARUKUNI, MD
Assistant Professor, Division of Adult Cardiothoracic Anesthesia, Department of Anesthesiology and Perioperative Medicine, Oregon Health and Science University, Portland, Oregon

MOHAMED ISMAIL, MB, BCh, MSc
Department of Anesthesia and Perioperative Medicine, London Health Sciences Centre, Schulich School of Medicine and Dentistry, Western University, London, Ontario, Canada

AJAY KUMAR, MD, FACP, SFHM
Chief, Division of Hospital Medicine, Hartford Hospital, Hartford, Connecticut

ELIZABETH A. MARTINEZ, MD, MHS
Director of Quality and Safety, Department of Anesthesia, Critical Care and Pain Medicine, Associate Professor, Massachusetts General Hospital, Harvard Medical School, Boston, Massachusetts

ANAND R. MEHTA, MD
Staff, Cardiothoracic Anesthesiology, Assistant Professor of Anesthesiology, Cleveland Clinic Lerner College of Medicine of Case Western Reserve University, Cleveland Clinic, Cleveland, Ohio

EMAD B. MOSSAD, MD
Professor of Anesthesiology and Pediatrics, Baylor College of Medicine; Director of Pediatric Cardiovascular Anesthesia, Texas Children's Hospital, Houston, Texas

PABLO MOTTA, MD
Assistant Professor of Anesthesiology and Pediatrics, Baylor College of Medicine; Director of Pediatric Cardiovascular Anesthesia, Texas Children's Hospital, Houston, Texas

GEORGHIOS NICOLAOU, MB, BCh, FRCPC
Department of Anesthesia and Perioperative Medicine, London Health Sciences Centre, Schulich School of Medicine and Dentistry, Western University, London, Ontario, Canada

KARTHIK RAGHUNATHAN, MD, MPH
Assistant Professor, Department of Anesthesiology, Duke University Medical Center/ Durham VAMC, Durham, North Carolina

VALERIE SERA, MD, DDS
Clinical Associate Professor and Division Chief, Fellowship Program Director, Division of Adult Cardiothoracic Anesthesia, Department of Anesthesiology and Perioperative Medicine, Oregon Health and Science University, Portland, Oregon

ANDREW SHAW, MB, FRCA, FCCM
Associate Professor, Department of Anesthesiology, Duke University Medical Center/ Durham VAMC, Durham, North Carolina

STANTON K. SHERNAN, MA, FAHA, FASE
Department of Anesthesiology, Perioperative and Pain Medicine, Brigham and Women's Hospital, Harvard Medical School, Boston, Massachusetts

NICHOLAS G. SMEDIRA, MD
Professor, Department of Cardiovascular Surgery, Cleveland Clinic, Cleveland, Ohio

LARS G. SVENSSON, MD
Staff, Cardiothoracic Surgery, Professor of Surgery, Cleveland Clinic Lerner College of Medicine and Case Western Reserve University, Cleveland Clinic, Cleveland, Ohio

AVERY TUNG, MD, FCCM
Professor and Quality Chief for Anesthesia, Department of Anesthesia and Critical Care, University of Chicago, Chicago, Illinois

DAVID F. VENER, MD
Associate Professor of Anesthesiology and Pediatrics, Baylor College of Medicine; Director of Pediatric Cardiovascular Anesthesia, Texas Children's Hospital, Houston, Texas

WILLIAM VERNICK, MD
Assistant Professor, Department of Anesthesiology and Critical Care, The Perelman School of Medicine at the University Hospital of Pennsylvania, Philadelphia, Pennsylvania

ANDREA WORTHINGTON, BA
Department of Anesthesiology, Perioperative and Pain Medicine, Brigham and Women's Hospital, Harvard Medical School, Boston, Massachusetts

Contents

> The future of cardiothoracic anesthesia, simply stated, depends on establishing and maintaining a unique and differentiated quality and identity that promotes and contributes positive value to patients, surgical colleagues, and health system administrators who are all also responsible for seeking value. Cardiovascular anesthesiologists must therefore be prepared to define their value through demonstrating that unique quality. To do this, they must codify and continue to push the leading edge in education, research, and clinical innovation for the subspecialty of anesthesia and thereby ensure a role in defining true value as the best.

> Cardiac interventions are among the most quantitatively studied therapies. It is important for all involved with cardiac interventions to understand how information generated from observations made during patient care is transformed into data suitable for analysis, to appreciate at a high level what constitutes appropriate analyses of those data, to effectively evaluate inferences drawn from those analyses, and to apply new knowledge to better care for individual patients.

> After more than a decade of attention, the risks inherent in cardiac surgery have been well documented, but examples of effective interventions to reduce this risk remain scarce. The need is great, because the patient population is vulnerable and the potential consequences of poor outcomes are ever present and significant. This article reviews a decade of discussion surrounding quality and safety issues in cardiac surgery, and concludes with examples of strategies that have shown great promise for improving cardiac surgery quality and safety.

> The crystalloid-colloid debate has raged for decades, with the publication of many meta-analyses, yet no consensus. There are important differences between colloids and crystalloids, and these differences have direct relevance for cardiac surgical patients. Rather than asking crystalloid or

colloid, we believe better questions to ask are (1) High or low chloride content? and (2) Synthetic or natural colloid? In this paper we review the published literature regarding fluid therapy in cardiac surgery and explain the background to these two important and unanswered questions.

Ischemic mitral regurgitation (IMR) is a subcategory of functional rather than organic, mitral valve (MV) disease. Whether reversible or permanent, left ventricular remodeling creates IMR that is complex and multifactorial. A comprehensive TEE examination in patients with IMR may have important implications for perioperative clinical decision making. Several TEE measures predictive of MV repair failure have been identified. Current practice among most surgeons is to typically repair the MV in patients with IMR. MV replacement is usually reserved for situations in which the valve cannot be reasonably repaired, or repair is unlikely to be tolerated clinically.

The transition of mitral valve surgery away from the traditional sternotomy approach toward more minimally invasive strategies continues to evolve. The use of telemanipulative robotic arms with near 3-dimensional valve visualization has allowed for near complete endoscopic robotic-assisted mitral valve surgery, providing increased patient satisfaction and cosmesis. Studies have shown rapid recovery times without sacrificing perioperative safety or the durability of surgical repair. Although a steep learning curve exists as well as high fixed and disposable costs, continued technological development fueled by increasing patient demand may allow for further expansion in the use of robotic-assisted minimal invasive surgery.

Although cardiac transplant remains the gold standard for the treatment of end-stage heart failure, limited donor organ availability and growing numbers of eligible recipients have increased the demand for alternative therapies. Limitations of first-generation left ventricular assist devices for long-term support of patients with end-stage disease have led to the development of newer second-generation and third-generation pumps, which are smaller, have fewer moving parts, and have shown improved durability, allowing for extended support. The HeartMate II (second generation) and HeartWare (third generation) are 2 devices that have shown great promise as potential alternatives to transplantation in select patients.

The percutaneous transcatheter aortic valve replacement (TAVR) procedure, introduced in 2002, has emerged as a successful and comparable treatment option for many patients with aortic stenosis. Balanced general anesthesia or monitored anesthesia care in addition to local anesthesia have been used during transfemoral and transapical approaches. The results of different TAVR registries and the PARTNER trial have shown excellent success and survival rates, but stroke and paravalvular insufficiency represent major concerns. The key for successful procedural outcome involves thorough preparedness and knowledge of the pertinent procedural details.

Perioperative anesthetic management for cardiac transplantation is reviewed. Recent developments in adult cardiac transplantation are noted. This review includes demographics and historical results, recipient and donor selection and evaluation, mechanical circulatory support and heart transplantation techniques, and patient management immediately postimplantation.

There are currently in North America more adults with congenital heart disease than children. This article discusses the anesthetic considerations in adults with single-ventricle physiology and prior repairs who present for Fontan conversion surgery as a demonstration of the challenges of caring for adults undergoing interventions for the repair of congenital heart defects. The care of these patients requires an understanding of the impact of passive pulmonary blood flow and single systemic ventricular physiology. The perioperative morbidity in this patient population remains high.

As the spectrum of cardiac surgeries has grown, the diversity and complexity of postoperative cardiac surgical care has also increased. This article examines 4 areas in critical care where clinical practice is evolving rapidly. Among these are management of mechanical ventilation, thresholds for blood transfusion, strategies for hemodynamic monitoring, and processes for central line insertion. Also reviewed are current approaches to common dilemmas in postoperative cardiac care: diagnosis of tamponade, and the diagnosis and management of low cardiac output states in patients with a ventricular assist device.

Blood management is a system-based comprehensive approach that uses evidence-based medicine to facilitate an environment to encourage an appropriate use of blood products in the hospital setting. The ultimate goal of a blood-management program is to improve patient outcomes by integrating all available techniques to ensure safety, availability, and appropriate allocation of blood products. It is a patient-centered, multidisciplinary, multimodal, planned approach to the management of patients and blood products.

Thoracic endovascular aortic repair (TEVAR) has revolutionized thoracic aortic surgery and has increased the options available to the aortic specialist in treating thoracic aortic disease. TEVAR is less invasive, and is associated with a decrease in perioperative morbidity and mortality when compared with open surgical repair. The dramatic expansion of TEVAR activity has necessitated a better definition for the indications, contraindications, and limitations of this new technology. Ideally TEVAR should be performed in specialized aortic centers providing a full range of diagnostic and treatment options, using a multidisciplinary team approach.

The array of diagnostic and therapeutic procedures performed in the cardiology electrophysiology laboratory has expanded rapidly. Increasingly more facilities and cardiologists are performing these procedures, and the number of patients for whom these procedures are indicated is expanding. Because of the complexity of the procedures and associated patient comorbidity, anesthesia providers will become more involved in providing care in the electrophysiology laboratory. Therefore, anesthesia providers must be prepared to handle a broad range of case complexity. This article addresses the implications of providing anesthesia safely and effectively in the electrophysiology laboratory.

ANESTHESIOLOGY CLINICS

FORTHCOMING ISSUES

September 2013
Obstetric Anesthesia
Robert Gaiser, MD, *Editor*

December 2013
Transplantation
Claus Niemann, MD, *Editor*

RECENT ISSUES

March 2013
Trauma
Yoram G. Weiss, MD, MBA, FCCM and
Micha Y. Shamir, MD, *Editors*

December 2012
Thoracic Anesthesia
Peter Slinger, MD, FRCPC, *Editor*

September 2012
Postanesthesia Care Unit
Scott A. Falk, MD, *Editor*

RELATED INTEREST

Cardiology Clinics, November 2012 (Volume 30, Issue 4)
Emergency Cardiac Care 2012: From the ED to the CCU
Amal Mattu and Mandeep R. Mehra, *Editors*

Foreword

Cardiac Anesthesia

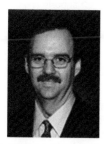

Lee A. Fleisher, MD, FACC, FAHA
Consulting Editor

Anesthesia for patients undergoing cardiac procedures has advanced greatly in the past several decades. It is one of the areas in which anesthesiologists have partnered closely with their surgical colleagues to advance patient care. With the development of less invasive procedures, especially in the electrophysiology laboratory, our role in the care has increased. In this issue of *Anesthesiology Clinics*, the guest editor has assembled an outstanding group of investigators to discuss a wide range of procedures. Additionally, she has outlined advances in patient management leading to improvement in patient safety.

I was fortunate to recruit Colleen G. Koch, MD, MS, MBA as guest editor for this issue. Dr Koch received her Medical Degree from the University of Cincinnati College of Medicine followed by an anesthesia residency at Brigham and Women's Hospital. She also completed a Masters Degree in Clinical Research Design and Statistics from the University of Michigan School of Public Health and a Masters in Business Administration from Case Western Reserve University. She is currently Professor of Anesthesiology and Vice Chair of Research and Education Department of Cardiothoracic Anesthesia at the Cleveland Clinic and holds a Joint Appointment Quality and Patient Safety Institute, Research, and Education. She is also a member of the Board of Directors of the Society of Cardiovascular Anesthesiologists. She is therefore well qualified to assemble a great group of leaders within cardiovascular anesthesia to discuss these important topics.

Lee A. Fleisher, MD, FACC, FAHA
Perelman School of Medicine
University of Pennsylvania
Philadelphia, PA 19104, USA

E-mail address:
lee.fleisher@uphs.upenn.edu

Anesthesiology Clin 31 (2013) xiii
http://dx.doi.org/10.1016/j.anclin.2013.03.001   **anesthesiology.theclinics.com**
1932-2275/13/$ – see front matter © 2013 Published by Elsevier Inc.

Preface

Cardiac Anesthesia

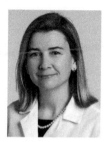

Colleen G. Koch, MD, MS, MBA
Editor

While health care debate has been the rage, real changes in health care are taking place at the patient level, which are affected by the changing demographics of the baby boomer generation, the evolution of surgical and anesthetic techniques, and refinements in quality and appropriateness, going beyond even complicated economic considerations. Over the past 20 years, I have had the privilege to provide anesthesia for cardiovascular surgical patients. Since that time, the landscape has changed considerably. Advances in the field have been rapid, exciting, and remarkable. Development and innovations in technology in the cardiovascular field have changed the practice of cardiovascular surgery and anesthesia. Patient comorbidity, coupled with procedural complexity, has underscored the importance of multidisciplinary teamwork and collaboration to ensure successful outcomes. There is more emphasis on quality, patient safety, and patient experience; these are now measurable outcomes used to rank hospitals and, in some cases, are tied to reimbursement. There are more demands to not only understand and be facile with the new technology but also be more involved in extending care outside the operating theater. Our specialty will continue to place greater emphasis on team dynamics and interdisciplinary care.

This edition on Cardiac Anesthesia is not intended to be a comprehensive review of the field but rather to serve as a focused reference and update on advances in the specialty for those who provide care for patients with cardiovascular disease.

I would like to thank Dr Lee Fleisher for the invitation to edit this volume of *Anesthesiology Clinics*. I would also like to thank our contributing authors for their contributions to this edition. They bring their clinical expertise and wealth of knowledge to the contents of these articles. Finally, I would like to thank Pamela Hetherington from

http://dx.doi.org/10.1016/j.anclin.2013.01.006
1932-2275/13/$ – see front matter

Elsevier for her expert assistance with this edition. I am delighted and honored to be guest editor for this edition of *Anesthesiology Clinics*.

Colleen G. Koch, MD, MS, MBA
Professor of Anesthesiology
Cleveland Clinic
Lerner College of Medicine
of Case Western Reserve University
Department of Cardiothoracic Anesthesia
and The Quality and Patient Safety Institute
Cleveland Clinic
9500 Euclid Avenue
Cleveland, OH 44195, USA

E-mail address:
kochc@ccf.org

The Future of Cardiothoracic Anesthesia

Anne Cherry, MD, Solomon Aronson, MD, MBA*

KEYWORDS

- Cardiothoracic anesthesia • Cardiovascular anesthesia • Reperfusion
- Stem cell therapy • Genomics • Future

"It is not the strongest of the species that survives, nor the most intelligent that survives. It is the one that is the most adaptable to change."

—*Charles Darwin*

"The line it is drawn The curse it is cast The slow one now will later be fast as the present now will later be past The order is rapidly fadin' and the first one now will later be last for the times they are a-changin'."

—*Bob Dylan*

These quotes hint that the future of any specialty lies in adaptation to change. Cardiothoracic anesthesiologists will certainly experience, and preferably effect, change in the health care system in the coming years. The specialty will simultaneously be presented with continuing changes in scientific knowledge, patient comorbidity burden, and novel surgical procedures that will challenge these practitioners to operate within an ever-expanding team of perioperative clinicians. The practice of cardiothoracic anesthesia will continue to evolve in parallel with those changes in technology, patient selection, and advanced procedures, and will also be affected by changes in standards of training, certification, and health care policy. Cardiovascular anesthesiologists already recognize that they have an important role in caring for the increasingly complex patients who will present in the future; it is one of the things that is most appealing about the specialty. It is the evolving complexity of perioperative management that will emphasize the importance of the practitioner's development of effective communication and systems-based practice and of maintaining their place at the table where health care policy decisions are made.

TRANSLATION OF BASIC SCIENCE RESEARCH

The most fundamental predictor of the future success of cardiovascular anesthesiology as a specialty lies in adaptation of the results of basic science research in

Division of Cardiac Thoracic Anesthesia, Department of Anesthesiology, Duke University Medical Center, DUMC 3094, Durham, NC 27710, USA
* Corresponding author.
E-mail address: solomon.aronson@duke.edu

Anesthesiology Clin 31 (2013) 207–216
http://dx.doi.org/10.1016/j.anclin.2012.12.001   anesthesiology.theclinics.com
1932-2275/13/$ – see front matter Published by Elsevier Inc.

a way that will benefit patients and change daily practice. These practitioners are fortunate to have, within the subspecialty and in their cardiovascular medicine and surgical colleagues, a remarkable group of scientists who are asking the right questions and performing groundbreaking research that will continue to advance the practice.

Preconditioning and Intermittent Reperfusion

A large number of surgical procedures involve temporary interruption of blood supply to vital organs, causing ischemia and potential tissue damage. Virtually all cardiac and thoracic surgeries, particularly those involving cardiopulmonary bypass, deep hypothermic circulatory arrest, or organ transplantation, involve ischemia and reperfusion of the heart and lungs. Methods of protection during these periods of ischemia and reperfusion are of great interest and have been the focus of decades of research. Cardiac protection began with the invention of cardiopulmonary bypass, the application of hypothermia, and the performance of antegrade and retrograde cardioplegia. Despite these measures, global and focal cardiac injury, the resulting functional impairment, and ischemic injury to other vital organs, continue to be major concerns for cardiovascular anesthesiologists.

In 1986, the first evidence was reported of a novel concept in protection: that of conditioning for prolonged cardiac ischemia through prior application of shorter cycles of ischemia.[1] This initial study of ischemic preconditioning involved intermittent left anterior descending coronary artery occlusion followed by a longer episode of ischemia (40 minutes) in dogs. Infarction size was markedly reduced when compared with a control group that experienced only a single long episode of ischemia. Direct translation of the method to the clinical arena within cardiac surgery has been challenging. Studies of intermittent cross-clamping of the aorta before prolonged cross-clamping have shown a reduction in arrhythmias, inotropic support, and intensive care unit (ICU) length of stay after coronary artery bypass grafting (CABG).[2] However, significant concern remains with the broad application of a technique that requires repeated clamping and unclamping of the aorta in a patient population known to be at risk for cerebral embolization with cross-clamp application.[3] The search for methods of conditioning that can be more easily applied, such as preconditioning using anesthetics, normobaric or hyperbaric hyperoxia, hypoxia, helium, or low-dose carbon monoxide, has gained momentum in recent years. Lastly, investigators have suggested that reperfusion injury might be attenuated by intermittent or slow reperfusion, particularly of transplanted organs.[1,4]

Perhaps the most intriguing of all these methods is the possibility of remote ischemic conditioning, wherein intermittent ischemia of a limb confers protection from ischemia for vital organs. The technique has been applied in a variety of settings, including after subarachnoid hemorrhage,[5] before abdominal aortic aneurysm repair,[6] and even in athletic training.[7] Pilot studies initially indicated that this treatment had some benefit in adult patients undergoing CABG, but subsequent trials showed mixed results. Explanations for the inconsistency vary, but in all, results suggest that subsets of the patient population and certain surgical procedures may exist for which remote conditioning would be of benefit. Two large, multicenter, randomized controlled studies are currently underway to help resolve these issues (Effect of Remote Ischemic Preconditioning on Clinical Outcomes in Patients Undergoing Coronary Artery Bypass Graft Surgery, to be completed in 2013; and Remote Ischemic Preconditioning for Heart Surgery, to be completed in 2014). As of October 19, 2012, 29 additional studies for perioperative cardiac surgery match the search term "Cardiac Remote Preconditioning" in the ClinicalTrials.gov database.

In pediatric cardiac surgery, however, the results are far more promising, with an initial study indicating that children treated with remote conditioning required less inotropic support and experienced less myocardial injury.[8] Direct ischemic postconditioning (intermittent release and reapplication of the aortic cross-clamp at the time of reperfusion) has also shown benefit in the pediatric cardiac surgical population in several studies.[9,10] This pediatric population, in contrast to an adult population with known cardiovascular disease, may have an improved risk/benefit profile with regard to repeated cross-clamping of the aorta, making this postconditioning treatment a viable option. In general, the pediatric population also benefits from a markedly lower burden of coexisting diseases, such as diabetes[11] and hypertension,[12] which may influence the magnitude of effect of conditioning stimuli. In all, these results suggest that preconditioning or postconditioning may be clinically applied to subsets of patients in the near future, pending results of ongoing trials.

Stem Cell Therapy

A second therapy that may be nearing implementation in cardiac surgical patients is stem cell therapy. The common result of myriad cardiac diseases is local or global fibrosis of myocardial tissue and a reduction in contractility, resulting in impaired function and cardiac output. The delivery of stem cells within myocardial tissue could, in theory, prevent remodeling and fibrosis caused by injury and maintain cardiac function. The exact mechanism for improvement is not yet clear, but evidence shows that increased cell differentiation, myocardial angiogenesis, and a direct paracrine effect on the extracellular matrix may all play a role.[13] The therapy has been applied in humans after myocardial infarction, and a meta-analysis indicates that there were small but statistically significant improvements in ventricular volumes, infarct size, and left ventricular ejection fraction.[14] Additional trials have shown reductions in mortality and readmission for heart failure,[15] but others have also shown an initial benefit that disappeared after 6 months.[16]

It has been suggested that persistence of effect is highly dependent on cell type and isolation technique,[17] along with the method of delivery of the cells in question. A significant body of work has been generated investigating the ideal type of stem cell, each with advantages and disadvantages primarily involving ease of differentiation and separation of cell types, proliferation and survival of cells, and side effects of implantation.[13] The most striking side effect noted to date has been teratoma formation at the site of injection with undifferentiated embryonic stem cells in mice,[18] an issue that is avoided through implantation of differentiated cells. Delivery methods, perhaps of particular interest to the cardiovascular anesthesiologist, include percutaneous (intravascular, intracoronary, transvenous injection into coronary veins, or transendocardial delivery) or surgical (transepicardial cell or tissue-engineered) options, each meant to balance the risk and benefit of precise delivery with increasing invasiveness for each given patient.[17]

Perioperative Genomics

The field of perioperative genomics, particularly for patients undergoing cardiac surgery and cardiopulmonary bypass, has been an area of considerable growth in the past decade. Research in the area primarily aims to identify and associate single nucleotide polymorphisms (SNPs) or sets of nearby SNPs (haplotypes) with various relevant outcomes. Identification is initially made through simultaneous evaluation of numerous SNPs within chromosomes and mitochondrial DNA (or even the entire genome) of individuals known to have had or not had the outcome of interest, and identifying SNPs or haplotypes that are found primarily in one group but not the other.

The concept is also often applied to elements downstream of the DNA: to the RNA, proteins (proteomics), or metabolic products of a cell (metabolomics). A positive association between a SNP, altered protein (structure or function), or metabolite and a disease or outcome can then be used as a hypothesis for more careful investigation of that element's value as a predictor of risk, disease progression, response to therapy, or even as a therapeutic target.

Associations discovered using genome-wide analysis that are relevant to cardiac surgery and anesthesia include SNPs or haplotypes that relate to atrial fibrillation,[19] metabolism of and response to warfarin,[20] likelihood of restenosis after percutaneous coronary intervention,[21] and propensity to develop thoracic aortic aneurysms (TAAs) and dissections.[22] Five SNPs have been found to be associated with left ventricular size and aortic root diameter.[23]

Further evaluation of the data from genome-wide association studies (GWAS) analyses will be an ongoing task. One variant identified through GWAS as being associated with coronary artery disease and myocardial infarction has been confirmed as being independently associated with perioperative myocardial injury and mortality after CABG, and was shown to improve the prognostic value of the European System for Cardiac Operative Risk Evaluation (euroSCORE).[24] A commercial test is available for the genetic variants associated with atrial fibrillation, and is expected to be of use in risk profiling for selected patients.[19] The SNP associated with TAAs happened to be located within a gene (FBN1) that, when mutated, is well-known to cause Marfan syndrome, confirming that a genome-wide analysis can bring into focus mutations in genes with considerable clinical significance.[22]

With the recent and ongoing dramatic reduction in the cost of genetic analysis, whole GWAS for SNPs and haplotypes are becoming more common (**Figs. 1** and **2**). An enormous amount of hypothesis-generating data has been and will continue to be produced by these analyses. Academic cardiac anesthesiologists are increasingly involved in research implementing genomics, proteomics, and metabolomics to ask

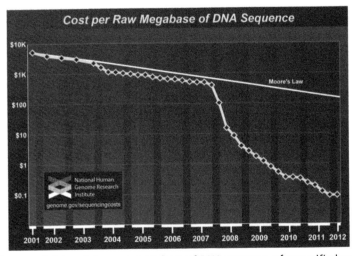

Fig. 1. The cost of determining one megabase of DNA sequence of a specified quality over time, which has been dramatically reduced over the last several years. (*From* Wetterstrand KA. DNA sequencing costs: data from the NHGRI Genome Sequencing Program (GSP). National Institutes of Health. Available at: www.genome.gov/sequencingcosts. Accessed October 11, 2012; with permission.)

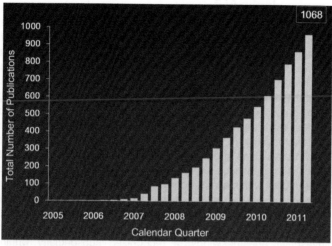

Fig. 2. Published genome-wide association reports, 2005–2009/2011. (*Courtesy of* Teri Manolio, MD, PhD, Bethesda, MD.)

questions that were, until now, unanswerable using traditional laboratory methods. All cardiac anesthesiologists and clinicians involved in the perioperative care of the cardiac surgical patient will certainly use data derived using these new tools for risk stratification and treatment in the near future.

FELLOWSHIPS, TRAINING, AND CERTIFICATION

In response to the exciting challenges in this subspecialty, its future lies in enhancing the training for cardiovascular anesthesiologists. The first cardiac anesthesia fellowships were initiated more than 40 years ago, with Accreditation Council for Graduate Medical Education (ACGME) accreditation beginning in 2006. In the 2012–13 academic year, 74 fellowships are available in the United States, 58 of which are ACGME-accredited. Current ACGME requirements for adult cardiothoracic fellowship training include minimum numbers of valve, CABG, and thoracic aortic procedures; training in TEE; and time spent in the ICU setting with options in other related areas (perfusion, invasive cardiology, outpatient cardiology or pulmonary medicine, research, or pediatric cardiothoracic anesthesia). These requirements are meant to ensure adequate training to prepare individuals to confidently and safely perform and supervise perioperative care for a variety of cardiac and thoracic surgical procedures. However, a thorough knowledge of perioperative care for the patients seen in 2013 will not necessarily translate to care for the patients who will be seen in 2042 (or even in 2015); likewise, the knowledge gained by the first fellows 40 years ago is largely irrelevant to treatment of the patients they see today. What remains relevant, and what is likely to be increasingly relevant in the future, are the less-tangible skills acquired during the year of working within the subspecialty. Those skills, practice-based learning and improvement, systems-based practice, interpersonal and communication skills, and professionalism are identified by the American Board of Anesthesiologists and the ACGME as a part of the "core competencies" of all successful trainees. As surgical procedures and patient disease presentations and comorbidities become more complicated, the organization of the team of professionals involved in perioperative care also becomes more complex. Consider the example of a transcatheter aortic valve implantation procedure in a hybrid operating room. The multidisciplinary team within the operating room consists of nursing staff, radiology technicians, surgical attendants, anesthesia technicians, anesthesiologists, cardiac surgeons, cardiologists, device representatives, cardiovascular perfusionists, and the patient. The success of the procedure relies on technical skills but, equally important, each individual's ability to work effectively with diverse team members.

With regard to the more tangible skills a cardiovascular anesthesiologist demonstrates, the establishment of fellowships in the subspecialty led inevitably toward accreditation of those fellowships. Recent history has shown that accreditation of a fellowship often leads to the implementation of subspecialty board examination for certification, particularly for those subspecialties in areas of practice that overlap substantially with physicians in other fields of medicine, such as pain, critical care, sleep medicine, and transesophageal echocardiography. Board certification, as a tool to gain credibility within a larger community of practitioners, has not previously been encouraged for subspecialties of anesthesiology without such competition (pediatric, cardiothoracic, and obstetric anesthesiology). These standards become increasingly necessary as national health care policy is reevaluated. With this precedent, cardiovascular anesthesiology, a recognized subspecialty within ACGME accredited fellowships and therefore with readily defined standards for training, will likely join others in instituting board examinations for certification in the near future. An important question regarding specialty training in the face of greater emphasis on efficiency and cost-effectiveness will be how academic programs can fulfill their educational mission and remain competitive?

CHANGES AND OPPORTUNITIES IN US HEALTH CARE

Finally, it is clear that change will soon occur on a system-wide scale, and that the ability of cardiovascular anesthesiologists to adapt on all fronts will be tested. Changes and therefore opportunities in US health care have not been more apparent at the national and global level since the institution of Medicare more than 5 decades ago. The Patient Protection and Affordable Care Act will change the landscape of medical care, including the practice of anesthesiology. In the United States, while the national debate over government spending continues, the business reality of health care, with underlying issues surrounding health care cost and quality, remains constant. Many important issues remain unresolved, and many models of care redesign and care management have been and are being proposed to help solve these issues. Fee for service is giving way to capitation at a varying pace depending on regional market pressure. Along the way, performance and value are giving way to bundling and shared savings and risk. It is argued that the fiscal solvency of the Federal government depends on the success of care redesign. For example, Don Berwick, former Centers for Medicare and Medicaid Services administrator, has outlined a $2 trillion dollar opportunity in the US health care market between now and 2020 through the elimination of non–value-added costs.

The consequence of health is equally striking. Estimates show that the prevalence of obesity in Americans will grow from 35% to 42% by 2030. This national endemic is projected to lead to a decrease in life expectancy for the first time ever in the United States. Furthermore, this condition will be associated with significant economic costs from diabetes, osteoarthritis, hypertension, and the other clinical derivatives. Health and health care are global issues (eg, polio and maternal mortality in Nigeria, developing hospital systems in India, health insurance schemes in China). Everywhere in the world governments are addressing questions about the financing and delivery of health care in the face of increasing demands and limited resources.

Regardless of politics, legislation, or policy, health care in the United States is rapidly becoming a value-based economy in a manner not seen in more than 5 decades. In a value-base economy, value is defined by unique and differentiating quality.

"Quality is not what you put into a product; quality is what the customer gets out of it."

—Peter Drucker

Going forward it is likely that the value proposition of specialty care and specialists will be defined differently: value (V) = quality (Q) × service (S)/cost (C). Critical questions will need to be asked and answered, such as whether specialists can justify higher marginal costs with higher marginal quality, and whether specialists will shift up the quality axis or down the cost axis, or both. How cardiovascular anesthesiologists respond will shape the specialty. Data-driven evidence will build perceptions and realities of best practice decisions and policy. Only through collecting and sharing outcomes data can meaningful assessment and comparison be possible through comparative effectiveness research.

Specialists and primary care physicians will need to increase integration to increase efficiency and focus on reducing complications, such as readmissions. The subspecialty of cardiovascular anesthesia will need to distinguish itself as critical to this value proposition in this changing environment (eg, they already do this in preoperative clinics, which, in the absence of a universal electronic medical record [EMR], collects outside records before admission for surgery and can avoid duplicate testing and provide valuable succinct information for the anesthesiologist).

Cardiovascular anesthesia, having a distinct and unique body of knowledge within anesthesiology, will lead ways to explore opportunities for clinical integration with partners in medicine and surgery. Value opportunities for cardiovascular anesthesiology to assume leadership positions in tomorrow's care redesign include developing teamwork training and safety standards for the cardiac operating room, patient transition of care and hand-off processes, and patient transport standards. The specialty of cardiovascular anesthesiology must take the lead in the science of safety to improve cross-disciplinary communication through identifying opportunities to reduce the risk of error and improve patient outcomes.

Diagnostic perioperative TEE has and will continue to distinguish the subspecialty of cardiovascular anesthesiology. TEE is recommended in the Practice Guidelines for Perioperative Echocardiography by the American Society of Anesthesiologists and Society of Cardiac Anesthesiologists (SCA) for all patients undergoing open chamber cardiac or thoracic aortic surgery in the absence of contraindications. Use during coronary artery bypass surgery is also suggested. In addition, intraoperative TEE has been shown to be beneficial during noncardiac surgery when high-risk cardiovascular disease and surgery might lead to life-threatening hemodynamic, pulmonary, or neurologic compromise. These recommendations for TEE use during cardiac and noncardiac surgery are mirrored in the recent guidelines from the European Association of Echocardiography and the European Association of Cardiothoracic Anaesthesiologists. The use of ultrasound in intensive care and emergency medicine has also evolved. In the future, surface ultrasound will be integrated into the everyday clinical practice as ultrasound-assisted examination and ultrasound-guided procedures. The SCA has led and must continue to be out front in the development of criteria for clinical application on TEE use based on research. Furthermore, specific criteria for perioperative TEE training have and are based on clinical research largely performed by cardiovascular anesthesiologists.

In addition, cardiovascular anesthesiology should assume leadership within the health system for blood management and take a leadership role in the coagulation laboratory. In the United States, unneeded services, inefficient delivery, and/or missed opportunities have been estimated to represent nearly 300 billion of the 2.8 trillion dollars spent on health care per year. The lack of guideline adaptation and variability in clinician practice has also been reported to continue to lead to the inappropriate use of blood components. More than 16,000,000 units of red blood cells and more than 5,000,000 units of plasma are transfused per year, with more than 60,000 adverse reactions reported, or 0.25% events per component administered. Blood transfusion continues to be 1 of the top 5 fastest growing procedures in medicine today. Blood transfusions occur in 1 of 10 of all hospital stays that involve a procedure. On the other end of the continuum, bleeding continues to be a major problem and contributor of morbidity in high-risk cardiac and aortic surgery. Knowledge of coagulation medicine and coagulation pharmacology falls easily within the domain of the subspecialty of cardiovascular anesthesiology. The role and value of cardiovascular anesthesia in blood management is self-evident.

Finally, going forward, rapid response management and postcardiac surgery critical care must be defined and shaped by both cardiac anesthesiologists along with cardiac surgeons when appropriate, in this country.

CLOSING THOUGHTS

The future of cardiothoracic anesthesia, simply stated, depends on establishing and maintaining a unique and differentiated quality and identity that promotes and contributes positive value to patients, surgical colleagues, and health system administrators who are all also responsible for seeking value. Cardiovascular anesthesiologists must therefore be prepared to define their value through demonstrating their unique qualities. To do this, they must codify and continue to push the leading edge in education, research, and clinical innovation for the subspecialty of anesthesia, and thereby ensure a role in defining true value as the best. Their value will be based on their ability to accept the challenge to differentiate themselves from others. They face a time in heath care of great change with great opportunity.

REFERENCES

1. Murry CE, Jennings RB, Reimer KA. Preconditioning with ischemia: a delay of lethal cell injury in ischemic myocardium. Circulation 1986;74(5):1124–36.
2. Walsh SR, Tang TY, Kullar P, et al. Ischaemic preconditioning during cardiac surgery: systematic review and meta-analysis of perioperative outcomes in randomised clinical trials. Eur J Cardiothorac Surg 2008;34(5):985–94.
3. Hausenloy DJ, Boston-Griffiths E, Yellon DM. Cardioprotection during cardiac surgery. Cardiovasc Res 2012;94(2):253–65.
4. Vinten-Johansen J, Shi W. Preconditioning and postconditioning: current knowledge, knowledge gaps, barriers to adoption, and future directions. J Cardiovasc Pharmacol Ther 2011;16(3–4):260–6.
5. Gonzalez NR, Hamilton R, Bilgin-Freiert A, et al. Cerebral hemodynamic and metabolic effects of remote ischemic preconditioning in patients with subarachnoid hemorrhage. Acta Neurochir Suppl 2013;115:193–8.
6. Ali ZA, Callaghan CJ, Lim E, et al. Remote ischemic preconditioning reduces myocardial and renal injury after elective abdominal aortic aneurysm repair: a randomized controlled trial. Circulation 2007;116(Suppl 11):I98–105.

7. Jean-St-Michel E, Manlhiot C, Li J, et al. Remote preconditioning improves maximal performance in highly trained athletes. Med Sci Sports Exerc 2011; 43(7):1280–6.

8. Cheung MM, Kharbanda RK, Konstantinov IE, et al. Randomized controlled trial of the effects of remote ischemic preconditioning on children undergoing cardiac surgery: first clinical application in humans. J Am Coll Cardiol 2006;47(11): 2277–82.

9. Li B, Chen R, Huang R, et al. Clinical benefit of cardiac ischemic postconditioning in corrections of tetralogy of Fallot. Interact Cardiovasc Thorac Surg 2009;8(1): 17–21.

10. Luo W, Li B, Lin G, et al. Postconditioning in cardiac surgery for tetralogy of Fallot. J Thorac Cardiovasc Surg 2007;133(5):1373–4.

11. Lu R, Hu CP, Peng J, et al. Role of calcitonin gene-related peptide in ischaemic preconditioning in diabetic rat hearts. Clin Exp Pharmacol Physiol 2001;28(5–6): 392–6.

12. Moro L, Pedone C, Mondi A, et al. Effect of local and remote ischemic preconditioning on endothelial function in young people and healthy or hypertensive elderly people. Atherosclerosis 2011;219(2):750–2.

13. Elnakish MT, Kuppusamy P, Khan M. Stem cell transplantation as a therapy for cardiac fibrosis. J Pathol 2013;229:347–54.

14. Lipinski MJ, Biondi-Zoccai GG, Abbate A, et al. Impact of intracoronary cell therapy on left ventricular function in the setting of acute myocardial infarction: a collaborative systematic review and meta-analysis of controlled clinical trials. J Am Coll Cardiol 2007;50(18):1761–7.

15. Assmus B, Rolf A, Erbs S, et al. Clinical outcome 2 years after intracoronary administration of bone marrow-derived progenitor cells in acute myocardial infarction. Circ Heart Fail 2010;3(1):89–96.

16. Meyer GP, Wollert KC, Lotz J, et al. Intracoronary bone marrow cell transfer after myocardial infarction: eighteen months' follow-up data from the randomized, controlled BOOST (BOne marrOw transfer to enhance ST-elevation infarct regeneration) trial. Circulation 2006;113(10):1287–94.

17. Templin C, Luscher TF, Landmesser U. Cell-based cardiovascular repair and regeneration in acute myocardial infarction and chronic ischemic cardiomyopathy-current status and future developments. Int J Dev Biol 2011; 55(4–5):407–17.

18. Nussbaum J, Minami E, Laflamme MA, et al. Transplantation of undifferentiated murine embryonic stem cells in the heart: teratoma formation and immune response. FASEB J 2007;21(7):1345–57.

19. Milan DJ, Lubitz SA, Kaab S, et al. Genome-wide association studies in cardiac electrophysiology: recent discoveries and implications for clinical practice. Heart Rhythm 2010;7(8):1141–8.

20. Johnson JA, Gong L, Whirl-Carrillo M, et al. Clinical Pharmacogenetics Implementation Consortium Guidelines for CYP2C9 and VKORC1 genotypes and warfarin dosing. Clin Pharmacol Ther 2011;90(4):625–9.

21. Sampietro ML, Trompet S, Verschuren JJ, et al. A genome-wide association study identifies a region at chromosome 12 as a potential susceptibility locus for restenosis after percutaneous coronary intervention. Hum Mol Genet 2011;20(23): 4748–57.

22. Lemaire SA, McDonald ML, Guo DC, et al. Genome-wide association study identifies a susceptibility locus for thoracic aortic aneurysms and aortic dissections spanning FBN1 at 15q21.1. Nat Genet 2011;43(10):996–1000.

23. Vasan RS, Glazer NL, Felix JF, et al. Genetic variants associated with cardiac structure and function: a meta-analysis and replication of genome-wide association data. JAMA 2009;302(2):168–78.
24. Muehlschlegel JD, Liu KY, Perry TE, et al. Chromosome 9p21 variant predicts mortality after coronary artery bypass graft surgery. Circulation 2010; 122(Suppl 11):S60–5.

Generating New Knowledge in Cardiac Interventions

Eugene H. Blackstone, MD

- Data • Analysis • Clinical research • Cardiac • Cardiac interventions

KEY POINTS

- Understand how information generated from observations made during patient care is transformed into data suitable for analysis.
- Appreciate at a high level what constitutes appropriate analyses of those data.
- Effectively evaluate inferences drawn from those analyses.
- Apply new knowledge to better care for individual patients.

INTRODUCTION

Cardiac interventions are among the most quantitatively studied therapies in medicine.[1] These studies reveal a complex, multifactorial, and multidimensional interplay among patient characteristics, variability of the heart disease, effect of the disease on the patient, conduct of the intervention, and response of the patient to it. The introduction of medical report cards made it evident that multiple factors influencing results of therapy must be taken into account to make fair comparisons of outcomes. Thus, it is important for all involved with cardiac interventions to (1) understand how information generated from observations made during patient care is transformed into data suitable for analysis, (2) appreciate at a high level what constitutes appropriate analyses of those data, (3) effectively evaluate inferences drawn from those analyses, and (4) apply new knowledge to better care for individual patients.

This article should be read by (1) cardiac anesthesiologists, to improve their comprehension of the medical literature and to hone their skills in its critical appraisal; (2) trainees and junior faculty interested in becoming clinical investigators, who need instruction on how to pursue successful clinical research, (3) mature physician-investigators and their collaborating statisticians, mathematicians, and computer scientists, who will benefit from some of the philosophic ideas; and (4) data managers of larger clinical research groups, who need to fully appreciate their pivotal role in successful research: the knowledge-generating team (**Box 1**).

Large portions of this article are contained in section I of chapter 6 of Kirklin/Barratt-Boyes, *Cardiac Surgery,* 4th edition.
Clinical Investigations, Heart and Vascular Institute, Cleveland Clinic, 9500 Euclid Avenue, JJ40, Cleveland, OH 44195, USA
E-mail address: blackse@ccf.org

Anesthesiology Clin 31 (2013) 217–248
http://dx.doi.org/10.1016/j.anclin.2012.12.006
1932-2275/13/$ – see front matter © 2013 Elsevier Inc. All rights reserved.

Box 1
Knowledge-generating team

Structure

Regardless of whether the same individuals are involved, clinical research generally includes 2 fundamentally different activities: (1) continuous registry and database activity and (2) individual clinical studies activity. The registry activity involves gathering and entering data for a prescribed set of core data elements for every case. The individual clinical studies activity can be categorized roughly into 2 classes that require different skill sets: (1) clinical trials (either intramurally funded or extramurally sponsored by government or industry) and (2) studies of clinical experience (cohort studies).

Roles

Clinician-Investigator

The clinical investigator (with collaboration of key individuals in data management, statistics, and study coordination) must develop the clinical question (aims, objectives), define the study group of interest, identify variables and end points (outcomes) of interest, review the literature, and develop all elements of a study protocol. They must adjudicate data quality, gather values for variables in addition to the core data elements, help interpret the analyses performed, position findings in a clinical context, present the findings to colleagues, and write articles.

Data Manager

There is no more key support person than the data manager. They are at the interface between data gathering and data analysis. Assembly of data for meaningful analysis is often complex, requiring information to be retrieved from a variety of electronic sources. Data managers usually need formal training in computer science and specifically in database construction and management. They must master an effective data query language.

Their most valuable skill, perhaps inborn rather than developed, is attention to the smallest detail of the data. Physicians are usually not of the temperament for this kind of work, and statisticians by training are big-picture–oriented; if physicians see the forest, data managers must see the trees. Thus, data management is not simply skill in formulating databases, writing and executing query logic, and documenting these in detail (although these are important); rather, it is skill in examining the data, finding errors in them, finding inconsistencies and deviation from the norm that should be verified, verifying what appear as outliers, and assessing quality of data for every variable.

The physician-investigator and data manager organize the variables for analysis. If time-related or longitudinal outcomes are being assessed, the data manager must become expert in forming intervals and assessing time-related data (time zero, events, intervals), 2 of the most demanding and essential tasks for such analyses.

For larger clinical quality and research organizations, a statistical programmer must convert data from database format into analysis data sets that make sense to the statistician.

Data Gatherers

Persons skilled in data gathering for data entry fall into a hierarchy. For gathering some variables, expert medical knowledge is essential. Other data elements can be extracted by individuals with little formal training other than in medical terminology. Essential ingredients are accuracy and integrity. Accuracy may be inborn and is indispensable; it can be assessed prospectively by testing and maintained by quality management and education.

Education/Quality

If large quantities of data are maintained, 1 or more individuals must assess the quality of the data and from these findings educate the data gatherers. Such individuals must have expert medical knowledge. In large organizations, this role includes maintaining clinical documentation of the database, keeping current with procedural trends, and pruning variables that no longer are of value or are of questionable quality.

Statistician

Most serious clinical research efforts require equally serious collaboration with 1 or more statisticians. The applied statistician needs to become expert, facile, and experienced in many methods, including time-related events analysis; binary, ordinal, and polytomous regression; longitudinal mixed-model (hierarchical) data analysis; multivariable analysis; case-matching analysis; cluster randomized trials; diagnostic accuracy; and classification algorithms. The applied statistician must also engage in ongoing statistical methodological research. Many studies, perhaps most, use analytical methods that answer specific questions, but the questions answered may not precisely match the ones that are medically relevant (because of assumptions or lack of more appropriate methods). Encountering these difficulties should stimulate development of more appropriate methodology.

Other Professionals

Other professionals may be part of the team, depending on the nature of the research. These professionals include mathematicians (who develop mathematical models that attempt to capture known mechanistic relations within the data, in contrast to the statistician, who takes a more empiric approach), computer scientists (such as those in bioinformatics, computational biology, data mining, or algorithmic data analysis), human factors psychologists (for investigation of human error), ontologists (who maintain the meaning of data), experts in artificial intelligence, and many others. Indispensable is the editorial assistant, who helps with preparation of articles, ensures proper grammar and style, and manages references.

Infrastructure

Some individuals are shared by several groups. They maintain computer networks, computers, and software; enter and verify data; perform patient follow-up; perform financial analysis; write grants; produce medical illustrations or computer graphics; and engage in many other support roles.

It may be more comfortable and convenient for the investigator to have a single point of contact among these individuals. However, a collaborative team with a multitude of skills is often needed, with data flowing progressively (often iteratively) from the information through analysis phases, forcing the investigator to leave comfort and convenience behind and become immersed in multidisciplinary and transdisciplinary efforts.

The potential obstacle for all is language. For the anesthesiologist, the languages of statistics, mathematics, data management, and computer programming pose a daunting obstacle of symbols, numbers, and algorithms. For collaborating statisticians, mathematicians, and computer scientists, the Greek and Latin language of medicine is equally daunting. This article attempts to surmount the language barrier by translating ideas, philosophy, and unfamiliar concepts into words.

Because this article is intended for a mixed audience, it focuses on the most common points of intersection between cardiac intervention and quantitative science, with the goal of establishing sufficient common ground for effective and efficient collaboration. It is not a substitute for statistical texts or academic courses, nor a substitute for the physician-investigator to establish a collaborative relationship with biostatisticians, nor is it intended to equip anesthesiologists with sufficient statistical expertise to conduct highly sophisticated data analyses themselves. It serves as a brief overview to the more detailed discussion contained in the first section of chapter 6 of the Kirklin/Barratt-Boyes text, *Cardiac Surgery*.[2]

The organizational basis for this article is the Newtonian inductive method of discovery.[3] It begins with information about a microcosm of medicine, proceeds to translation of information into data and analysis of those data, and ends with new knowledge about a small aspect of nature. This organizational basis emphasizes the phrase, "Let the data speak for themselves."[4]

Information

In health care, information is a collection of material, documentation of work flow, and recorded observations. Information may be recorded in paper-based medical records or in electronic (computer) format.

Data

Data consist of organized values for variables, usually expressed symbolically (eg, numerically) by means of a controlled vocabulary.[5] Characterization of data includes descriptive statistics that summarize parts or all of the data and express their variability from patient to patient.

Analysis

Analysis is a process, often prolonged and repeated (iterative), that uses a large repertoire of methods by which data are explored, important findings are revealed and unimportant ones suppressed, and relations are clarified and quantified.

Knowledge

Knowledge is the synthesis of information, data, and analyses arrived at by inductive reasoning. However, generation of new knowledge does not occur in a vacuum; an important step is assimilating new knowledge within the body of existing knowledge.

New knowledge may take the form of clinical inferences, which are simple summarizing statements that synthesize information, data, and analyses, drawn with varying degrees of confidence that they are true. It may take the form of speculations, which are statements suggested by the data or by reasoning, often about mechanisms, without direct supportive data. Ideally, it takes the form of new hypotheses, which are testable statements suggested by reasoning or inferences from the information, data, and analyses.

New knowledge can be applied to many processes in health care, including (1) generating new concepts, (2) making individual patient care decisions, (3) obtaining informed consent from patients, (4) improving outcomes of interventions, (5) assessing the quality and appropriateness of care, and (6) making regulatory decisions.

DRIVING FORCES OF NEW KNOWLEDGE

Many forces drive the generation of new knowledge in cardiac interventions, including the economics of health care, need for innovation, clinical research, procedure success and failure, and awareness of medical error.

Economics

The economics of health care are driving changes in practice toward what is hoped to be less expensive, more efficient, yet higher quality care. Interesting methods for testing the validity of these claims have become available in the form of cluster randomized trials.[6,7] In such trials, patients are not randomized, but physicians are. This situation leads to inefficient studies, which nevertheless can be effective with proper design and a large enough pool of physicians.[7,8] It is a study design in which the unit of randomization (physician) is not the unit of analysis (individual patient outcome).[9]

Innovation

Innovation is often at odds with cost reduction and is perceived as being at odds with traditional research. However, in all areas of science, injection of innovation is the enthalpy that prevents entropy, stimulating yet more research and development and more innovation. Without it, cardiac surgery and interventional cardiology would be unable to adapt to changes in managing ischemic heart disease, potential reversal of the atherosclerotic process, percutaneous approaches to valvar and congenital heart disease, and other changes directed toward less invasive, safer, more effective, and more appropriate therapy.

What is controversial is (1) when and if it is appropriate to subject innovation to formal clinical trial and (2) the ethics of innovation in interventions, for which standardization is difficult.[10-13]

Reducing the Unknown

New knowledge in cardiac interventions has been driven from its inception by a genuine quest to fill voids of the unknown, whether by clinical research or laboratory research. Clinical research has historically followed 1 of 2 broad designs: randomized clinical trials and nonrandomized studies of cohorts of patients (clinical practice). However, increasing emphasis is being placed on translational research, that is, bringing basic research findings to the bedside. John Kirklin, a pioneer of heart surgery, called this the "excitement at the interface of disciplines." Part and parcel of the concept of the incremental risk factor is that it is an essential link in a feedback loop that starts with procedure failure, and proceeds to identifying risk factors, drawing inferences about specific gaps in knowledge that need to be addressed by basic science, generating fundamental knowledge, and bringing these full circle to the clinical arena through testing and assessing the value of the new knowledge generated for improving medical care.[14]

Intervention Success and Failure

Results of intervention in heart disease, particularly surgical failure, have driven much of the new knowledge generated by clinical research. In the late 1970s and early 1980s, a useful concept arose about surgical failures applicable to any failure of an intervention. That is, in the absence of natural disaster or sabotage, there are 2 principal causes of failure of interventions to provide a desired outcome for an individual patient: (1) lack of scientific progress and (2) human error.

The usefulness of this concept is that it leads to the programmatic strategies of research on the one hand and development on the other. Thus, lack of scientific progress is gradually reduced by generating new knowledge (research), and human error is reduced in frequency and consequences by putting available knowledge into practice (development), a process as vital in medicine as it is in the transportation and manufacturing sectors.[15,16]

Error

Increased awareness of medical error drives the generation of new knowledge just as it drives increasing regulatory pressure and medicolegal litigation.[17] Human error also places it into the context of cognitive sciences, human factors, and safety research.[18,19] This interface of disciplines is essential for facilitating substantial reduction in injury from medical errors.

Philosophy

Clinical research as emphasized in this article consists largely of patient-oriented investigations motivated by a serious quest for new knowledge to improve clinical results, that is, to increase early and long-term survival; reduce complications;

enhance quality of life; extend appropriate interventions to more patients, such as high-risk subsets; and devise and evaluate new beneficial procedures.

This inferential activity, aimed at improving clinical results, is in contrast to pure description of experiences. Its motivation also contrasts with those aspects of outcomes assessment motivated by regulation or punishment, institutional promotion or protection, quality assessment by outlier identification, and negative aspects of cost justification or containment. These coexisting motivations stimulated Kirklin and me to identify, articulate, and contrast philosophies that underlie serious clinical research.[2] It is these philosophies that should inform the approach to analysis of clinical experiences for generating new knowledge.

Deduction Versus Induction

Let the data speak for themselves.[4]

Arguably, Sir Isaac Newton's greatest contribution to science was a novel intellectual tool: a method for investigating the nature of natural phenomena.[20] His method had 2 strictly ordered aspects, which for the first time were systematically expressed: a first, and extensive, phase of data analysis, whereby observations of some small portion of a natural phenomenon are examined and dissected, followed by a second, less emphasized, phase of synthesis, whereby possible causes are inferred and a small portion of nature revealed from the observations and analyses.[3] This was the beginning of the inductive method in science: valuing first and foremost the observations made about a phenomenon, then letting the data speak for themselves in suggesting possible natural mechanisms.

This represented the antithesis of the deductive method of investigation, which had been so successful in the development of mathematics and logic. The deductive method begins with what is believed to be the nature of the universe (referred to by Newton as "hypothesis"), from which logical predictions are deduced and tested against observations. If the observations deviate from logic, the data are suspect, not the principles behind the deductions. The data do not speak for themselves.

Newton realized that it was impossible at any time or place to have complete knowledge of the universe. Therefore, a new methodology was necessary to examine portions of nature, with less emphasis on synthesizing the whole. The idea was heralded as liberating in nearly all fields of science.

Determinism Versus Empiricism

Determinism is the philosophy that everything (events, acts, diseases, decisions) is an inevitable consequence of causal antecedents: "Whatever will be will be." If disease and patients' response to disease and to disease treatment were clearly deterministic and inferences deductive, there would be no need to analyze clinical data to discover their general patterns. Great strides are being made in linking causal mechanisms to predictable clinical response.[21,22] Yet, many areas of cardiovascular medicine remain nondeterministic and incompletely understood. In particular, the relation between a specific patient's response to complex therapy such as a cardiac operation and known mechanisms of disease seems to be predictable only in a probabilistic sense. For these patients, therapy is based on empiric recognition of general patterns of disease progression and observed response to therapy.

Generating new knowledge from clinical experiences consists, then, of inductive inference about the nature of disease and its treatment from analyses of ongoing, empiric observations of clinical experience that take into account variability, uncertainty, and relationships among surrogate variables for causal mechanisms.

Collectivism Versus Individualism

Are you a lumper or splitter: woods or trees?[23] When generating new knowledge about the nature of heart disease and its treatment, it is important both to examine groups of patients (the woods) and to investigate individual therapeutic failures (the trees). Both views give valuable insights into nature. Statistical methods emphasizing probabilities and general inferences tend to apply to the former, and those emphasizing optimum discrimination for identifying individual patients at risk tend to apply to the latter.[21,22]

Continuity Versus Discontinuity in Nature

When we turn our focus from a specific patient experiencing an intervention failure to groups of patients, data analysis becomes mandatory to discover relationships between outcome and items that differ in value from patient to patient (called variables). A challenge immediately arises: many of the variables related to outcome are measured either on an ordered clinical scale (ordinal variables), such as New York Heart Association (NYHA) functional class, or on a more or less unlimited scale (continuous variables), such as age. Perhaps as an adaptive function of our brains, humans have a tendency to dichotomize: normal versus abnormal, for example.[24] What the investigator must embrace is a key concept in the history of ideas: continuity in nature. The idea has emerged in mathematics, science, philosophy, history, and theology.[25] The common practice of stratifying age and other more or less continuous variables into 2 or just a few discrete categories is lamentable, because stratifying loses the power of continuity (some statisticians call this "borrowing power"). Focus on small, presumed homogenous, groups of patients also loses the power inherent in a wide spectrum of heterogeneous, but related, cases: any trend observed over an ever-narrower framework looks more and more like no trend at all. Modern methods of machine learning that use classification methods may seem to stumble at this point, but repetition of analyses over thousands of sampled data sets combined with averaging achieves a close approximation to continuity in nature.[26,27]

Single Versus Multiple Dimensionality

Univariable (1 variable at a time) statistics are attractive, because they are simple to understand. However, most clinical problems are multifactorial. At the same time, clinical data contain enormous redundancies that need to be taken into account (eg, height, weight, body surface area, and body mass index are highly correlated and relate to the conceptual variable "body size"). Multivariable analysis permits multiple factors to be examined simultaneously, takes into account redundancy of information among variables (covariance), and identifies a parsimonious set of variables, which, in cardiovascular disease, have been called risk factors.[28] These are not cause-effect relations, but associations with underlying causal mechanisms. The relationships that are found may be spurious, fortuitous, hard to interpret, and even confusing because of the degree of correlation among variables. For example, women may be at a higher risk of mortality after certain cardiac procedures, but female gender may not be a risk factor, because other factors, such as body mass index, may be the more general variable related to risk, whether in women or men. Even so, it is simultaneously true that (1) being female is not per se a risk factor, but (2) women are at higher risk because on average they are smaller than men. This means that a close collaboration must exist between statistical experts and investigators, particularly in organizing variables for analysis.

Linearity Versus Nonlinearity

Risk factor methodology introduces another complexity besides increased dimensionality. The probability space is bounded by 0 at the bottom and 1 at the top, a floor and ceiling constraint. An important mathematical relationship between a continuous scale of risk and the probability of an adverse event occurring is the logistic equation.[29,30] It is a symmetric S-shaped curve, which expresses the relationship between a scale of risk, called logit units, and a corresponding scale of absolute probability of experiencing an event (**Fig. 1**). This nonlinear relationship makes medical sense. Imagine a risk factor with a logit unit coefficient of 1.0. If all other things position a patient far to the left on the logit scale, a 1-logit-unit increase in risk results in a trivial increase in the probability of experiencing an event. As other factors move a patient closer to the center of the scale (0 logit units, corresponding to a 50% probability of an event), a 1-logit-unit increase in risk makes a huge difference. This finding is consistent with the medical perception that some patients experiencing the same disease, trauma, or complication respond differently. Some are medically robust, because they are far to the left (low-risk region) on the logit curve before the event occurred. Others are medically fragile, because their age or comorbid conditions place them close to the center of the logit curve. For the latter, a 1-logit-unit increase in risk can be the straw that breaks the camel's back. It is this kind of relation that makes it difficult to show, for example, the benefit of bilateral internal thoracic artery grafting in young adults followed for even a couple of decades, but easy in patients who have other risk factors.[31] Other types of analysis such as survival analysis have a similar S-shaped relation of outcome and risk, although the relationship might not be symmetric.

Raw Data Versus Models of Data

Because logistic regression and other statistical models generate an equation based on raw data (or an algorithm as from machine learning[21]), it can be solved for a given

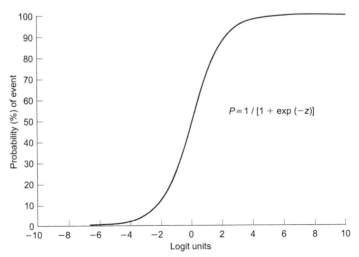

$$P = 1 / [1 + \exp(-z)]$$

Fig. 1. Fundamental logistic relation of a scale of risk (logit units) to absolute probability of an event. Logistic relation, shown when risk factors are translated into logit units,[28] is depicted along horizontal axis and probability of the outcome event along vertical axis. Logistic equation is inserted, where *exp* is the natural exponential function.

set of values for risk factors. Whenever possible and appropriate, the results of clinical data analyses should be expressed in a form that can be solved after plugging in values for an individual patient's risk factors to estimate absolute risk and its confidence limits. Equations are compact and portable, so that with the ubiquitous computer, they can be used to advise individual patients.[32–34]

It can be argued that equations do not represent raw data. But in most cases, are we really interested in raw data? Archaeologists are interested in the past, but the objective of most clinical investigation is not to predict the past, but to draw inferences based on observations of the past that can be used in treating future patients. Thus, equations derived from raw data about the past are more useful than raw, undigested data.

Nihilism Versus Predictability

One of the important advantages of generating equations is that they can be used to predict future results for either groups of patients or individual patients. We recognize that when speaking of individual patients, we are referring to a prediction concerning the probability of events for that patient; we generally cannot predict exactly who will experience an event or when an event will occur.

Of course, the nihilist may say, "You can't predict anything." There are an increasing number of models for predicting institutional results of cardiac interventions, and many of these are narrowly focused on more or less homogenous subsets of patients. For many individuals with complex heart disease and comorbidities, these predictions may fall short of true risk because they do not account for all the complexities that a patient may bring.[35]

Blunt Instruments Versus Fine Dissecting Instruments

A related use of predictive equations is in comparing alternative therapies: comparative effectiveness research. Some argue that the only believable comparisons are those based on randomized trials, and that clinical experience is irrelevant and misleading.[36] However, many randomized trials are homogenous and focused and are analyzed by blunt instruments, such as an overall effect. On the other hand, real-world clinical experience involves patient selection that is difficult to quantify, may be a single-institution experience with limited generalizability except to other institutions of the same variety, is not formalized unless there is prospective gathering of clinical information into registries, and is less disciplined. Nevertheless, analyses of clinical experiences can yield a fine dissecting instrument in the form of equations that are useful for comparing alternative treatments and advising patients.

Parsimony Versus Complexity

Although clinical data analysis methods and results may seem complex at times, as in the large number of risk factors that must be assessed for comparing treatment strategies in ischemic heart disease, an important philosophy behind such analysis is parsimony (simplicity). Parsimony is needed because clinical data contain inherent redundancy, and 1 purpose of multivariable analysis is to identify that redundancy and simplify the dimensionality of the problem. Parsimony also aids assimilation of new knowledge by extracting the essence of the data. Thus, clinical inferences are often more simple than the multivariable analyses.

Simplicity is a virtue based on philosophic, not scientific, grounds. The concept was introduced by William of Ocken in the early fourteenth century as a concept of beauty: beauty of ideas and theories.[37] Nevertheless, it is pervasive in science.

However, there are dangers associated with parsimony and beauty. The human brain seems to assimilate information in the form of models, not data.[38] Thus, new ideas, innovations, breakthroughs, and new interpretations of the same data often hinge on discarding past paradigms.[24] There are other dangers in striving for simplicity. Important relations may be missed because the threshold for detecting them is too high. Complex clinical questions may be reduced to simple but inadequate questions that we know how to answer.

New Knowledge Versus Selling Shoes

The philosophies described so far focus on the challenge of generating new knowledge from clinical experiences. However, clinical data have other uses.

Clinical data may be used as a form of advertising, just like selling shoes. Innovation stems less from purposefulness than from esthetically motivated curiosity, frustration with the status quo, sheer genius, fortuitous timing, favorable circumstances, and keen intuition. With innovation comes the need to promote, to sell the idea. However, promotional records of achievement should not be confused with serious study of safety, clinical effectiveness, and long-range appropriateness of interventions.

Of growing importance is the use of clinical information for regulation or to gain institutional competitive advantage (3 stars). Using clinical outcomes data to rank institutions or individual doctors has become popular in the United States.[39,40] Many perceive clinical report cards as a means for punishment or regulation. What is troubling is that their use is based on a questionable quality-control model of outlier identification. Because doctors are people and not machines, this approach generates counterproductive ethical side effects, including defensiveness and hiding the truth.[41] It hinders candid, nonculpable, serious examination of medical processes for the express purpose of improving patient care.

Critics of clinical report cards charge that to improve their rankings, some institutions refuse to operate on sicker patients.[42–44] However, risk-adjusted mortality may remain high even for low-risk cases.

With the intense focus on institutional performance, another undesirable side effect of data analysis, decried years ago, has crept back in: undue emphasis on hospital mortality and morbidity. Studies of hospital events have the advantage of readily available data for extraction, but early events may be characterized incompletely. After repair of many congenital and acquired heart diseases, early risk of surgery extends beyond the hospital stay.[45] This has led to reflection on the effect of time frame on studies of clinical experiences. Use of intermediate-term data is likely to characterize the early events well, but requires cross-sectional patient follow-up.[45] Long-term follow-up is essential to establish appropriateness of therapy, but it is expensive and runs the risk of being criticized as being of historical interest only.

Clinical information is also used for profit or corporate advantage. At present, the philosophies of scientific investigation and business are incompletely reconciled.[46–48] One thrives on open dissemination of information, the other on proprietary information offering a competitive advantage. In an era of dwindling public resources for research and increasing commercial funding, we may be seeing the beginning of the end of open scientific inquiry.

Past Versus Future

Is there a future for quantitative analysis of the results of therapy, as there was in the developmental phase of cardiac surgery and interventional cardiology? If treatment of heart disease requires complex procedures, and if most are palliative in the life history of chronic disease, there is a need to understand more fully the nature of the disease, its treatment, and its optimal management. This requires approaches to data that are inescapably philosophic.

CLINICAL RESEARCH

In response to the American Medical Association's Resolution 309 (I-98), a Clinical Research Summit and an ongoing Institute of Medicine Clinical Research Roundtable have sought to define and reenergize clinical research.[49] The most important aspects of the definition of clinical research are that (1) it is but 1 component of medical and health research aimed at producing new knowledge; (2) the knowledge produced should be valuable for understanding the nature of disease, its treatment, and prevention; and (3) it embraces a wide spectrum of types of research. Here, we highlight 2 examples on that spectrum: clinical trials with randomly assigned treatment and clinical studies with nonrandomly assigned treatment, both of which are an integral part of clinical effectiveness research.

Clinical Trials with Randomly Assigned Treatment

Clinical trials in which cardiac interventions and medical therapy have been randomly assigned have made major contributions to our knowledge of treatment and outcomes of heart disease.[50–54] Randomization of treatment assignment has 3 valuable and unique characteristics:

- It eliminates selection factors (bias) in treatment assignment (although this can be defeated at least partially by enrollment bias).
- It distributes patient characteristics equally between groups, whether they are measured or not, known or unknown.[55–58]
- It meets assumptions of statistical tests used to compare end points.[57]

Randomized clinical trials are also characterized by concurrent treatment, high quality and complete compilation of data gathered according to explicit definitions, and proper follow-up evaluation of patients. These operational by-products may have contributed nearly as much new knowledge as the random assignment of treatment.

It has become ritualistic for some to dismiss out of hand all information, inferences, and comparisons relating to outcome events derived from experiences in which treatment was not randomly assigned.[36] If this attitude were valid, then much of the information used to manage patients with cardiac disease would need to be dismissed and ignored. However, moral justification (equipoise) may not be present for a randomized comparison of procedures and protocols that clinical experience strongly suggests, for at least some physicians, lead to important difference in outcomes.[56] When Benson and Hartz[59] investigated differences between randomized trials and observational comparisons over a broad range of medical and surgical interventions, they found "little evidence that estimates of treatment effects in observational studies reported after 1984 are consistently larger than or qualitatively different from those obtained in randomized controlled studies." (However, see the rebuttal by Pocock and Elbourne.[60]) These findings were confirmed by Concato and colleagues.[61] Nevertheless, many acknowledge a hierarchy of clinical research study designs, and the randomized trial generates the most secure information about treatment differences.[62]

Trials in which treatment is randomly assigned are testing a hypothesis, and hypothesis testing, in general, requires a yes or no answer unperturbed by uncontrollable factors. Thus, ideally, the study is of short duration, with all participants blinded and with a treatment that can be well standardized. However, in many clinical situations involving patients with heart disease, the time-relatedness of freedom from an unfavorable outcome event is important and can jeopardize interpretation of the trial.[63] This is because (1) individual patients assign different values to different durations of time-related freedoms (long-term benefit may be more important than short-term risk and vice versa), (2) differing severities of disease (and corresponding differences in natural history) affect different time frames, and (3) the longer the trial, the more likely there will be crossovers (such as from medical to interventional therapy).[64] Also, the greater the number of risk factors associated with the condition for which treatment is being evaluated, the greater the potential heterogeneity (number of subsets) of patients with that condition and the greater the likelihood that a yes-no answer applies only to certain subsets of patients. In such situations, a randomized trial may have the disadvantage of including only a limited number of subsets or it may apply to no subset, because the average patient for whom the answer is derived may not exist except as a computation. Trials have addressed this problem by basing the randomization on subsets[65] or by later analyzing subsets by stratification (but see concerns raised by Guillemin[66]) or by multivariable analysis.[67]

These considerations, in addition to ethical concerns,[12,68,69] have fueled the debate on whether surgery and invasive intervention in general are an appropriate arena for randomized trials of innovation, devices, and operations.[59,70–72] Some argue strongly that randomization should be required at the outset of introducing a new therapy.[69] In 3 related articles arising from the Balliol Colloquium held at the University of Oxford between 2007 and 2009, clinicians and anesthesiologists sought to clarify the issues surrounding surgical clinical trials.[73–75] They recognized important stages in developing a surgical technique, starting with innovation and progressing through development, exploration, assessment, and long-term outcomes. They then explored options for evaluative studies and barriers to each, including sham operations and nonoperative treatment alternatives.[74] They ended with an IDEAL model for surgical development (idea, development, exploration, assessment, long-term study), and the role of feasibility randomized trials in exploration, definitive trials in assessment, and registries in long-term surveillance.[75]

Moses[76] and others[62,70,77] present the case for a balance between randomized clinical trials and observational clinical studies. However, observational studies are beset with problems of selection bias and skill variance; thus, not to be overlooked are the development and rapid introduction of powerful new methods for drawing causal inferences from nonrandomized trials.[78,79]

Clinical Studies with Nonrandomly Assigned Treatment

Clinical studies with nonrandomly assigned treatment produce little new knowledge when improperly performed and interpreted. Because this is often the case, many investigators have a strong bias against these studies. However, when properly performed and interpreted, and particularly when they are multi-institutional or externally validated, clinical studies of real-world experience can produce secure knowledge.

The fundamental objection to using observational clinical data for comparing treatments is that many uncontrolled variables affect outcome.[80] Thus, attributing outcome differences to just 1 factor (alternative treatments) stretches credibility. Even a cursory glance at the characteristics of patients treated 1 way versus another usually reveals that they are, on average, different groups. This should be expected, because treatment has been selected by experts who believe that they know what is best for a given patient. The accusation that apples and oranges are being compared is justified![81] Multivariable adjustment for differences in outcome is valuable but not guaranteed to be effective in eliminating selection bias as the genesis of a difference in outcome (a form of confounding).[79,82,83]

Balancing Scores

Apples-to-apples nonrandomized comparisons of outcome can be achieved, within certain limitations, by use of balancing scores, of which the propensity score is the simplest.[78] Balancing scores are a class of multivariable statistical methods that identify patients with similar chances of receiving 1 or the other treatment. Patients with similar balancing scores are well balanced with respect to nearly all patient, disease, and comorbidity characteristics taken into account in forming the balancing score. This balancing of characteristics permits the most reliable nonrandomized comparisons of treatment outcomes available. Developers of balancing score methods claim that the difference in outcome between patients who have similar balancing scores but receive different treatments provides an unbiased estimate of the effect attributable to the comparison variable of interest.[78] That is technical jargon for saying that the method can identify the apples from among the mixed fruit of clinical practice variance, transforming an apples-to-oranges outcomes comparison into an apples-to-apples comparison.[84–87]

Randomly assigning patients to alternative treatments in clinical trials balances both patient characteristics (at least in the long run) and number of subjects in each treatment arm. In a nonrandomized setting, neither patient characteristics nor number of patients is balanced for each treatment. A balancing score achieves local balance of patient characteristics at the expense of unbalancing n. **Tables 1** and **2** show local balance of patient characteristics achieved by using a specific balancing score known as the propensity score. **Table 1** shows that patients on long-term aspirin therapy have dissimilar characteristics from those not on this therapy. Unadjusted comparison of outcomes in these 2 groups is invalid (an apples-to-oranges comparison).[81] Therefore, multivariable logistic regression analysis was performed to identify factors predictive of treatment received (chronic aspirin therapy vs not).[88] The resulting logistic equation was solved for each patient's probability of being on long-term aspirin therapy. This probability is 1 expression of what is known as a propensity score (in this case, the propensity to be on chronic aspirin therapy). Patients were then sorted according to the balancing (propensity) score and divided into 5 equal-size groups, called quintiles, from low score to high.[78] Patients in each quintile had similar balancing scores (see **Table 2**).

Table 1
Selected patient characteristics according to long-term aspirin use in patients undergoing stress echocardiography for known or suspected coronary artery disease[a]

Patient Characteristic	ASA	No ASA	P
n	2455	4072	
Men (%)	49	56	.001
Age (mean ± SD y)	62 ± 11	56 ± 12	<.0001
Smoker (%)	10	13	.001
Resting heart rate (beats/min)	74 ± 13	78 ± 14	<.0001
Ejection fraction (%)	50 ± 9	53 ± 7	<.0001

Abbreviations: ASA, long-term aspirin use; SD, standard deviation.
[a] Table shows that patient characteristics differ importantly, making direct comparisons of outcome invalid. As shown in original article, many other patient characteristics differed between the 2 groups.
Data from Gum PA, Thamilarasan M, Watanabe J, et al. Aspirin use and all-cause mortality among patients being evaluated for known or suspected coronary artery disease: A propensity analysis. JAMA 2001;286:1187–94.

Table 2
Selected patient characteristics according to long-term aspirin use in patients undergoing stress echocardiography for known or suspected coronary artery disease: stratified by propensity score for aspirin use[a]

Patient Characteristic	Quintile									
	I		II		III		IV		V	
	ASA	No ASA	ASA	No ASA	ASA	No ASA	ASA	No ASA	ASA	No ASA
n	113	1092	194	1111	384	922	719	586	1045	261
Men (%)	22	22	57	63	74	71	78	78	88	87
Age (y)	55	49	56	55	61	61	62	64	63	65
Smoker (%)	15	13	15	15	12	11	11	13	7	9
Resting heart rate (beats/min)	84	83	79	79	76	76	76	76	71	73
Ejection fraction (%)	53	54	54	54	53	53	49	49	49	48

Abbreviation: ASA, long-term aspirin use.
[a] Table shows that balancing patient characteristics by the propensity score comes at the expense of unbalancing number of patients within comparable quintiles.
Data from Gum PA, Thamilarasan M, Watanabe J, et al. Aspirin use and all-cause mortality among patients being evaluated for known or suspected coronary artery disease: a propensity analysis. JAMA 2001;286:1187–94.

Simply by virtue of having similar balancing scores, patients within each quintile were found to have similar characteristics (except for age in quintile I). As might be expected, patient characteristics differed importantly from 1 quintile to the next. For example, most patients in quintile I were women; most in quintile V were men. Except for unbalanced n, these quintiles look like 5 individual randomized trials with differing inclusion and exclusion criteria, which is what balancing scores are intended to achieve. Thus, the propensity score balanced essentially all patient characteristics within localized subsets of patients, in contrast to randomized clinical trials, which balance both patient characteristics and n globally within the trial.

To achieve this balance, a widely dissimilar number of patients received long-term aspirin therapy from quintile to quintile. Quintile I contained only a few patients who received long-term aspirin therapy, whereas quintile V had few not receiving aspirin.

Propensity score
The most widely used balancing score is the propensity score.[78] It provides for each patient an estimate of the propensity toward (probability of) belonging to 1 group versus another (group membership). The following sections describe (1) designing the nonrandomized study, (2) constructing a propensity model, (3) calculating a propensity score for each patient using the propensity model, and (4) using the propensity score in various ways to achieve a balanced comparison.

Designing the nonrandomized study The essential approach to a comparison of treatment outcomes in a nonrandomized setting is to design the comparison as if it were a randomized clinical trial and to interpret the resulting analyses as if they emanated from such a trial. This essential approach is emphasized in Rubin's 2007 article, "The design versus the analysis of observational studies for causal effects: parallels with the design of randomized trials."[79]

As noted by Rubin, "I mean all contemplating, collecting, organizing, and analyzing data that takes place before seeing any outcome data." He emphasizes by this statement his thesis that a nonrandomized set of observations should be conceptualized as "a broken randomized experiment…with a lost rule for patient allocation, and specifically for the propensity score, which the analysis will attempt to construct." For example, the investigator should ask, "Could each patient in all comparison groups be treated by all therapies considered?" If not, this constitutes specific inclusion and exclusion criteria. If this were a randomized trial, when would randomization take place? Variables must be used to construct a propensity score that would be known only at the time randomization would have occurred, not after that; this means that variables chosen in the propensity score analysis are not those that could be affected by the treatment.

Constructing a propensity model For a 2-group comparison, typically, multivariable logistic regression is used to identify factors predictive of group membership.[78] In most respects, this is what clinical investigators have done for years: find correlates of an event. In this case, it is not risk factors for an outcome event, but rather correlates of membership in 1 or the other comparison group of interest.

I recommend initially formulating a parsimonious multivariable explanatory model that identifies common denominators of group membership.[81] Once this traditional modeling is completed, a further step is taken to generate the propensity model, which augments the traditional model by other factors, even if not statistically significant. Thus, the propensity model is not parsimonious.[86] The goal is to balance patient characteristics by whatever means possible, incorporating all information recorded that may relate to either systematic bias or simply bad luck, no matter the statistical significance. It is important to use as many continuous variables as possible to represent these patient characteristics because it produces a fine, as opposed to coarse, set of values when the propensity score is calculated.

When taken to the extreme, forming the propensity model can cause problems, because medical data tend to have many variables that measure the same thing (redundancy). The solution is to pick 1 variable from among a closely correlated cluster of variables as a representative of the cluster. An example is to select 1 variable representing body size from among height, weight, body surface area, and body mass index.

Calculating a propensity score Once the propensity modeling is completed, a propensity score is calculated for each patient. A logistic regression analysis, as used for the propensity model, produces a coefficient or numeric weight for each variable. The coefficient maps the units of measurement of the variable into units of risk. Specifically, a given patient's value for a variable is transformed into risk units by multiplying it by the coefficient. If the coefficient is 1.13 and the variable is "male" with a value of 1 (for "yes"), the result is 1.13 risk units. If the coefficient is 0.023 for the variable "age" and a patient is 61.3 years old, 0.023 times 61.3 is 1.41 risk units.

One continues through the list of model variables, multiplying the coefficient by the specific value for each variable. When finished, the resulting products are summed. To this sum is added the intercept of the model, and the result is the propensity score. Technically, the intercept of the model, which is constant for all patients, does not have to be added; however, in addition to using the propensity score in logit risk units as described here, it may be used as a probability, for which the intercept is necessary.

Using the propensity score for comparisons Once the propensity model is constructed and a propensity score is calculated for each patient, 3 common types of comparison are used: matching, stratification, and multivariable adjustment.[89]

The propensity score can be used as the sole criterion for matching pairs of patients (**Table 3**).[84,90,91] Although several matching strategies have been used by statisticians

Table 3
Comparison of patient characteristics according to long-term aspirin use in propensity-matched pairs[a]

Patient Characteristic	ASA	No ASA
n	1351	1351
Men (%)	49	51
Age (y)	60	61
Smoker (%)	50	50
Resting heart rate (beats/min)	77	76
Ejection fraction (%)	51	51

Abbreviation: ASA, long-term aspirin use.
[a] Table shows ability of the propensity score to produce what appears to be a randomized study balancing both patient characteristics and n.
Data from Gum PA, Thamilarasan M, Watanabe J, et al. Aspirin use and all-cause mortality among patients being evaluated for known or suspected coronary artery disease: a propensity analysis. JAMA 2001;286:1187–94.

for many years, new optimal matching algorithms have arisen within computer science and operations research. These algorithms have been motivated by the need to optimally match volume of intranet and Internet traffic to computer network configurations.[92,93] In addition, (Rubin, personal communication, 2008) has suggested matching with replacement versus the usual "greedy" matching, which removes matched patients from further consideration. Matching can be bootstrapped, creating multiple matched comparison groups, over which outcome can be averaged.[94]

Exact matches are rarely found. Instead, a patient is selected from the smaller of the 2 groups being compared with a propensity score nearest to that of a patient in the larger group. If multiple patients are close in propensity scores, optimal selection among these candidates can be used.[84] Problems of matching on multiple variables disappear by compressing all patient characteristics into a single score (compare **Table 3** with unmatched data in **Table 1**).

Matching works well. The comparison data sets have all the appearances of a randomized study. The average effect of the comparison variable of interest is assessed as the difference in outcome between the groups of matched pairs. However, unlike a randomized study, the method does not balance unmeasured variables well, and this may be fatal to the inference.

Once patients are matched, it is important to diagnostically test the quality of matching. This test can be accomplished visually by graphs of standardized differences, defined as the difference in mean value between groups divided by the pooled standard deviation. This quantity is similar to the test statistic in a t-test (**Fig. 2**).[84] Differences that were substantial should virtually disappear. If they do not, it is possible that interaction terms (multiplicative factors rather than additive factors) may be required.

A graph of propensity scores for the groups is instructive (**Fig. 3**). The scores for 2 treatments may nearly overlap, as they would for a randomized trial. On the other hand, there may be little overlap, as in **Fig. 4**, and the comparison focuses on the center part of the spectrum of propensity scores, where there is substantial overlap (the region of virtual equipoise).

Outcome can be compared within broad groupings of patients, called strata or subclasses, according to propensity score.[86] After patients are sorted by propensity score, they are divided into equal-sized groups. For example, they may be split into

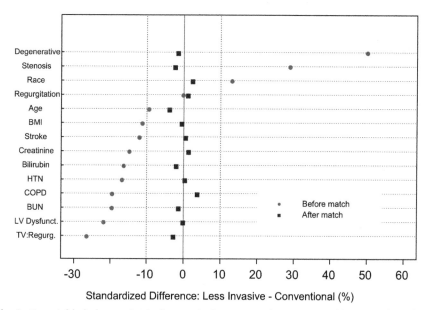

Fig. 2. Covariable balance plot before and after propensity score matching on selected co-variables. Symbols depict percent standardized differences for covariables between patients in less invasive and conventional groups. BMI, body mass index; BUN, blood urea nitrogen; COPD, chronic obstructive pulmonary disease; Dysfunct., dysfunction; HTN, hypertension; LV, left ventricular; Regurg., regurgitation; TV, tricuspid valve. (*Data from* Johnston DR, Atik FA, Rajeswaran J, et al. Outcomes of less invasive J-incision approach to aortic valve surgery. J Thorac Cardiovasc Surg 2012;144:852–8.e3.)

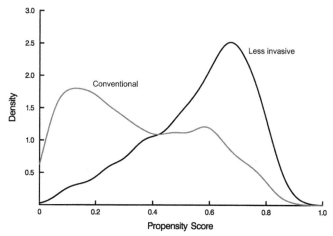

Fig. 3. Distribution of propensity scores for conventional and less invasive approaches for aortic valve replacement. (*Data from* Johnston DR, Atik FA, Rajeswaran J, et al. Outcomes of less invasive J-incision approach to aortic valve surgery. J Thorac Cardiovasc Surg 2012;144:852–8.e3.)

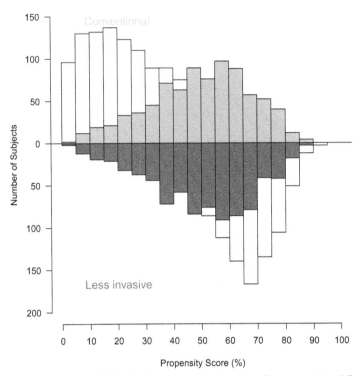

Fig. 4. Mirrored histogram of distribution of propensity scores for conventional (bars above zero line) and less invasive (bars below zero line) approaches for aortic valve replacement. Darkened area represents matched patient pairs, showing that they cover the complete spectrum of cases, but predominate in the central area (area of virtual equipoise). (*Data from* Johnston DR, Atik FA, Rajeswaran J, et al. Outcomes of less invasive J-incision approach to aortic valve surgery. J Thorac Cardiovasc Surg 2012;144:852–8.e3.)

5 groups, or quintiles (see **Table 2**; **Table 4**), but fewer or more groups may be used, depending on the size of the study. Comparison of outcome for the comparison variable of interest is made within each stratum. If a consistent difference in outcome is not observed across strata, intensive investigation is required. Usually, something is discovered about the characteristics of the disease, the patients, or their clinical condition that results in different outcomes across the spectrum of disease. For example, in their study of ischemic mitral regurgitation, Gillinov and colleagues[95] discovered that the difference in survival between those undergoing valve repair versus replacement progressively narrowed as complexity of the pattern of regurgitation increased and condition of the patient worsened (**Fig. 5**). Apparent anomalies such as this give important insight into the nature of the disease and its treatment.

The propensity score for each patient can be included in a multivariable analysis of outcome.[83] Such an analysis includes both the comparison variable of interest and the propensity score. The propensity score adjusts the apparent influence of the comparison variable of interest for patient selection differences not accounted for by other variables in the analysis.

Occasionally, the propensity score remains statistically significant in such a multivariable model. This constitutes evidence that adjustment for selection factors by multivariable analysis alone is ineffective, something that cannot be ignored.[83] It may mean

Table 4 Balance in patient and selection characteristics achieved by unbalancing number of cases in each propensity-ranked group in 3 separate studies		
Study	Factor Present (n)	Factor Absent (n)
Long-Term Aspirin Use		
Quintile 1	113	1192
Quintile 2	194	1111
Quintile 3	384	922
Quintile 4	719	586
Quintile 5	1045	261
Natural Selection: Preoperative AF in Degenerative MV Disease		
Quintile 1	2	225
Quintile 2	13	214
Quintile 3	32	195
Quintile 4	78	149
Quintile 5	162	66
OPCAB vs On-Pump		
Quintile 1	40	702
Quintile 2	71	671
Quintile 3	61	682
Quintile 4	90	652
Quintile 5	219	524

Abbreviations: AF, atrial fibrillation; MV, mitral valve; OPCAB, off-pump coronary artery bypass grafting.

that not all variables important for bias reduction have been incorporated into the model, such as when a simple set of variables is used. It may mean that an important modulating or synergistic effect of the comparison variable occurs across propensity scores, as noted in **Fig. 5** (eg, the mechanism of disease may be different within quintiles). It may mean that important interactions of the variable of interest with other variables have not been accounted for, leading to a systematic difference identified by the propensity score. The collaborating statistician must investigate and resolve these possibilities. Understanding aside, this statistically significant propensity score has performed its intended function of adjusting the variable representing the group difference.

In some settings in which the number of events is small, the propensity score can be used as the sole means of adjusting for the variable representing the groups being compared.[92]

Oranges

The propensity score may reveal that a large number of patients in 1 group do not have scores close to patients in the other.[31] Thus, some patients may not be matched. If stratification is used, quintiles of patients may have hardly any matches at 1 or the other, or both, ends of the propensity spectrum, and these remaining may not be well matched.

The knee-jerk reaction is to infer that these unmatched patients represent apples and oranges unsuited for direct comparison.[96] However, the most common reason for lack of matches is that a strong surrogate for the comparison group variable has

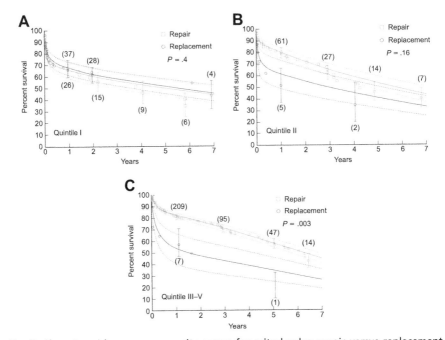

Fig. 5. Changing risk across propensity scores for mitral valve repair versus replacement. Because of small numbers of patients with mitral valve replacement in quintiles III through V, these quintiles are grouped together. Patient profiles are similar in each quintile, but differ across quintiles. Each symbol represents a death according to the Kaplan-Meier estimator. Vertical bars enclose asymmetric 68% confidence limits (CL); solid lines enclosed within dashed 68% CLs represent parametric survival estimates; numbers in parentheses are numbers of patients traced beyond that point. *P*-values are for log-rank test. (*A*) Quintile I. (*B*) Quintile II. (*C*) Quintiles III through V. (*From* Gillinov AM, Wierup PN, Blackstone EH, et al. Is repair preferable to replacement for ischemic mitral regurgitation? J Thorac Cardiovasc Surg 2001;122:1131.)

been included inadvertently in the propensity score. This variable must be removed and the propensity model revised. If this is not the case, the analysis may have identified truly unmatchable cases (mixed fruit). In some settings, they represent a different end of the spectrum of disease, for which different therapies have been applied systematically.[95,97] Often, the first clue to this anomaly is finding that the influence of the comparison variable of interest is inconsistent across quintiles.[95] This finding emphasizes the nature of comparisons with balancing score methodology: the comparisons relate only to the subset of patients who are apples-to-apples. Comparing these apples with the remaining oranges with respect to outcomes is not valid. The oranges result from systematic selection of patients for one versus the other treatment.

Thus, when apples and oranges (and other mixed fruit) are revealed by a propensity analysis, investigation should be intensified rather than the oranges being set aside.[81] After the investigations are complete, comparisons among the well-matched patients can proceed with known boundaries within which valid comparisons are possible.

Limitations

Some investigators claim that balancing score methods are valid only for large studies, citing Rubin.[98] It is true that large numbers facilitate certain uses of these scores, such as stratification. However, experience suggests that there is considerable latitude in matching that still reduces bias; the method seems to work even for modest-sized data sets.

Another limitation is having few variables available for propensity modeling. The propensity score is seriously degraded when important variables influencing selection have not been collected.[82] A corollary to this is that unmeasured variables cannot be reliably balanced. If these variables are influential on outcome, a spurious inference may be made.[99]

The propensity score may not eliminate all selection bias.[100] This may be attributed to limitations of the modeling itself imposed by the linear combination of factors in the regression analysis that generates the balancing score. If the comparison data sets are comparable in size, it may not be possible to match every patient in the smaller of the 2 data sets, because closely comparable patients have been used up, unless bootstrap sampling with replacement has been used.

Perhaps the most important limitation is inextricable confounding. Suppose on-pump coronary artery bypass grafting is to be compared with off-pump operations. A study is designed to compare the results of institution A, which performs only off-pump bypass, with those of institution B, which performs only on-pump bypass. Even after careful application of propensity score methods, it remains impossible to distinguish between an institutional and a treatment difference, because they are inextricably intertwined (confounded); that is, the values for institution and treatment are 100% correlated.

Extension

At times, a comparison of more than 2 groups may be wanted. Under this circumstance, multiple propensity models are formulated,[85] such as by fully conditional multiple logistic regression.[101]

Most applications of balancing scores have been concerned with dichotomous (yes-no) comparison group variables. However, balancing scores can be extended to a multiple-state ordered variable (ordinal) or even a continuous variable.[102] An example of the latter is use of correlates of heart valve prosthesis size as a balancing score to isolate the possible causal influence of valve size on outcome.

Logistic regression is not the only way to formulate propensity scores. A nonparametric machine learning technique (random forests) can be used and has been found by Lee and colleagues[94] to better balance groups, with reduced bias. Our group has formulated a generalized theorem as an extension of the work of Imai and van Dyk[103] for propensity scores and devised a data-adaptive, random-forest, nearest-neighbor algorithm that simultaneously matches patients and estimates the treatment effect from thousands of bootstrap samples and simultaneously refines the characteristics of true oranges (noncomparable patients).

TECHNIQUE FOR SUCCESSFUL CLINICAL RESEARCH

Marbán and Braunwald, in reflecting on training the clinician-investigator, provide guiding principles for successful clinical research.[104] Among these:

- Choose the right project
- Embrace the unknown
- Use state-of-the-art approaches
- Do not become the slave of a single technique
- Never underestimate the power of the written or the spoken word

Because of increasingly limited resources for conducting serious clinical research, a deliberate plan is needed to successfully carry a study through from inception to publication.[105] The following sections outline such a plan for study of a clinical question for which clinical experience (a patient cohort) provides the data. This plan appears as a linear work flow (**Fig. 6**); in reality, most research efforts do not proceed linearly but rather iteratively, with each step more refined and usually more focused, right up to the last revision of the article.

Research Proposal

Every serious clinical study needs a formal proposal that clarifies the question. A common mistake is to ask questions that are unfocused, uninteresting, unimportant, or overworked. Marbán and Braunwald write, "Ask a bold question…about which you can feel passionate."[104] Brainstorming with collaborators is essential.

The next step is to define the inclusion and exclusion criteria for the study group. A common mistake is to define this group too narrowly, such that cases are overlooked or homogenerity precludes discovering trends. Inclusive dates should be considered carefully. Readers are suspicious if the dates are not whole years or at least half-years. Similarly, suspicion arises when a study considers a neat number of patients, such as "the first 1000 aortic valve procedures."

In defining the study group, particular care should be taken to include a denominator or comparison group to put events into context. A retrospective study is a study of only numerators, such as only patients who have required renal dialysis after an intervention. If the denominator is included, it is a prospective or cohort study. If the cohort is placed in the context of alternative approach to the disease, it is a comparative effectiveness study.

End points (results, outcomes) must be clearly defined in a reproducible fashion. Generally, every event should be accompanied by its date of occurrence. A common failing is that repeated end points (eg, thromboembolism or assessments of functional status) are recorded only the first or most recent time that they occur. Techniques are available to analyze repeated end points.

Careful attention must be paid to the variables that are studied. They should be pertinent to the study question. A common failing is to collect values for too many variables such that quality suffers. This error is understandable: the clinical investigator reasons that because the patient's records must be reviewed, several other variables should also be abstracted at that time. Or, realizing the complexity of the clinical setting, the investigator feels compelled to collect information on all possible ramifications of the study, even if it is peripheral to the focus of the study. This is termed the "Christmas tree effect", meaning adding ornament on ornament until they dominate what once was a fine tree. There needs to be a balance between so sparse a set of variables that little can be done by way of risk factor identification or balancing characteristics of the group, and so rich a set of variables that the study flounders or insufficient care is given to the quality and completeness of relevant variables.

Study feasibility must then be assessed. A common failing is forgetting that if an outcome event is the end point, the effective sample size is the number of events observed. A study may have 1000 patients, but if only 10 events are observed, one cannot find multiple risk factors for those events.

Investigators should plan data analysis at the beginning of a study. Often, the setup for the analysis data set is specific to the methods of analysis. This needs to be communicated to the data managers (see **Box 1**).

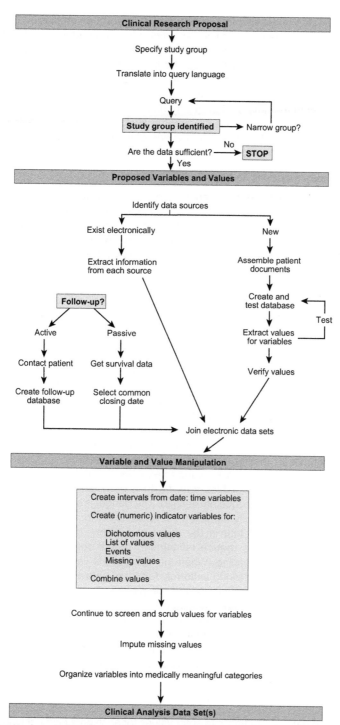

Fig. 6. Linearized work flow for a clinical research study: Transforming information to data suited for analysis.

A necessary step is review of the literature. Sifting through articles is often painful, but it should result in identifying a few key articles that are pertinent to the study. The search is too often confined to recent literature, and this may result in duplication.

A realistic timeframe with deliverables should be established with collaborators. A common failing is not providing sufficient time for data verification and other aspects of data management that are the heart of a high-quality study. Analysis of data may consume one-tenth the time of high-quality data preparation.

The completed formal research proposal is likely to be updated throughout the course of a study, facilitated by online tracking of each study, with periodic updates of the protocol as necessary.

Database Development and Verification

The next step for successful research is careful attention to the data themselves. If electronically available data are to be used, every variable must be defined both medically and at the database content level. If data are to be collected de novo, then an appropriate database must be developed (see **Fig. 6**). Every variable must be in a format of 1 value per variable. These variables must follow a controlled vocabulary for analysis, not free text.

Data Collection

A core set of variables should be collected for each patient. In cardiac surgical and interventional cardiology settings, these data elements are stipulated by regulatory agencies (eg, the state of New York) or societies (eg, Society of Thoracic Surgeons National Database, the American College of Cardiology National Cardiovascular Data Registry). They include demographics (it is essential to record patients' date of birth rather than age because age can be calculated from date of birth to any chosen time zero), cardiac procedure and clinical symptoms and status at time of procedure, cardiac medical history (particularly previous cardiac procedures), disease cause, coexisting cardiac defects, coexisting noncardiac morbidity (such as diabetes), laboratory measurements known to be consistently associated with clinical outcomes, findings of diagnostic testing, findings during the procedure, support techniques during the procedure, and factors related to experience (such as date of procedure).

Investigators also need variables specific to a particular study. These variables should be identified and reproducibly defined. The danger is specifying too many variables; however, a thoughtfully compiled list adds depth to a study. Further, experienced investigators realize that in the midst of a study, it occasionally becomes evident that some variables require refinement, others collecting de novo, others rechecking, and others redefining. When this occurs, the variables must be refined, collected, rechecked, or redefined uniformly for every patient in the study.

Clinical studies are only as accurate and complete as the data available in patients' records.[106] Therefore, physician-investigators seriously interested in scientific progress must ensure that their preintervention, intervention, and postintervention records are clear, organized, precise, and extensive, so that information gathering can be complete and meaningful. Records should emphasize description; although records may contain the conclusions of the moment, descriptions of basic observations become useful in later analyses.

Verification

The first step in data verification is to enter values for each data element (variable) for 5 to 10 patients only. These values reveal problems of definition, incomplete pick lists, missed variables, difficult-to-find variables that may not be worth the effort to locate, poor-quality variables, inconsistent recording, and questionable quality of observations. Once these issues are addressed, general data abstraction may proceed.

When all values for variables are in a computer database, formal verification commences. This verification can take 3 general forms: (1) value-by-value checking of recorded data against primary source documents, (2) random quality checking, and (3) automatic reasonableness checking. If a routine activity of recording core data-elements is used, it is wise to verify each element initially to identify those that are rarely in error (these can be spot checked by a random process) and those that are more often in error. The latter are usually a small fraction of the whole and are often values requiring interpretation. These values may require element-by-element verification.

When it is thought that data are correct (this is an iterative process with verification), they are checked for reasonableness of ranges, including discovery of inconsistencies among correlated values. For example, the database may indicate that a patient had a quadrangular resection of the mitral valve, but someone had failed to record that the posterior leaflet was prolapsing and had ruptured chordae, or the database records that a patient is 60 cm tall and weighs 180 kg; this is likely a problem of confused units of measurement.

Data Conversion for Analysis

An often underappreciated, unanticipated, and time-consuming effort is the conversion of data elements residing in a database to a format suitable for data analysis. Even if the day comes when all medical information is recorded as values for variables in a computer-based patient record,[107] this step is unavoidable. Statistical procedures require data to be arranged in columns and rows, with each column representing values for a single variable (often in numeric format), and each row either a separate patient or multiple records on a single patient (as in many-to-1 repeated-measures longitudinal data analysis). This conversion process may involve redundancy, such as the necessity to again document all variables and provide a data key to the possible values for each.

This process nearly always involves creating additional variables from a single variable, such as a separate variable for each mutually exclusive cause of cardiomyopathy. These polytomous variables (lists) are then converted to a series of dichotomous variables (best expressed as 0 for absence and 1 for presence of the listed value).

Some categorical variables are ordinal, such as NYHA functional classes. These variables may need to be reformulated as an ordered number sequence (eg, 1–4). Variables recorded with units (eg, weight in kilograms, weight in pounds) must be converted to a common metric.

Calculated variables are also formed. These variables include body surface area and body mass index from height and weight, z values from measured cardiac dimensions, ejection fraction from systolic and diastolic ventricular volumes, intervals between date and time variables for which event indicator variables are created, and many other calculations. Because data conversion, creation of derived variables, and formation of calculated variables is time consuming and error prone, groups that conduct a large number of studies often store trusted, well-verified computer code to perform these operations on a repetitive basis.

Often information is gathered from multiple databases with queries, concatenations, and joining functions. These otherwise arduous functions can, under some circumstances, be automated. Alternatively, a data warehouse composed of multiple disparate electronic data sources can be implemented and maintained.

Managing sporadic missing data is important. If too many data are missing, the variable may be unsuitable for use in analyses. Otherwise, missing value imputation is necessary so that entire patients are not removed from analyses, the default option in many analysis programs.[108]

Data Analysis

The data analysis process should lead first to understanding of the raw data, often called exploratory data analysis.[109] This understanding is gleaned from simple descriptive statistics, correlations among variables, simple life tables for time-related events, cumulative distribution graphs of continuously distributed variables, and cluster analyses, whereby variables with shared information content are identified.

The analytical process then attempts to extract meaning from the data by various methods akin to pattern recognition.[21] Answers are sought for the following questions: which variables relate to outcome and which do not? What inference can be made about whether an association is or is not attributable to chance alone? Might there be a causal relationship? For what might a variable associated with outcome be a surrogate?

What will be discovered is that answering such questions in the most clinically relevant way often outstrips available statistical, biomathematical, and algorithmic methodology. Instead, a question is answered with available techniques, but not the question. One of the purposes of this article is to stimulate collaboration between physician-investigators and data analysis experts so that data are analyzed thoroughly and with appropriate methodology.

Interpreting Analyses

It is one thing for a statistician to provide a statistical inference; it is another for the physician-investigator to draw meaningful interpretations that affect patient care (clinical inferences).

The most successful way to embark on this interpretive phase of clinical research is to write down the truest 2 or 3 sentences that capture the essence of the findings (and no more).[110] This important exercise produces an ultramini abstract for an article (whether or not it is required by a journal) and provides the roadmap for writing the article.[111]

Communicating the Findings

A common error of the physician-investigator is to summarize the data instead of drawing meaningful clinical inferences from the data and analyses by asking the following questions: (1) What new knowledge has been gleaned from the clinical investigation? (2) How can this new knowledge be incorporated into better patient care? (3) What do the data suggest in terms of basic research that needs to be stimulated? (4) How can I best communicate information to my colleagues? (5) How can I best present this information to the cardiologic world at large?

Meaningful new knowledge may not be generated because the statistical inferences from data analyses are accepted as the final result. Results need to be studied carefully. Often, this leads to additional analyses that increasingly illuminate the message that the data are trying to convey. Graphic depictions are of particular importance in transforming numbers into insight. Depictions must lead beyond statistical inference to clinical inference. What have the data revealed about how to better care for patients? This question is the one best linked to the original purpose of the study. If the study has suggested ways to improve patient care, the next step is to put what has been learned into practice.

Most studies generate more new questions than they answer. Some of these new questions require additional clinical research. Others require the physician-investigator to stimulate colleagues in the basic sciences to investigate fundamental mechanisms of the disease process.

Because most physician-investigators are part of a group, an important facet of generating new knowledge is discussing with colleagues the results, statistical and clinical inferences, and implications of a study. Multiple points of view nearly always clarify rather than obscure their interpretation.

Clinical research is not a proprietary activity. Yet, too often research does not result in an article. One reason may be that an abstract was not accepted for a meeting, perhaps because the data were not thoroughly digested before its submission. Although abstract deadlines may be important mechanisms for wrapping up studies, they too often stifle a serious and contemplative approach to generating new knowledge. A second reason articles do not get written is that the physician-investigator views the task as overwhelming. Possibly they have not developed an orderly strategy for writing. A third barrier to writing is time demands on the physician-investigator. Usually, this situation results from not making writing a priority in their professional life. This is a decision that should be made early in one's medical career. If dissemination of new knowledge is a desire, then writing must be made a high priority part of one's life style.

REFERENCES

1. ACC/AHA guidelines and indications for coronary artery bypass graft surgery. A report of the American College of Cardiology/American Heart Association Task Force on Assessment of Diagnostic and Therapeutic Cardiovascular Procedures (Subcommittee on Coronary Artery Bypass Graft Surgery). Circulation 1991;83:1125–73.
2. Kouchoukos NT, Blackstone EH, Hanley FL, et al. Cardiac surgery. 4th edition. Philadelphia: Elsevier; 2012. p. 251–352.
3. Newton I. Philosophiae naturalis principia mathematica.1687.
4. Blackstone EH. Let the data speak for themselves? Semin Thorac Cardiovasc Surg Pediatr Card Surg Annu 2004;7:192–8.
5. Kirklin JW, Vicinanza SS. Metadata and computer-based patient records. Ann Thorac Surg 1999;68:S23–4.
6. Bland JM, Kerry SM. Statistics notes. Trials randomised in clusters. BMJ 1997; 315:600.
7. Donner A, Klar N. Design and analysis of cluster randomization trials in health research. New York: Oxford University Press; 2000.
8. Bland JM. Sample size in guidelines trials. Fam Pract 2000;17:S17–20.
9. Divine GW, Brown JT, Frazier LM. The unit of analysis error in studies about physicians' patient care behavior. J Gen Intern Med 1992;7:623.
10. Antman K, Lagakos S, Drazen J. Designing and funding clinical trials of novel therapies. N Engl J Med 2001;344:762–3.
11. Edwards SJ, Braunholtz DA, Lilford RJ, et al. Ethical issues in the design and conduct of cluster randomised controlled trials. BMJ 1999;318:1407–9.
12. Margo CE. When is surgery research? Towards an operational definition of human research. J Med Ethics 2001;27:40–3.
13. McKneally MF. A bypass for the Institutional Review Board: reflections on the Cleveland Clinic study of the Batista operation. J Thorac Cardiovasc Surg 2001;121:837–9.

14. Blackstone EH, Kirklin JW. Rational decision-making in paediatric cardiac surgery. In: Godman M, editor. Paediatric cardiology, vol. 4. Edinburgh (United Kingdom): Churchill Livingstone; 1981. p. 334–44.
15. Lawrence AC. Human error as a cause of accidents in gold mining. J Safety Res 1974;6:78.
16. Wigglesworth EC. A teaching model of injury causation and a guide for selecting countermeasures. Occup Psychol 1972;46:69–78.
17. Kohn L, Corrigan J, Donaldson M, editors. To err is human: building a safer health system. Washington, DC: National Academy Press; 1999.
18. Rizzoli G, Blackstone EH, Kirklin JW, et al. Incremental risk factors in hospital mortality rate after repair of ventricular septal defect. J Thorac Cardiovasc Surg 1980;80:494–505.
19. de Leval MR, Francois K, Bull C, et al. Analysis of a cluster of surgical failures. Application to a series of neonatal arterial switch operations. J Thorac Cardiovasc Surg 1994;107:914–23 [discussion: 923–4].
20. Guerlac H. Theological voluntarism and biological analogies in Newton's physical thought. J Hist Ideas 1983;44:219–29.
21. Breiman L. Statistical modeling: the two cultures. Stat Sci 2001;16:199–231.
22. Hastie T, Tibshirani R, Friedman JH. The elements of statistical learning: data mining, inference, and prediction. New York: Springer-Verlag; 2001.
23. Blackstone EH, Rice TW. From trees to wood and back: perspective on clinical data analysis in thoracic surgery. Thorac Surg Clin 2007;17:309–27.
24. Hrushesky WJ. Triumph of the trivial. Perspect Biol Med 1998;41:341.
25. Bochner S. Continuity and discontinuity in nature and knowledge. In: Wiener PP, editor. Dictionary of the history of ideas: studies of selected pivotal ideas, vol. 1. New York: Charles Scribner's Sons; 1968. p. 492.
26. Breiman L. Random forests. Mach Learn 2001;45:5–32.
27. Ishwaran H, Kogalur UB. Random survival forest 3.0.1. R package. 2008. Available at: http://cran.r-project.org. Accessed November 20, 2012.
28. Kannel WB, Dawber TR, Kagan A, et al. Factors of risk in the development of coronary heart disease–six year follow-up experience. The Framingham Study. Ann Intern Med 1961;55:33–50.
29. Berkson J. Why I prefer logits to probits. Biometrics 1951;7:327–39.
30. Kirklin JW. A letter to Helen (presidential address). J Thorac Cardiovasc Surg 1979;78:643–54.
31. Lytle BW, Blackstone EH, Loop FD, et al. Two internal thoracic artery grafts are better than one. J Thorac Cardiovasc Surg 1999;117:855–72.
32. Levy WC, Mozaffarian D, Linker DT, et al. The Seattle Heart Failure Model: prediction of survival in heart failure. Circulation 2006;113:1424–33.
33. Allen LA, Yager JE, Funk MJ, et al. Discordance between patient-predicted and model-predicted life expectancy among ambulatory patients with heart failure. JAMA 2008;299:2533–42.
34. Lughezzani G, Briganti A, Karakiewicz PI, et al. Predictive and prognostic models in radical prostatectomy candidates: a critical analysis of the literature. Eur Urol 2010;58:687–700.
35. Pettersson GB, Martino D, Blackstone EH, et al. Advising complex patients who require complex heart operations. J Thorac Cardiovasc Surg, in press.
36. Byar DP. Problems with using observational databases to compare treatments. Stat Med 1991;10:663–6.

37. Formigari L. Chain of being. In: Wiener PP, editor. Dictionary of the history of ideas: studies of selected pivotal ideas, vol. 1. New York: Charles Scribner's Sons; 1968. p. 325.
38. Reason JT. Human error. Cambridge (United Kingdom): Cambridge University Press; 1990.
39. Hannan EL, Kumar D, Racz M, et al. New York State's Cardiac Surgery Reporting System: four years later. Ann Thorac Surg 1994;58:1852–7.
40. Malcolm JA Jr. Plans proceed to publish physician-specific data. Pa Med 1992; 95:18–9.
41. Burack JH, Impellizzeri P, Homel P, et al. Public reporting of surgical mortality: a survey of New York State cardiothoracic surgeons. Ann Thorac Surg 1999; 68:1195–200 [discussion: 1201–2].
42. Hannan EL, Siu AL, Kumar D, et al. Assessment of coronary artery bypass graft surgery performance in New York. Is there a bias against taking high-risk patients? Med Care 1997;35:49–56.
43. Omoigui NA, Miller DP, Brown KJ, et al. Outmigration for coronary bypass surgery in an era of public dissemination of clinical outcomes. Circulation 1996;93:27–33.
44. Peterson ED, DeLong ER, Jollis JG, et al. The effects of New York's bypass surgery provider profiling on access to care and patient outcomes in the elderly. J Am Coll Cardiol 1998;32:993–9.
45. Osswald BR, Blackstone EH, Tochtermann U, et al. The meaning of early mortality after CABG. Eur J Cardiothorac Surg 1999;15:401–7.
46. Coyle SL. Physician-industry relations. Part 1: individual physicians. Ann Intern Med 2002;136:396–402.
47. Coyle SL. Physician-industry relations. Part 2: organizational issues. Ann Intern Med 2002;136:403–6.
48. Horrobin DF. Evidence-based medicine and the need for non-commercial clinical research directed towards therapeutic innovation. Exp Biol Med (Maywood) 2002;227:435–7.
49. Association of American Medical Colleges Task Force on Clinical Research. In: For the health of the public: ensuring the future of clinical research, vol. 1. Washington, DC: AAM; 1999. p. 16.
50. Yusuf S, Zucker D, Peduzzi P, et al. Effect of coronary artery bypass graft surgery on survival: overview of 10-year results from randomised trials by the Coronary Artery Bypass Graft Surgery Trialists Collaboration. Lancet 1994; 344:563–70.
51. Eleven-year survival in the Veterans Administration randomized trial of coronary bypass surgery for stable angina. The Veterans Administration Coronary Artery Bypass Surgery Cooperative Study Group. N Engl J Med 1984;311: 1333–9.
52. National Heart, Lung, and Blood Institute Coronary Artery Surgery Study. A multicenter comparison of the effects of randomized medical and surgical treatment of mildly symptomatic patients with coronary artery disease, and a registry of consecutive patients undergoing coronary angiography. Circulation 1981;63: I1–81.
53. Varnauskas E. Twelve-year follow-up of survival in the randomized European Coronary Surgery Study. N Engl J Med 1988;319:332–7.
54. Frye RL, Sopko G, Detre KM. The BARI trial: baseline observations. The BARI Investigators. Trans Am Clin Climatol Assoc 1992;104:26–30.

55. Burdette WI, Gehan EA. Planning and analysis of clinical studies. Springfield (IL): Charles C Thomas; 1970.
56. Birnbaum Memorial Symposium. Medical research: statistics and ethics. Science 1977;198:677.
57. Byar DP, Simon RM, Friedewald WT, et al. Randomized clinical trials. Perspectives on some recent ideas. N Engl J Med 1976;295:74–80.
58. Weinstein MC. Allocation of subjects in medical experiments. N Engl J Med 1974;291:1278–85.
59. Benson K, Hartz AJ. A comparison of observational studies and randomized, controlled trials. N Engl J Med 2000;342:1878–86.
60. Pocock SJ, Elbourne DR. Randomized trials or observational tribulations? N Engl J Med 2000;342:1907–9.
61. Concato J, Shah N, Horwitz RI. Randomized, controlled trials, observational studies, and the hierarchy of research designs. N Engl J Med 2000;342:1887–92.
62. Hannan EL. Randomized clinical trials and observational studies: guidelines for assessing respective strengths and limitations. JACC Cardiovasc Interv 2008;1:211–7.
63. Feinstein AR. T. Duckett Jones Memorial Lecture. The Jones criteria and the challenges of clinimetrics. Circulation 1982;66:1–5.
64. Lee YJ, Ellenberg JH, Hirtz DG, et al. Analysis of clinical trials by treatment actually received: is it really an option? Stat Med 1991;10:1595–605.
65. Feinstein AR, Landis JR. The role of prognostic stratification in preventing the bias permitted by random allocation of treatment. J Chronic Dis 1976;29:277–84.
66. Guillemin F. Primer: the fallacy of subgroup analysis. Nat Clin Pract Rheumatol 2007;3:407–13.
67. Wahlgren N, Ahmed N, Eriksson N, et al. Multivariable analysis of outcome predictors and adjustment of main outcome results to baseline data profile in randomized controlled trials: Safe Implementation of Thrombolysis in Stroke-MOnitoring STudy (SITS-MOST). Stroke 2008;39:3316–22.
68. Bonchek LI. Sounding board. Are randomized trials appropriate for evaluating new operations? N Engl J Med 1979;301:44–5.
69. Meier P. Statistics and medical experimentation. Biometrics 1975;31:511–29.
70. Grunkemeier GL, Starr A. Reply to correspondence on randomization in surgical studies. J Heart Valve Dis 1993;2:359–61.
71. Horton R. The clinical trial: deceitful, disputable, unbelievable, unhelpful, and shameful–what next? Control Clin Trials 2001;22:593–604.
72. Love JW. Drugs and operations. Some important differences. JAMA 1975;232:37–8.
73. Barkun JS, Aronson JK, Feldman LS, et al. Evaluation and stages of surgical innovations. Lancet 2009;374:1089–96.
74. Ergina PL, Cook JA, Blazeby JM, et al. Challenges in evaluating surgical innovation. Lancet 2009;374:1097–104.
75. McCulloch P, Altman DG, Campbell WB, et al. No surgical innovation without evaluation: the IDEAL recommendations. Lancet 2009;374:1105–12.
76. Moses LE. Measuring effects without randomized trials? Options, problems, challenges. Med Care 1995;33:AS8–14.
77. Grunkemeier GL, Starr A. Alternatives to randomization in surgical studies. J Heart Valve Dis 1992;1:142–51.
78. Rosenbaum PR, Rubin DB. The central role of the propensity score in observational studies for causal effects. Biometrika 1983;70:41–55.

79. Rubin DB. The design versus the analysis of observational studies for causal effects: parallels with the design of randomized trials. Stat Med 2007;26:20–36.
80. Rosenbaum PR. Observational studies. New York: Springer-Verlag; 1995.
81. Blackstone EH. Comparing apples and oranges. J Thorac Cardiovasc Surg 2002;123:8–15.
82. Drake C. Effects of misspecification of the propensity score on estimators of treatment effect. Biometrics 1993;49:1231.
83. Drake C, Fisher L. Prognostic models and the propensity score. Int J Epidemiol 1995;24:183–7.
84. D'Agostino RB Jr. Propensity score methods for bias reduction in the comparison of a treatment to a non-randomized control group. Stat Med 1998;17: 2265–81.
85. Little RJ, Rubin DB. Causal effects in clinical and epidemiological studies via potential outcomes: concepts and analytical approaches. Annu Rev Public Health 2000;21:121–45.
86. Rosenbaum PR, Rubin DB. Reducing bias in observational studies using subclassification on the propensity score. J Am Stat Assoc 1984;79:516–24.
87. Rosenbaum PR. From association to causation in observational studies: the role of tests of strongly ignorable treatment assignment. J Am Stat Assoc 1984;79:41.
88. Gum PA, Thamilarasan M, Watanabe J, et al. Aspirin use and all-cause mortality among patients being evaluated for known or suspected coronary artery disease: a propensity analysis. JAMA 2001;286:1187–94.
89. Austin PC, Mamdani MM. A comparison of propensity score methods: a case-study estimating the effectiveness of post-MI statin use. Stat Med 2006;25: 2084–106.
90. Bergstralh EJ, Konsanke JL. Computerized matching of cases to controls. Technical report No. 56. Department of Health Science Research. Rochester (MN): Mayo Clinic; 1995.
91. Rubin DB. The use of matched sampling and regression adjustment to remove bias in observational studies. Biometrics 1973;29:185–203.
92. Rosenbaum PR. Optimal matching for observational studies. J Am Stat Assoc 1985;84:1024–32.
93. Li YP. Balanced risk set matching. J Am Stat Assoc 2001;96:870.
94. Lee BK, Lessler J, Stuart EA. Improving propensity score weighting using machine learning. Stat Med 2010;29:337–46.
95. Gillinov AM, Wierup PN, Blackstone EH, et al. Is repair preferable to replacement for ischemic mitral regurgitation? J Thorac Cardiovasc Surg 2001;122: 1125–41.
96. Rosenbaum PR, Rubin DB. The bias due to incomplete matching. Biometrics 1985;41:103–16.
97. Beach JM, Mihaljevic T, Svensson LG, et al. Coronary artery disease and outcomes of aortic valve replacement for severe aortic stenosis. J Am Coll Cardiol, in press.
98. Rubin DB. Estimating causal effects from large data sets using propensity scores. Ann Intern Med 1997;127:757–63.
99. Deeks JJ, Dinnes J, D'Amico R, et al. Evaluating non-randomised intervention studies. Health Technol Assess 2003;7:1–186.
100. Heckman JJ, Ichimura H, Smith J, et al. Sources of selection bias in evaluating social programs: an interpretation of conventional measures and evidence on the effectiveness of matching as a program evaluation method. Proc Natl Acad Sci U S A 1996;93:13416–20.

101. Hosmer DW, Lemeshow S. Applied logistic regression. 2nd edition. New York: Wiley-Interscience; 1989.
102. Robins JM, Mark SD, Newey WK. Estimating exposure effects by modelling the expectation of exposure conditional on confounders. Biometrics 1992;48: 479–95.
103. Imai K, van Dyk DA. Causal inference with general treatment regimes: generalizing the propensity score. J Am Stat Assoc 2004;99:854–66.
104. Marban E, Braunwald E. Training the clinician investigator. Circ Res 2008;103: 771–2.
105. Blackstone EH. Planning the research. In: Penson DF, Wei JT, editors. Clinical research methods for surgeons. New York: Humana Press; 2006. p. 3–29.
106. Feinstein AR. Clinical biostatistics. XX. The epidemiologic trohoc, the ablative risk ratio, and "retrospective" research. Clin Pharmacol Ther 1973;14:291–307.
107. Dick RS, Steen EB, editors. The computer-based patient record: an essential technology for health care. Washington, DC: The National Academy Press; 1991.
108. Rubin DB. Multiple imputation for non-response in surveys. New York: Wiley; 1987.
109. Tukey JW. Exploratory data analysis. Reading (MA): Addison-Wesley; 1977.
110. Kirklin JW, Blackstone EH. Notes from the editors: ultramini-abstracts and abstracts. J Thorac Cardiovasc Surg 1994;107:326.
111. Blackstone EH, Rice TW. Clinical-pathologic conference: use and choice of statistical methods for the clinical study, "superficial adenocarcinoma of the esophagus". J Thorac Cardiovasc Surg 2001;122:1063–76.

Quality, Patient Safety, and the Cardiac Surgical Team

Elizabeth A. Martinez, MD, MHS

KEYWORDS

- Quality • Patient safety • Cardiac surgery • Continuous quality improvement
- Registries • System redesign • Collaboratives • Interventions

KEY POINTS

- The patient safety literature has evolved from a quality-assurance focus to quality improvement using multidisciplinary teams that review the continuum of care: structure, process, and outcomes.
- Recent publications regarding patient safety in cardiac surgery consider teamwork and collaboration to be integral to improving patient safety.
- Cardiac surgery has a rich history in patient safety, including the use of benchmarking, public reporting, collaboratives, and systems redesign.
- Effective interventions use tools to ensure collaboration, such as briefings, checklists, and handoff protocols.

BACKGROUND

The need for quality improvement (QI), coupled with increased safety and efficiency, continues to be at the forefront of health care discussions. To accomplish these goals, clinical leaders need to be proficient in the principles of QI, identification and mitigation of hazards, and redesign of care process. The practice of quality evaluation has evolved from primarily an external review of practice (such as accreditation, board certification, and licensing) to an internalized process of ensuring QI, and an increasing focus on outcomes. This evolution denotes the growing (and arguably obvious) recognition that quality cannot be improved by focusing on structure, process, or outcomes independently; rather, the entire continuum of care must be considered. Recent efforts to infuse industrial process innovations into health care, coupled with a national

Funding Sources: Dr Martinez is currently receiving funding from the Agency for Healthcare Research and Quality, The Commonwealth Fund and the Massachusetts General Hospital Clinical Innovations award.
Conflict of interest: None.
Department of Anesthesia, Critical Care and Pain Medicine, Massachusetts General Hospital, Harvard Medical School, GRB 444, 55 Fruit Street, Boston, MA 02114, USA
E-mail address: Martinez.Elizabeth@mgh.harvard.edu

Anesthesiology Clin 31 (2013) 249–268
http://dx.doi.org/10.1016/j.anclin.2013.01.004
1932-2275/13/$ – see front matter © 2013 Elsevier Inc. All rights reserved.

agenda to improve the quality of care and reduce costs, have solidified a commitment to continuous QI (CQI). The trend towards more intensive self-evaluation is supported by partnerships with physicians to conduct QI, which is now a required element by licensing and accreditation bodies.

Cardiac surgery remains an area of focus for quality and safety efforts, because of its prevalence, high cost, and high-risk nature. There is a long history of quality work in cardiac surgery, but there is residual room for improvement. Early research seemed to indicate that volume was inversely correlated with outcomes: surgeons and centers that performed more operations tended to have lower mortality. Volume was initially accepted as a surrogate for quality and was adopted as a quality measure by the Leapfrog group.[1] However, it has since been shown that volume, when appropriately risk adjusted, is not the most important driver, or even a proxy for, quality in cardiac surgery. Thus, although practice (high volume) is important, other factors are amenable to improvements that influence patient safety, such as better teamwork and collaboration combined with a systems approach to proactively identify hazards and near-misses to correct or mitigate them.

This review introduces the reader to the principles of research in QI and the science of safety, followed by a targeted review of several decades of discussion surrounding quality and safety issues in medicine, and then presents a focused review of efforts to improve quality and safety in cardiac surgery, specifically. The review concludes with recommendations for future research regarding effective interventions to improve quality and safety of cardiac surgery.

INTRODUCTION TO QUALITY AND SAFETY
Perceptions of Quality and Safety

Patients and clinicians tend to agree that patient safety and health care quality are not yet where they need to be. In 1999, the Institute of Medicine's (IOM's) report *To Err is Human*[2] reinvigorated the focus on the state of patient safety in US medicine. Although this oft-cited report got the nation's attention, the problem was not new. The practice of assessing quality began more than 4 decades ago with the publication in 1966 of Avedis Donabedian's[3] article on the evaluation of quality in health care. One of the concepts introduced in this seminal work is the notion of assessing quality from 3 vantage points: (1) structure (staffing patterns, personnel training, organization, tools, and technology), (2) process (the degree to which care practices are evidence-based, timely, safe, and followed), and (3) outcomes (such as mortality, functional improvement, and patient satisfaction).[4] Donabedian's framework reflects the interrelatedness of these concepts (**Fig. 1**). Furthermore, in 1991, Brennan and Leape[5] noted that approximately 3% of hospitalized patients suffered a medical error, resulting in 44,000 to 98,000 deaths per year and billions in excess costs.

Several years later, a 1997 survey by the National Patient Safety Foundation found that 1 in 3 US adults have reported that they have been personally involved with a medical mistake with a permanent negative effect on health, and only half reported being very satisfied with their latest experience with a health care professional.[6,7] In the intervening years, opinion has not improved measurably, even among clinicians. In a nationwide survey in 2001 of health professionals,[8] 58% reported that health care in the United States was not very good, with as many as 95% of physicians reporting that they had witnessed a serious medical error. Four of 5 professionals stated that they believed that fundamental changes were needed in the American health care system. The problem continues to be grave. In a recent survey of 1034 Americans, 66% gave "the quality of health care in the country as a whole" a grade of C or lower.[9]

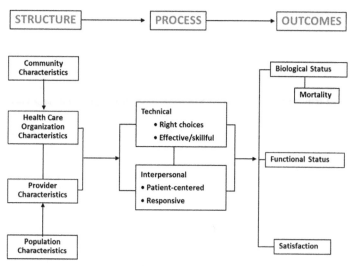

Fig. 1. Structure-process-outcome model for QI.

Improving patient safety is important, because it is the right thing to do. But there are economic imperatives as well; mistakes are costly. Purchasers and insurers are keen on making value-based decisions. Regulators, both governmental agencies and not-for-profit accreditation organizations, have developed improvement projects with built-in incentives for adoption, some of which may result in improved reimbursement, and others that are linked to a disincentive, such as nonpayment for certain hospital-acquired conditions (eg, development of a pressure ulcer or a nosocomial infection). To this end, safety data have been collected and analyzed to identify trends, compare and reward institutions, and promote accountability.

Twelve-year trend analysis of patient perception of health care quality shows that patients are increasingly aware of the existence of such reports, and are taking an active role in ensuring quality and coordination of care. Health care decisions are more likely to be based on information about provider quality, such as expert ratings, than in previous years.[6] Most (70%) patients double-check prescriptions for accuracy, and 2 in 3 call to follow up on tests. However, hospital decisions continue to be primarily driven by referrals from family and friends, and more than 90% of respondents were unaware of a new government Web site providing hospital comparison data (http://www.hospitalcompare.hhs.gov/). These data suggest that patients and providers are beginning to accept their joint role in monitoring and improving quality and safety. Yet these data raise as many questions as they answer. With continued vigilance on safety and ever-more information about inherent risks, why are there still safety issues? And what can be done about them?

Why Are Quality and Safety Poor?

Although this progress toward a more vigilant public and provider community is encouraging, some experts contend that the decade that has elapsed since the IOM report has not seen enough improvement in the quality and safety of clinical care. Adverse events continue to happen, many of which are deemed preventable,[10,11] and this may be particularly true for cardiovascular procedures, which are inherently complex and multidisciplinary, requiring attention to detail, adherence to protocols, and careful coordination. Yet such adherence is difficult to establish and sustain. In 2 evaluations of 12 different geographically located communities, McGlynn and colleagues[12,13] reported that although some disparities in quality of care exist between regions and demographic subgroups, none of the gaps in care was as large as the deviations from standards of care. These investigators identified that, on average, patients are receiving the recommended practices only 54.9% (95% confidence interval [CI] 54.3%–55.5%) of the time, and 60% (95% CI 64.2%–71.8%) for coronary artery disease.[12] Such systemic deficiencies in safety and quality indicate that attention needs to be directed toward errors of omission. This strategy may be particularly relevant to those working to improve quality and safety in cardiac surgery, in which adherence to standards of care and streamlining operating room (OR) procedures can have a real impact on patient safety, every day. In the highly technical and demanding surgical suite, attention should remain focused on identifying latent hazards that contribute to errors and adverse events.

Types of Errors and How They Jeopardize Safety

Although the patient safety literature has expanded since the IOM report, with nearly 3 times[14] as many articles published and research awards granted in subsequent years, it is unclear whether this proliferation of attention in the journals came with any attendant change in frontline provider awareness or modifications to basic processes. Stelfox and colleagues[14] suggest that despite the popularity of Reason's Swiss cheese paradigm[15,16] of latent and active failures in complex systems (**Fig. 2**), many providers cannot accurately describe what the model means. For many providers, the holes in the cheese are perceived to be caused solely by systems issues (latent failures), not potentially active failures (or departures from standards of care) by an individual.

In Reason's model, the vulnerable system syndrome is created by the inadvertent alignment of both active and latent failures. Active failures have an immediate and adverse effect. Latent errors arise from managerial and organizational decisions (or the lack thereof) that shape working conditions. These latent errors often result from production pressures. Damaging consequences may not be evident until a triggering event occurs. Thus, the perception may be that chance is still largely responsible for adverse events. In the cycle of blame and denial typical of a vulnerable system, Reason argued, individual workers cannot be expected to pursue excellence. To

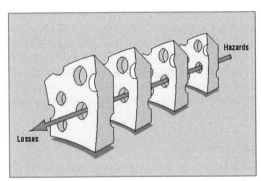

The Swiss cheese model of how defences, barriers, and safeguards may be penetrated by an accident trajectory

Fig. 2. James Reason's Swiss cheese model of latent and active failures. (*Reproduced from* Reason J. Human error: models and management. BMJ 2000;320(7237):768–70; with permission.)

combat this perception, a culture of safety must be created by implementing systems to identify hazards and the structural issues that contribute to them, as opposed to blaming individuals after the fact. Perhaps the emerging recognition that teamwork and good communication are central to improving quality and safety will galvanize efforts to create systems that better support the humans performing difficult tasks under intense conditions.

IMPROVING QUALITY AND SAFETY

Creating a viable safety culture requires cognizance of both the inherent hazards in processes of care as well as structural adaptations to prevent or minimize risk. In its continued effort to provide guidance to hospitals, 4 of the 6 2013 Joint Commission National Patient Safety Goals[17] are aimed at reducing errors (medication, patient identification, surgical mistakes, and infection); the remaining 2 are to improve communication and to identify patient safety risks (eg, reducing suicide). The last decade has seen more robust and multidisciplinary examinations of both structural and process-related factors with respect to their impact on outcomes. These efforts are reviewed in the next section.

Evolution of QI Methods in Medicine

Goal setting starts with definition. What is good quality of care? "Quality of care is the degree to which health services for individuals and populations increase the likelihood of desired health outcomes and are consistent with current professional knowledge."[18] In 2001, 2 years after its initial report, the IOM developed a 4-tiered approach to improving quality and safety by: (1) establishing a national focus on safety leadership and knowledge; (2) identifying and learning from errors; (3) setting performance standards and expectations for safety; (4) implementing safety systems in health care organizations. Six specific aims for improving quality were developed (**Box 1**):

The quality literature has evolved, as have quality efforts. The term quality assurance (QA) was first used to describe quality initiatives. However, QA derives from a regulatory perspective: assurance that organizations or products and services are meeting minimum standards. The use of the term QA has since fallen out of favor, because it has traditionally been linked to just meeting the minimum standard. QI, on the other hand, invokes movement toward a goal. Accreditation bodies, such as The Joint Commission, seek to merge the 2 philosophies by both measuring quality and promoting standards of care delivery.

Box 1
The 6 IOM aims for quality

1. Safe: avoids injuries to patients from the care that is intended to help them
2. Effective: provides services based on scientific knowledge to all who could benefit, and refrains from providing services to those not likely to benefit
3. Patient-centered: provides care that is respectful of and responsive to individual patient preferences, needs, and values
4. Timely: minimizes waits and sometimes harmful delays
5. Efficient: avoids waste
6. Equitable: provides care that does not vary in quality because of personal characteristics such as gender, ethnicity, geographic location, and socioeconomic status

Numerous frameworks for assessing and improving quality have been proposed. Donabedian's[3] structure/process/outcome model (see **Fig. 1**) is still relevant more than 4 decades later. Structure comprises the stable elements of a system in which care is delivered via certain processes and interactions, which result in an outcome. Although both are useful and informative, there are important differences between process measures and outcome measures.

Process measures may be collected quickly and provide immediate feedback on how well the system is working to deliver care according to prescribed standards. Outcome measures are more meaningful to patients, clinicians, and insurers, but they are more difficult to measure and require risk-adjustment methods to adequately control for differences in the health status of patients. When selecting process measures, strong evidence must be available that shows that the process is linked to the desired outcome. Outcome measures are important to patients, physicians, and insurers, but they are imprecise. In a recent study, Shahian and colleagues[19,20] reported that when comparing 4 different methods of assessing hospital mortality, 4 different rates were calculated. However, when outcomes are appropriately and accurately measured, comparing them can drive QI efforts by identifying differences that illuminate the complex interaction between structure and process and suggest problems in the implementation of care processes.

Once these hazards are identified, implementing improvements based on the principles of QI and patient safety are imperative. Such principles include the use of CQI methods, which includes plan-do-study-act (PDSA) cycles or similar rapid-cycle approaches to change, standardization of care, use of checklists, and other measures to introduce redundancy (reminders) into the system. Because cardiac surgery is one of the most prevalent surgical procedures in the United States, it provides an excellent proving ground for putting these principles into action. The impact of care redesign can be seen readily, and performance against recommendations can be compared across institutions to further motivate improvement.

Safety in Cardiac Surgery

Of the 357,000 patients undergoing a coronary artery bypass graft (CABG) or valve procedure in the United States each year, nearly 8% experience an adverse event[21]; half of these events may be preventable,[22,23] and 1 in 3 deaths may be avoidable.[24] A recent focused literature review performed by the LENS (Locating Errors Through Networked Surveillance) research team[25] supported by the Society of Cardiovascular Anesthesiologists Foundation (SCAF)[26] synthesized nearly 4 dozen studies of such events to gain insights into hazards in cardiac surgery. The investigators found that most of the studies published were retrospective; only 3 identified at that time investigated observational interventions aimed at improving safety. One recently published study attempted to prospectively gather data on hazards using direct observation and contextual inquiry.[27] More than 160 hours and 20 cardiac surgeries were observed and 84 contextual inquiries were captured. The team identified 59 hazard categories and grouped these according to the following system: care providers, tasks, tools and technologies, physical environment, organization, and processes (**Box 2**). This multicenter observational study[25,27] provides numerous contemporary examples of hazards in cardiac surgery. The direct observational nature of the study afforded the investigators rich detail, making their findings actionable.

Among the latent failures identified by Martinez and colleagues,[26] lack of a vigorous QA program to monitor and detect problems stands out as a key organizational deficiency exemplified in 2 pediatric cardiac mortality series that gained widespread attention in the late 1980s. The first was at Bristol Infirmary (Bristol, UK)[28,29] and the

Box 2
Direct observation of hazards in the cardiac OR

- Care provider
  - Inadequate/insufficient knowledge or skills
  - Inadequate/lack of professionalism such as not respecting other providers
  - Nonstandardized approach to care delivery or task performance caused by habits, preferences, education, and previous experiences of individual care providers, which may not be based on the current evidence
- Task
  - Avoidable time pressure and unexpected changes
  - Ambiguities caused by different preferences of care providers
  - Nonvalue adding tasks
- Tools and technologies
  - Poor usability (eg, nonintuitive interface design, inconsistency in design, poor visibility of system status)
  - Poor fit or misalignment of safety features with users' needs or work as intended (eg, too many alarms without prioritization)
  - Use of tools, technologies, and supplies with different design characteristics and brands across different sectors of the work environment (eg, ORs and intensive care units [ICUs])
  - Delay in availability of tool and technology at the point and time of need (such as surgical equipment not sterilized in a timely manner)
- Physical environment
  - Poor planning and design of work area in relation to other parts of the OR suite and the hospital (proximity of OR suites to each other, to the storage areas and laboratories, and to the ICU)
  - Insufficiency of size and poor layout design of the ORs
  - Nonstandardization of work-space designs across different ORs
  - Poor configuration of work spaces leading to clutter, inadequate storage, and poor organization of tools, equipment, furniture, and cables
- Organization
  - Focus on productivity in expense of patient safety
  - Lack of or poorly organized policies and protocols for care and other processes
  - Inadequate discussion, training, and dissemination of protocol and policy changes
  - Exclusion of frontline providers' input to purchasing decisions that can potentially affect safety of care
  - Lack of or insufficient reinforcement of policies and protocols
- Care processes
  - Noncompliance with the recommended guidelines and practices
  - Lack of standardization in care processes
- Other processes
  - Ineffective supply chain management processes, resulting in unavailability of supplies and equipment in a timely manner

Reproduced from Gurses AP, Kim G, Martinez EA, et al. Identifying and categorising patient safety hazards in cardiovascular ORs using an interdisciplinary approach: a multisite study. BMJ Qual Saf 2012;21(10):813; with permission.

second was in Winnipeg, Canada.[30–32] During a 6-year period (1988–1994), Bristol Infirmary providers' concerns about 29 pediatric deaths initially went unheeded. Eventually, public outcry resulted in a moratorium on pediatric cardiac surgery while a full investigation was conducted. The investigators recommended systemic organizational changes to place a priority on QA, including feedback from patients and families. The investigators specifically recommended a centralized quality department with an audit function[28,29,33] to detect issues and monitor progress after interventions. In Winnipeg, the pediatric cardiac surgery service experienced 12 deaths over the course of a year (1994). On investigation, issues with the QA program of the organization were again identified as contributors. In addition, the low volume of cases was implicated as a contributor to the clinicians' lack of expertise in both series.

Just more than a decade after these 2 important cases occurred, enough evidence has accumulated to refine our understanding of other contributors, such as organizational issues, poorly designed tools and technology, and teamwork and communication. In a study by Weigmann and colleagues,[34] poor teamwork and communication were found to be the only significant predictors of surgical errors (**Fig. 3**). Similar results have been found in studies by Hazelhurst and colleagues,[35] Wong and colleagues,[36,37] and others. Communication issues can be symptomatic of a hierarchical atmosphere in the cardiac OR. In an atmosphere that is not conducive to speaking up, small errors can compound, resulting in an inability of the team to compensate for major errors (**Fig. 4**).[38] These studies provide real-world perspective on the hazards inherent in cardiac surgery and the numerous opportunities to improve safety with relatively simple changes.

A HISTORY OF IMPROVING OUTCOMES IN CARDIAC SURGERY

Cardiac surgery has a rich history of QI. Despite older and more ill patients presenting for surgery, mortality has decreased significantly over time. In this next section, some

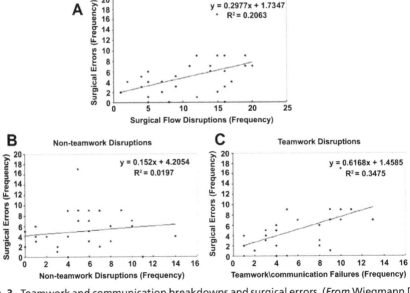

Fig. 3. Teamwork and communication breakdowns and surgical errors. (*From* Wiegmann DA, ElBardissi AW, Dearani JA, et al. Disruptions in surgical flow and their relationship to surgical errors: an exploratory investigation. Surgery 2007;142(5):662; with permission.)

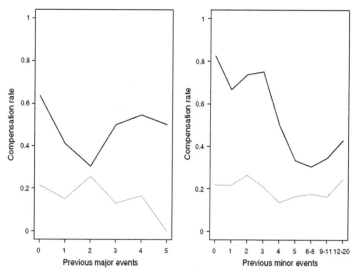

Fig. 4. Minor errors matter: ability of surgical team to compensate is eroded. (*Data from* Solis-Trapala IL, Carthey J, Farewell VT, et al. Dynamic modeling in a study of surgical error management. Stat Med 2007;26(28):5196.)

of the major efforts to improve cardiac surgical care and some recent examples of focused QI efforts are reviewed.

Registries

The Society of Thoracic Surgeons (STS) developed a national registry to capture important risk factors, processes of care, and outcomes. The STS database was introduced more than 20 years ago and has served as a source for national benchmarking and identification of variations in care processes. The results of findings from studies using the STS database have driven important QI efforts.[39] Furthermore, the database and its risk models serve as a gold standard[40] for other registries in health care. Nearly all cardiac surgical centers submit data to the STS or a state level registry (eg, New York State CABG Surgery Reporting System) and receive data reports that show their performance in relation to national peers. This feedback loop has served as a powerful impetus for both local and national improvement efforts. Development of credible reporting tools is an important component of improving quality; understanding current performance is integral to priority setting.

Report Cards and Public Reporting

Early in the 1990s, the states of New York and Pennsylvania began to publicly report surgeon and hospital outcomes in cardiac surgery. The goal of this public reporting was to help cardiac surgeons improve the quality of care they deliver and to allow patients to select care from high-performing surgeons.[41] Although cardiac surgical outcomes improved during the 1990s, controversy remains as to the impact, if any, this reporting had. However, it began to set the stage for transparency in health care[42] and currently cardiac surgical outcomes are publicly reported nationally; some centers have even been ranked in an article in *Consumer Reports* (Consumer Reports home page (http://www.consumerreports.org/health/home.htm).[43]

Collaboratives

In addition to report cards, there is a long history of collaboratives for continuous QI, 4 of which are presented here. The first large collaborative was the Northern New England Cardiovascular Disease Study Group, which consisted of 23 surgeons, representing 5 hospitals from Maine, New Hampshire, and Vermont.[44] These surgeons performed a pre-post analysis after implementation of a program designed to help the cardiac surgical centers learn from each other. The interventions consisted of 3 key elements: (1) feedback on outcome data, (2) CQI training, and (3) site visits. Beginning in 1990, each surgeon in the collaborative received a report on their data in addition to a report on the performance of their hospital and the regional data, to which the surgeons remained blind. These reports were distributed 3 times a year and were timed with regional face-to-face meetings to discuss the reports. All members of the group were exposed to CQI training at the start of the intervention period so that they could participate in local improvement initiatives. Multidisciplinary teams, which included an industrial engineer in addition to clinical staff, were invited to visit another site. During these site visits, teams would observe practices throughout the course of the CABG procedure, including preoperative catheterizations through postoperative care.[44] The teams returned with lessons learned and some of the findings inspired local QI projects.

After the intervention, which took place over 1 year, the collaborative team showed a 24% reduction in hospital mortality ($P = .001$), despite an increased complexity of the patient population. In an attempt to understand the drivers of this improvement, interviews with the management team at each center were conducted to identify what had changed. The list included modifications in technical aspects of care, the processes and organization of in-hospital care, personnel organization and training, and methods of evaluating care and in making treatment decisions.[44] This group has remained intact with varying membership and has maintained its CQI framework to achieve successful data-driven improvements.

Another well-known collaborative in Alabama[45] involved the state peer review organizations (PROs) as well as CABG practitioners and administrators from the 20 Alabama hospitals in which cardiac surgery was being performed at the time of the study. This collaborative intervention focused on 7 quality indicators (**Table 1**). Similar to the Northern New England collaborative, beginning in 1997 they included face-to-face meetings to introduce the project, its objectives, and baseline (preintervention)

Table 1 Alabama standardized care processes	
Care Process	**Standardized Approach**
Timing of operation	No elective patient is to be scheduled for surgery the day after cardiac catheterization
Preoperative briefing	Use of a robust checklist to review the care plan for the OR
Stroke prevention	Aortic imaging and cerebral oximetry were to be used in all cases
Prevention of atrial fibrillation	Standardized amiodarone and β-blocker protocol
Glycemic control	Use of standardized glycemic control protocol with clear glucose goals
Appropriate referral	Predefined complex cases were to be referred out

Data from Culig MH, Kunkle RF, Frndak DC, et al. Improving patient care in cardiac surgery using Toyota production system based methodology. Ann Thorac Surg 2011;91(2):394–9.

data. In addition, a representative from the Northern New England Cardiovascular Disease Study Group met the teams to review their implementation process and provide a forum for questions. The Alabama teams also held a teleconference in 1999 to discuss progress, and a member of the state PRO visited each of the sites to check in on the progress they were making. Similar to the Northern New England collaborative, teams were invited to carry out reciprocal site visits. If a site visit took place, each hospital received a written report of the assessment by their peer highlighting similarities and differences between the sites.[45] The collaborative showed that risk-adjusted mortality decreased in Alabama by 2% (4.9%–2.9%, P<.01). The collaborative also showed improvements in many of the targeted indicators; those that achieved statistical significance are highlighted in **Table 1**.

A third quality collaborative was developed by the Michigan Society of Thoracic and Cardiovascular Surgeons. This group partnered with the state's largest payer group (Blue Cross/Blue Shield of Michigan) to expand their quality work. The group comprised all of the cardiac surgical services in the state, and the funding by the payer group allowed for a more robust infrastructure, which helped support the efforts of the teams and facilitated opportunities to communicate, share data, and implement improvements. Improvement targets included: (1) internal mammary artery (IMA) usage, (2) preoperative intra-aortic balloon pump usage, (3) prolonged ventilation, (4) postoperative atrial fibrillation, and (5) CABG crude and risk-adjusted mortality. The teams met quarterly and reviewed their own performance in the context of the Michigan and national STS averages on the performance targets. IMA usage was targeted early because of the wide variation within the cohort and 7 notable outliers. As part of the improvement phase, surgeons were required to complete a form explaining why they did not use an IMA and fax it to the collaborative coordinating center; these were then shared with the teams at the next face-to-face meeting. Using this process, the 7 outliers improved their performance (**Fig. 5**), and the state's performance on this metric improved. Similar successes in reducing variation and rates of prolonged ventilation were achieved.[46] Site visits were also conducted at hospitals with risk-adjusted mortality that was consistently higher than the Michigan average. The visiting team then reported back to the site with an analysis of their findings and suggested opportunities for improvement.[46] This collaborative continues to be active and has since developed a focused review of all deaths in the state to continue the momentum.

The Cardiac Surgical Translational Study is a fourth collaborative, which incorporates the Comprehensive Unit-Based Safety Program[47] and evidence-based practices to reduce perioperative infections in a national cohort of cardiac surgical centers. Principal investigator Peter Pronovost plans to implement the same intervention design

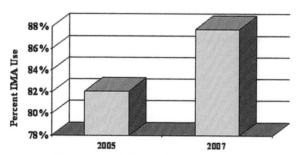

Fig. 5. Improvements in IMA use in Michigan. (*Reproduced from* Prager RL, Armenti FR, Bassett JS, et al. Cardiac surgeons and the quality movement: the Michigan experience. Semin Thorac Cardiovasc Surg 2009;21(1):24; with permission.)

that improved the rate of catheter-related blood steam infections in Michigan.[48] This study, supported by the Agency for Healthcare Research and Quality, and in collaboration with national professional societies including the SCAF, is under way and results are not yet available.

SCAF (http://scahqgive.org/; accessed January 13, 2013) has implemented the FOCUS (Flawless Operative Cardiovascular Unified Systems) project, with the goal of eliminating systems-based failures in cardiac surgical care.[49] SCAF partnered with researchers from Johns Hopkins University to identify hazards in cardiac surgery[25,27] and continues to serve as a member of the CSTS Collaborative. These investigators are working to build and solidify bridges between the national societies representing all of those individuals who care for cardiac surgical patients, including the American Society of Extracorporeal Technology, Association of Operating Room Nurses, National Center for Human Factors Engineering in Healthcare, and the STS. Only through unified approaches such as these can we make important and long-standing improvements in cardiac surgical care.

Process Redesign

The literature provides 2 good examples of a process redesign in cardiac surgical service to guide improvements in the care delivery process. The first implemented process improvement within a long-standing clinical program,[50] and the second incorporated quality and safety principles into plans for a new cardiovascular center.[51] The first, a program called ProvenCare, was implemented at Geisinger Health System, which is a large integrated health system in Pennsylvania. In 2005, the cardiac surgical service team set out to update the delivery of evidence-based care in cardiac surgery by implementing a program in 3 phases[52]: (1) review and validate best practice evidence, (2) redesign the process (of delivery), and (3) implement the new process. To accomplish phase 1, the team reviewed the literature, with a focus on the American College of Cardiology/American Heart Association class I and IIa recommendations for patients with CABG.[53] A leadership team distilled this information and presented it to the cardiac surgeons at Geisinger. Through discussions and consensus, 19 recommendations (which consisted of 40 process elements) were agreed on and standardized for inclusion in the program. During the redesign phase, the team identified the process flows for each surgeon so that they could identify local variation in care delivery and begin to formulate a new process flow that would be used to anchor their redesign efforts (**Fig. 6**).[52] This process map identified the points at which the

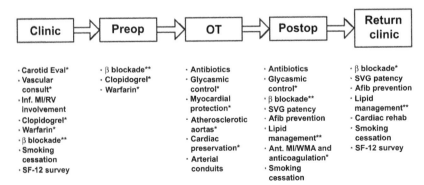

Fig. 6. Process map for care of the cardiac surgical patient. (*Reproduced from* Berry SA, Doll MC, McKinley KE, et al. ProvenCare: quality improvement model for designing highly reliable care in cardiac surgery. Qual Saf Health Care 2009;18(5):363; with permission.)

best practices should be integrated in the care delivery continuum. Integral to this process was a review of ways to leverage the electronic health record to facilitate the adoption of the 40 evidence-based processes. The teams undertook several PDSA cycles to settle on the ideal processes to incorporate standards and reduce redundancy.

Six months after the initiative began, ProvenCare was implemented. In the overall analysis, the investigators reported that performance improved on the 40 measures by 41%: at baseline, 59% of patients with elective CABG received all 40 elements compared with 100% during the last 6 months of the data collection period. Outcomes at 30 days are shown in **Table 2** and represent 137 patients in the preintervention phase and 117 in the postintervention phase. Although provable trends toward improvement were noted for many of the outcomes evaluated, the only statistically significant difference was the number of patients discharged home.[50]

The second example of a process redesign is reported by Culig and colleagues.[51] In this unique example of a proactive process design evaluation, the team reviewed all aspects of the cardiac service line before the introduction of a new cardiac service. The Toyota production system-based methodology (operational excellence) was used to inform the evaluation. The team began the training 2 months before a patient was treated, and the work continued for 2 years. The entire team (both clinical and administrative) was educated on the plans and methodology. A key to the redesign in this system was real-time problem solving: problems were identified daily and addressed by the team during daily reviews of the previous 24 hours. Plans for process changes were initiated immediately on review. In addition, the team standardized 6 care processes (**Box 3**). Other standardized protocols were implemented based on daily hazard identification.

Because a new service was being redesigned, baseline data were not available. However, the team did compare results with like patients within the same geographic region using the STS database. Reported mortality and complications rates were 61% and 57% lower than the comparator group, respectively. The team addressed more

Table 2 Outcomes after ProvenCare implementation			
Outcome Variable	Before ProvenCare	With ProvenCare	Improvement/ Reduction[a]
Average total length of stay (days)	6.2	5.7	–
30-d readmission rate (%)	6.9	3.8	↓44
Discharged home (%)	80	91	↑11[b]
Patients with any complication (%)	38	30	↓21
Patients with less than 1 complication (%)	7.6	5.5	↓28
Incidence of atrial fibrillation (%)	23	19	↓17
Neurologic complication (%)	1.5	0.6	↓60
Any pulmonary complication (%)	7	4	↓43
Received blood products (%)	23	18	↓22
Reoperation for bleeding (%)	3.8	1.7	↓55
Deep sternal wound infection (%)	0.8	0.6	↓25

[a] At 18 months.
[b] $P = .03$; the only statistically significant outcome.

Data from Casale AS, Paulus RA, Selna MJ, et al. "ProvenCareSM": a provider-driven pay-for-performance program for acute episodic cardiac surgical care. Ann Surg 2007;246(4):613–21 [discussion: 21–3].

> **Box 3**
> **Quality indicators for the Alabama collaborative**
>
> 1. IMA use
> 2. Aspirin therapy at discharge
> 3. Duration of intubation
> 4. Intraoperative use of intra-aortic balloon pump
> 5. Readmission to the ICU
> 6. Reoperation for bleeding
> 7. Readmission to hospital

than 900 perioperative issues identified by frontline staff at an estimated cost savings of greater than $884,900.[51] One of the limitations of this study is that 83% of the cases were performed by a single surgeon, making it potentially more difficult to generalize the effect of changes to a broader population of clinicians.

Teamwork, Communication, and Culture Change

Communication difficulties are consistently identified as the root cause of errors. According to data gathered by The Joint Commission, which monitors all reported sentinel events, communication breakdowns contribute to more than 60% of all sentinel events.[54] Several strategies can provide a way to structure communication such that oversights are not so common. Briefings are 1 way to provide information to all team members at the beginning of surgical cases, and have been shown to affect outcomes among general surgical cases.[55] In the cardiac surgical literature, Henrickson and colleagues[56] pilot-tested the impact of a cardiac surgery-specific briefing tool (**Fig. 7**), which was developed based on input from focus groups and survey data.

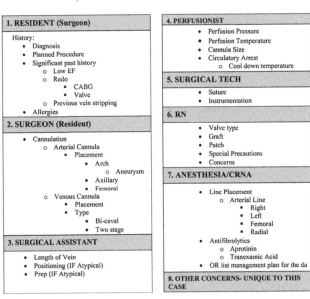

Fig. 7. Preoperative briefing template. (*Reproduced from* Henrickson SE, Wadhera RK, Elbardissi AW, et al. Development and pilot evaluation of a preoperative briefing protocol for cardiovascular surgery. J Am Coll Surg 2009;208(6):1117; with permission.)

The new briefing tool was implemented by a single surgeon at the institution and observational data were collected before intervention (10 operations) and after intervention (6 cases). Observations were made by a single individual to identify surgical flow disruptions, the number of trips made by the circulating nurse to the central core for equipment or other issues, and the time spent in the core.

After implementation of the tool, there was a statistically significant reduction in surgical flow disruptions (4.1–2.7 per case), procedural knowledge disruptions (4.1–2.17 per case), miscommunication events (2.5–1.17 per case), number of trips to the core (10–4.7 per case), and time spent in the core (397.4–172.3 seconds).[56] Minimizing disruption is important because it has been shown to affect outcomes[34]: disruption reduces the team's ability to compensate for minor errors and predisposes the surgical team to experiencing a major event.[38]

There are multiple examples of interventions to improve teamwork and communication during transitions of care. Two are highlighted in this section: 1 for pediatrics and 1 for adult cardiovascular patients. Among pediatric patients, Catchpole and colleagues[57] implemented a Formula 1 pit-stop model to reduce technical errors and omissions during handoffs to the ICU. Their model was successful, and did not increase handoff duration (**Fig. 8**). Petrovic and colleagues[58,59] performed a pre-post study of a handoff protocol from the OR to the cardiac surgical ICU. These investigators introduced a standardized template and required that all caregivers be present at the patient's bedside and focused on the patient with only 1 person speaking at a time. A decrease in the percentage of missed information in the surgical team's report

Summary of the new handover protocol

Phase 0: prehandover	The Patient Transfer Form is completed by the anesthetist and collected from theater at least 30 min before the patient is transferred to the ICU. The receiving nurse ensures the bed space is set up according to the monitoring, ventilation and other requirements specified on the Patient Transfer Form. The receiving doctor ensures that all appropriate paperwork is ready.
Phase 1: equipment and technology handover	On arrival the team transfers the patient ventilation, monitoring and support from portable systems used during the transfer to the ICU systems.
Phase 2: information handover	Safety check: the anesthetist checks the equipment and that the patient is appropriately ventilated and monitored and is stable. The receiving nurse and doctor are identified and confirm their readiness. The anesthetist, then the surgeon, speak alone and uninterrupted, providing the relevant information about the case, using the *Information Transfer Aid Memoir*. Safety check: the receiving nurse and doctor should use the *Information Transfer Aid Memoir* to check that all necessary information has been obtained, and ask appropriate questions.
Phase 3: discussion and plan	The surgeon, anesthetist and receiving team discuss the case as a group. The receiving physician manages the discussions, identifies anticipated problems, and anticipated recovery is discussed. The ICU team now has responsibility for patient care, and confirms the plans for the patient.

Fig. 8. Formula 1 pit-stop handover protocol. (*Reproduced from* Catchpole KR, de Leval MR, McEwan A, et al. Patient handover from surgery to intensive care: using Formula 1 pit-stop and aviation models to improve safety and quality. Paediatr Anaesth 2007;17(5):473; with permission.)

to the ICU from 26% to 16% ($P = .03$) was reported, and the percentage of ICU nurses who reported being satisfied with the report increased from 61% to 81% (**Fig. 9**).

A third example of improved teamwork and communication can be found in work carried out by the Concord Hospital in Concord, New Hampshire. This intervention focused on the ICU and introduced team-based, daily collaborative rounds using a structured communications protocol (Collaborative Care Model).[60] These investigators also introduced a biweekly forum to discuss the progress to date and address systems-level concerns. Key elements in the new process included rounds led by the nurse practitioner instead of the surgeon, dramatically changing the hierarchical playing field. Also novel is the fact that the patient and family members were invited to participate and share with the team anything that had not gone well ("system glitches", in the team's parlance) during the episode of care.[60] The researchers evaluated the impact of the intervention on mortality and staff quality of life, and reported improvements in both, with a decrease in the observed mortality compared with the expected mortality and an increase in scores on the staff quality of life survey.

In all these interventions, communications were standardized using new tools and processes that made the communication process more collaborative and less hierarchical, showing improved patient outcomes and staff satisfaction. These processes recognize the fallibility of the human element in communication and provide the tools (checklists, standardization) to guide the conversations and support good communication. With improved communication, the culture changes from fear of failure to a more progressive stance that promotes patient safety.

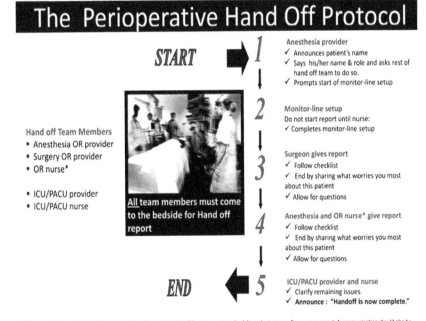

Fig. 9. Johns Hopkins medicine perioperative handoff protocol. (Copyright © 2009 The Johns Hopkins University. All rights reserved.)

SUMMARY

The literature shows how structural and process factors can predispose the cardiothoracic surgical team to experience errors while completing the complex series of tasks during the perioperative period. Successful completion of these tasks hinges on both technical work (completion of tasks in compliance with recommended standards) and adaptive work (organizational culture, teamwork, and provider characteristics).[26] A culture of collaboration is essential to ensuring that both the technical and adaptive work are performed in a manner conducive to safety. Good teamwork and communication are at the epicenter of patient safety reforms, because they create a culture of safety and collaboration.

Relatively simple tactics can deliver big gains in patient safety, such as those described in this review. Other industries, such as aviation and nuclear power, rely on systems approaches to optimize communication and prevent human error. Processes to standardize care, provide feedback on performance, and add redundancies as safety checks provide similar supports in medicine. High reliability depends on vigilance at every level and at every step in the care process. Martinez and colleagues[26] suggest 3 strategies to create such an environment: transparency (reporting systems and an atmosphere conducive to speaking up); teamwork (train team members in constructive communication skills to deconstruct the hierarchical nature of the OR); and task performance (keeping skills up to date and identifying weaknesses in tools and technology that compromise task performance). Individuals must share a mental model of the goals and methods for care, and this distributed cognition should extend to training in tools and technology. It is imperative that strategies that improve the safety and quality of care of the cardiac surgical patient population continue to be identified and quantified.

ACKNOWLEDGMENTS

This article greatly benefited from the thoughtful editing of Allison Krug, MPH.

REFERENCES

1. Shahian DM, Normand SL. The volume-outcome relationship: from Luft to Leapfrog. Ann Thorac Surg 2003;75(3):1048–58.
2. Kohn LT, Corrigan J, Donaldson MS. To err is human: building a safer health system. Washington, DC: National Academy Press; 2000.
3. Donabedian A. Evaluating the quality of medical care. Milbank Mem Fund Q 1966;44(Suppl 3):166–206.
4. Warrier S, McGillen B. The evolution of quality improvement. Med Health R I 2011; 94(7):211–2.
5. Brennan TA, Leape LL, Laird NM, et al. Incidence of adverse events and negligence in hospitalized patients. Results of the Harvard Medical Practice Study I. N Engl J Med 1991;324(6):370–6.
6. The Henry J. Kaiser Family Foundation. 2008 update on consumers' views of patient safety and quality information. 2008. Available at: http://www.kkf.org/. Accessed January 11, 2013.
7. Louis Harris & Associates for the National Patient Safety Foundation at the AMA. Public opinion of patient safety issues research findings. 1997. Available at: http://www.npsf.org/wp-content/uploads/2011/10/Public_Opinion_of_Patient_Safety_Issues.pdf. Accessed January 11, 2013.

8. Institute for Healthcare Improvement. U.S. health care providers say quality of care is 'unacceptable.' 2011. Boston; 2001. Available at: http://www.ihi.org/about/news/Documents/IHIPressRelease_USHealthcareQualityUnacceptable_May01.pdf. Accessed January 13, 2013.

9. Blendon R, Benson J, SteelFisher G, et al. Report on American's views on the quality of health care. Understanding Americans health agenda: a joint project of the Robert Wood Johnson Foundation and the Harvard School of Public Health. 2011. Available at: http://www.rwjf.org/content/dam/web-assets/2011/03/report-on-americans–views-on-the-quality-of-health-care. Accessed January 13, 2013.

10. Landrigan CP, Parry GJ, Bones CB, et al. Temporal trends in rates of patient harm resulting from medical care. N Engl J Med 2010;363(22):2124–34.

11. US Department of Health and Human Services Office of Inspector General. Adverse events in hospitals: national incidence among Medicare beneficiaries. OEI-06-09-00090. 2010. Available at: https://oig.hhs.gov/oei/reports/oei-06-09-00090.pdf.

12. McGlynn EA, Asch SM, Adams J, et al. The quality of health care delivered to adults in the United States. N Engl J Med 2003;348(26):2635–45.

13. Arthur ME, Castresana MR, Paschal JW, et al. Acute cerebellar stroke after inadvertent cannulation and pulmonary artery catheter placement in the right vertebral artery. Anesth Analg 2006;103(6):1625–6.

14. Stelfox HT, Palmisani S, Scurlock C, et al. The "To Err is Human" report and the patient safety literature. Qual Saf Health Care 2006;15(3):174–8.

15. Reason J. Human error: models and management. BMJ 2000;320(7237):768–70.

16. Reason J. The contribution of latent human failures to the breakdown of complex systems. Philos Trans R Soc Lond B Biol Sci 1990;327(1241):475–84.

17. The Joint Commission. The Joint Commission National Patient Safety Goals effective January 1, 2013. 2012. Available at: http://www.jointcommission.org/assets/1/18/NPSG_Chapter_Jan2013_HAP.pdf. Accessed January 13, 2013.

18. Lohr K. A strategy for quality assurance, vol. 1. Washington, DC: Institute of Medicine, The National Academies Press; 1990.

19. Shahian DM, Wolf RE, Iezzoni LI, et al. Variability in the measurement of hospital-wide mortality rates. N Engl J Med 2010;363(26):2530–9.

20. Shahian DM, Iezzoni LI, Meyer GS, et al. Hospital-wide mortality as a quality metric: conceptual and methodological challenges. Am J Med Qual 2012;27(2):112–23.

21. Lloyd-Jones D, Adams RJ, Brown TM, et al. Heart disease and stroke statistics–2010 update: a report from the American Heart Association. Circulation 2010; 121(7):e46–215.

22. Gawande AA, Thomas EJ, Zinner MJ, et al. The incidence and nature of surgical adverse events in Colorado and Utah in 1992. Surgery 1999;126(1):66–75.

23. Rebasa P, Mora L, Luna A, et al. Continuous monitoring of adverse events: influence on the quality of care and the incidence of errors in general surgery. World J Surg 2009;33(2):191–8.

24. Guru V, Tu JV, Etchells E, et al. Relationship between preventability of death after coronary artery bypass graft surgery and all-cause risk-adjusted mortality rates. Circulation 2008;117(23):2969–76.

25. Martinez EA, Marsteller JA, Thompson DA, et al. The Society of Cardiovascular Anesthesiologists' FOCUS initiative: locating errors through networked surveillance (LENS) project vision. Anesth Analg 2010;110(2):307–11.

26. Martinez EA, Thompson DA, Errett NA, et al. Review article: high stakes and high risk: a focused qualitative review of hazards during cardiac surgery. Anesth Analg 2011;112(5):1061–74.

27. Gurses AP, Kim G, Martinez EA, et al. Identifying and categorising patient safety hazards in cardiovascular operating rooms using an interdisciplinary approach: a multisite study. BMJ Qual Saf 2012;21(10):810–8.
28. Walshe K, Offen N. A very public failure: lessons for quality improvement in healthcare organisations from the Bristol Royal Infirmary. Qual Health Care 2001;10(4):250–6.
29. Coulter A. After Bristol: putting patients at the centre. BMJ 2002;324(7338): 648–51.
30. Davies JM. Painful inquiries: lessons from Winnipeg. CMAJ 2001;165(11):1503–4.
31. Sibbald B. Winnipeg inquest recommendation could leave young MDs in lurch, expert warns. CMAJ 2001;164(3):393.
32. Sibbald B. Why did 12 infants die? Winnipeg's endless inquest seeks answers. CMAJ 1998;158(6):783–9.
33. Fyle J, McGlynn AG. Bristol: still posing questions. RCM Midwives J 2002;5(7): 212–3.
34. Wiegmann DA, ElBardissi AW, Dearani JA, et al. Disruptions in surgical flow and their relationship to surgical errors: an exploratory investigation. Surgery 2007; 142(5):658–65.
35. Hazlehurst B, McMullen CK, Gorman PN. Distributed cognition in the heart room: how situation awareness arises from coordinated communications during cardiac surgery. J Biomed Inform 2007;40(5):539–51.
36. Wong DR, Torchiana DF, Vander Salm TJ, et al. Impact of cardiac intraoperative precursor events on adverse outcomes. Surgery 2007;141(6):715–22.
37. Wong DR, Vander Salm TJ, Ali IS, et al. Prospective assessment of intraoperative precursor events during cardiac surgery. Eur J Cardiothorac Surg 2006;29(4): 447–55.
38. Solis-Trapala IL, Carthey J, Farewell VT, et al. Dynamic modelling in a study of surgical error management. Stat Med 2007;26(28):5189–202.
39. Caceres M, Braud RL, Garrett HE Jr. A short history of the Society of Thoracic Surgeons national cardiac database: perceptions of a practicing surgeon. Ann Thorac Surg 2010;89(1):332–9.
40. Edwards FH. The STS database at 20 years: a tribute to Dr Richard E. Clark. Ann Thorac Surg 2010;89(1):9–10.
41. Epstein AJ. Do cardiac surgery report cards reduce mortality? Assessing the evidence. Med Care Res Rev 2006;63(4):403–26.
42. O'Rourke LM. Do quality report cards make a difference? The New York and Pennsylvania experience with releasing physician-specific outcomes. Qual Lett Healthc Lead 1993;5(6):2–11.
43. Ferris TG, Torchiana DF. Public release of clinical outcomes data–online CABG report cards. N Engl J Med 2010;363(17):1593–5.
44. O'Connor GT, Plume SK, Olmstead EM, et al. A regional intervention to improve the hospital mortality associated with coronary artery bypass graft surgery. The Northern New England Cardiovascular Disease Study Group. JAMA 1996; 275(11):841–6.
45. Holman WL, Allman RM, Sansom M, et al. Alabama coronary artery bypass grafting project: results of a statewide quality improvement initiative. JAMA 2001; 285(23):3003–10.
46. Prager RL, Armenti FR, Bassett JS, et al. Cardiac surgeons and the quality movement: the Michigan experience. Semin Thorac Cardiovasc Surg 2009;21(1): 20–7.

47. Sawyer M, Weeks K, Goeschel CA, et al. Using evidence, rigorous measurement, and collaboration to eliminate central catheter-associated bloodstream infections. Crit Care Med 2010;38(Suppl 8):S292–8.

48. Pronovost P, Needham D, Berenholtz S, et al. An intervention to decrease catheter-related bloodstream infections in the ICU. N Engl J Med 2006;355(26):2725–32.

49. Spiess BD, Wahr JA, Nussmeier NA. Bring your life into FOCUS! Anesth Analg 2010;110(2):283–7.

50. Casale AS, Paulus RA, Selna MJ, et al. "ProvenCareSM": a provider-driven pay-for-performance program for acute episodic cardiac surgical care. Ann Surg 2007;246(4):613–21 [discussion: 21–3].

51. Culig MH, Kunkle RF, Frndak DC, et al. Improving patient care in cardiac surgery using Toyota production system based methodology. Ann Thorac Surg 2011; 91(2):394–9.

52. Berry SA, Doll MC, McKinley KE, et al. ProvenCare: quality improvement model for designing highly reliable care in cardiac surgery. Qual Saf Health Care 2009;18(5):360–8.

53. Eagle KA, Guyton RA, Davidoff R, et al. ACC/AHA 2004 guideline update for coronary artery bypass graft surgery: a report of the American College of Cardiology/American Heart Association Task Force on Practice Guidelines (Committee to Update the 1999 Guidelines for Coronary Artery Bypass Graft Surgery). Circulation 2004;110(14):e340–437.

54. The Joint Commission. The Joint Commission's annual report on safety and quality. 2007. Available at: http://www.jointcommissionreport.org/. Accessed January 11, 2013.

55. Haynes AB, Weiser TG, Berry WR, et al. A surgical safety checklist to reduce morbidity and mortality in a global population. N Engl J Med 2009;360(5):491–9.

56. Henrickson SE, Wadhera RK, Elbardissi AW, et al. Development and pilot evaluation of a preoperative briefing protocol for cardiovascular surgery. J Am Coll Surg 2009;208(6):1115–23.

57. Catchpole KR, de Leval MR, McEwan A, et al. Patient handover from surgery to intensive care: using Formula 1 pit-stop and aviation models to improve safety and quality. Paediatr Anaesth 2007;17(5):470–8.

58. Petrovic MA, Aboumatar H, Baumgartner WA, et al. Pilot implementation of a perioperative protocol to guide operating room-to-intensive care unit patient handoffs. J Cardiothorac Vasc Anesth 2012;26(1):11–6.

59. Petrovic MA, Martinez EA, Aboumatar H. Implementing a perioperative handoff tool to improve postprocedural patient transfers. Jt Comm J Qual Patient Saf 2012;38(3):135–42.

60. Uhlig PN, Brown J, Nason AK, et al. John M. Eisenberg Patient Safety Awards. System innovation: Concord Hospital. Jt Comm J Qual Improv 2002;28(12): 666–72.

Fluid Management in Cardiac Surgery: Colloid or Crystalloid?

Andrew Shaw, MB, FRCA, FCCM*, Karthik Raghunathan, MD, MPH

KEYWORDS

- Crystalloids • Colloids • Cardiac surgery • Fluids

KEY POINTS

- Fluids are drugs.
- Integrity of the endothelial glycocalyx determines fluid distribution.
- Assessment of volume responsiveness and deficiency should precede fluid resuscitation.
- Starch solutions should probably be avoided during and after cardiac surgery.
- Balanced crystalloids have several advantages, including maintenance of renal blood flow, avoidance of metabolic acidosis, and possibly the reduction of Post operative atrial fibrillation (POAF).

INTRODUCTION

Intravenous (IV) fluid administration is ubiquitous to all patients undergoing cardiac surgery; therefore, it is essential that those who care for cardiac surgical patients have a good understanding of its physiology and pharmacology. These principles determine the effects of IV fluids on the patient (*pharmacodynamics*, because fluids are drugs) and the effects of patient and surgical characteristics on fluid disposition (*volume kinetics*). Optimal outcomes, such as short lengths of stay in both the intensive care unit (ICU) and hospital, reduced morbidity, and improved long-term quality of life can only result from careful planning that begins early in the preoperative period with attention to detail that continues through the intraoperative and postoperative periods. The ideal fluid management plan would avoid both hypovolemia and hypervolemia and would involve the use of the right combination of fluids given at the right time. Although widely used for resuscitation, intravenous crystalloids and colloids have generally been regarded as homogenous groups. The debate of crystalloids versus colloids over the decades has compared the 2 groups in a somewhat unfocused fashion.[1] In fact, within-group differences (eg, balanced crystalloids vs saline or starch solutions vs albumin) are significant, and there might be reason to consider each class

Conflicts of Interest: Baxter Healthcare (Consultant) (A.S.); None (K.R.).
Department of Anesthesiology, Duke University Medical Center/Durham VAMC, Erwin Road, Durham, NC 27710, USA
* Corresponding author.
E-mail address: Andrew.Shaw@duke.edu

Anesthesiology Clin 31 (2013) 269–280
http://dx.doi.org/10.1016/j.anclin.2012.12.007
1932-2275/13/$ – see front matter Published by Elsevier Inc.

of drug separately.[2] Despite this fact, large international surveys[3] show that the specific fluids that are used depend more on where the patient receives care rather than specific procedural/patient-related factors.

THEORETICAL FRAMEWORK
Body Fluid Composition, Physiology, and Surgery

For fluid balance and acid-base purposes, the human body may be considered to be made up of water, protein, fat, carbohydrate, and several electrolytes in solution. Total body water for the average 70-kg adult male is about 45 L, of which, 30 L (65%) is intracellular fluid and 15 L (35%) extracellular fluid (ECF). The ECF has traditionally been divided between the interstitial space (10 L) and the vascular compartment (5 L). By definition, all IV fluids are given into the vascular compartment, and their fate (and physiologic effects) thereafter depends on the:

- Electrolyte content
- Colloid content (if any)
- Integrity of the endothelial glycocalyx
- Volume context in which they are used
- Total quantity administered

There have been advances recently in our understanding of how crystalloids and colloids are dispersed throughout the body in health and disease,[4,5] and this new knowledge is changing the way perioperative physicians think about fluid therapy.

The terms *osmolality*, *osmolarity*, and *tonicity* are frequently used interchangeably when fluids and their effects are discussed, but this is incorrect, and a brief review of their correct definitions is in order. Osmolarity may be defined as the number of osmoles of solute per liter of (solvent + solute). As such, it is expressed as milliosmoles per liter. Osmolality is the concentration of solute per kilogram of solvent, and has units of milliosmoles per kilogram. This is the preferred unit for clinical practice because it is robust to the fat and protein content of plasma, whereas osmolarity is not. In humans, the extracellular osmolality is typically 290 ± 10 mOsm/kg. It is worth considering that osmotic pressure differences may have profound effects on fluid shifts in perioperative cardiac practice; an osmotic pressure gradient of 6 mOsm/L can move the same amount of water across a semipermeable membrane as the hydrostatic pressure generated by the heart.[6] Tonicity refers to the relative osmolality of one solution in reference to another; *isotonic* means the osmotic pressures of the fluids being compared are equivalent. Hypertonic solutions have a higher osmolality relative to plasma and hence increase the plasma and ECF osmolality in addition to promoting cellular dehydration.

The stress response to surgery is directly proportional to the magnitude of the surgical insult. This is related—albeit not exclusively—to the size of the incision and the mass of tissue that is traumatized. On-pump cardiac surgical patients have a substantially different experience than their off-pump peers in that they have a mandatory exposure to a significantly increased vascular compartment, namely, the cardiopulmonary bypass (CPB) circuit. The results of this intervention depend markedly on the fluids used to prime the circuit, the way the perfusionist manages the transition to extracorporeal circulation, the conduct of bypass itself, and the way in which pump blood is processed before return to the patient at the end of CPB. CPB induces a profound stress response also, because the circulating volume is exposed to an extracorporeal surface for up to several hours in some cases. Traditionally, there are ebb and flow phases described in which there is an initial shocklike state (soon after incision) associated with peripheral vasoconstriction, centralization of blood (ie, from the periphery to central organs), and a reduction of body temperature. This ebb phase is then followed by a flow phase in which there is a catecholamine surge leading to increased cardiac output, vasodilatation, pyrexia, and increased capillary permeability. When accompanied by fluid administration, this period can lead to significant loading of the extravascular compartment—volume that must be removed in the course of the next few days as the patient recovers. This volume load is affected by the type and extent of fluid resuscitation administered in the operating room and the ICU, and its removal is familiar to all those who work with cardiac surgical patients postoperatively.

Physiology of Fluid Disposition: Crystalloids Versus Colloids

Intravenous fluid disposition depends on factors well beyond those appreciated by the conventional Starling Model. The traditional view was that:

$$Jv = Kf[(Pc - Pi) - \sigma(\pi c - \pi i)]$$

where Jv is net fluid movement across capillary walls, Kf is the capillary filtration coefficient, $Pc - Pi$ is the capillary hydrostatic pressure minus interstitial hydrostatic pressure, σ is the reflection coefficient and $\pi c - \pi i$ the capillary oncotic pressure minus interstitial oncotic pressure. Under this premise, isotonic solutions would be expected to have volume efficacy for plasma volume expansion of only about 20%.[2] Colloids would be expected to produce a much larger volume effect. Classic predictions were for a 1:3 ratio for colloid to crystalloid volume expansion efficacy as described in major textbooks.[7] This view is discordant with the observed effects of fluid therapy in multiple large, randomized, controlled trials.[8–10] In fact, the observed colloid to crystalloid ratio for volume expansion effects seen in these trials involving thousands of patients seems to be closer to 1:1.2—1:1.4, that is, at most 30% greater efficacy for colloids in certain specific situations (discussed below) rather than the 300% greater efficacy that was previously taught. There are also some significant differences between observations regarding fluid kinetics made during studies in healthy volunteers compared with observations in the critically ill.[11] The revised Starling model emphasizes a central role for the endothelial glycocalyx layer (EGL) as a key determinant of fluid disposition.[12] In addition, volume context determines how fluids move after they are given intravenously. Patients undergoing cardiac surgical procedures are likely to handle crystalloids and colloids differently depending on the point at which such fluids are given during the hospital course.

Early during elective cardiac surgical procedures, before the initiation of surgical inflammation and injury to the EGL, it is likely that colloids will have slightly more favorable volume expansion effects versus crystalloids—at least in terms of their ability to augment circulation in a goal-directed setting.

In this setting, volume context[4,9,10] and a relatively intact EGL may favor colloids because capillary pressures are normal, and volume loading with crystalloids will produce greater dilutional effects on plasma oncotic pressure with consequently greater volume loading of the interstitial space with crystalloids.

In sick patients or those undergoing emergent procedures in whom hemodynamic instability is present, there is likely to be no difference in volume expansion efficacy between colloids and crystalloids. During critical illness, including the postcardiopulmonary bypass/postoperative state, EGL denudation is present with high transcapillary escape rates.[10] Loss of functional EGL leads to interstitial edema and reduced volume-expanding effects of exogenous fluid administration.

With low capillary pressure hypovolemic or hemorrhagic shock states, intravascular retention of crystalloids is enhanced as clearance is reduced.[13] In this setting, crystalloids are effective intravascular volume expanders, as they are retained within the circulation for considerably longer periods with marked reduction in clearance. In addition to marked hemodynamic stress, patients undergoing cardiac surgical procedures are subject to considerable activation of inflammatory and hemostatic pathways. Significant shedding of the EGL seems to occur during procedures involving conventional CPB and also during off-pump procedures.[14] Thus, there is no evidence that colloids are better than crystalloids when CPB is used versus when procedures are done off pump.

CLINICAL PRACTICE
Dosing: What Goals?

Although "what is the patient context?" is an important question, equally important is "what is the goal of fluid administration?" When guided by functional dynamic measures of volume responsiveness, such as pulse pressure variation, stroke volume variation, systolic pressure variation or similar parameters, outcomes are much improved.[15] Static conventional parameters such as central venous pressure, pulmonary artery occlusion pressure, or even mean arterial pressure and urine output do not reliably distinguish between patients that will and will not respond to fluid therapy with an improved cardiac output. Dynamic parameters are not reliable in some situations common to the cardiac surgical setting such as arrhythmias and open chest conditions.[16,17] To address the question of "will IV fluid therapy augment the circulation?," suggestions include the use of volume challenges or mini-challenges of as little as 200 mL given over 5 minutes.[18] The authors believe that clinicians ought to try and predict the effects of fluid administration before its liberal use.[2] Reversible maneuvers such as the passive leg raise have been shown to distinguish fluid responders from nonresponders under diverse conditions.[19]

There are major differences between the effects of fluid therapy in a goal-directed therapy setting versus when used in pragmatic critical care settings.

1. When flow-directed algorithms are applied either intraoperatively[20] or postoperatively[21] in cardiac surgical patients, colloid use is greater and vasopressor and catecholamine use is reduced.[22] Short-term complications and the length of hospital stay are reduced.
2. When one examines data from large, randomized, controlled trials in intensive care settings in which a pragmatic approach is used to guide fluid therapy,[6–8] there is no difference between the amounts of colloids or crystalloids used.
3. Giving either crystalloids or colloids without assessing for the presence of volume responsiveness exposes patients to undesirable and avoidable hypervolemia with fluid accumulation in the interstitial spaces.

COLLOIDS IN CARDIAC SURGERY

Broadly, 2 types of colloids are used in the perioperative period for cardiac surgical patients: albumin (human-derived) and hydroxyethyl starch (HES) solutions (synthetic). Crystalloid vehicles in which colloids are suspended may be isotonic 0.9% saline solution or buffered (lactated/acetated) electrolyte solutions. Relevance of the carrier solution will become clearer in the Crystalloids section later in this article. HES solutions may be further grouped into older high molecular weight, high degree of molar-substitution solutions (hetastarch dissolved in 0.9% saline or other carrier) versus modern lower molecular weight, and lower degree of molar-substitution solutions (tetrastarch). Although developed to enhance metabolism and elimination from the intravascular space thus improving safety versus older starches,[23,24] modern tetrastarches (130/~0.4) have been shown to have significant risks in the intensive care unit setting.[7,8] Whether HES is suspended in saline[7] or in buffered electrolyte solution,[8] patients with higher mortality risks at baseline are at particularly increased risk of renal injury even when resuscitated with modern starch solutions. On average, 42% of the nearly 7000 patients in the CHEST study were surgical patients,[9] making it reasonable to extend findings to cardiac surgical patients.

The pattern of kidney injury from tetrastarch use seems related to pinocytosis of metabolites into renal proximal tubular cells after glomerular filtration.[25,26] Increased uptake into renal tissue occurs as plasma half-life decreases with the newer starches versus the older starches.[27] Starch-associated bleeding risks are not explained by hemodilution effects.[28,29] Thromboelastographic differences are apparent consistent with impaired fibrin polymerization and decreased levels of factors VIII, vWF, and XIII.[26] The authors believe the combination of plausible biologic basis for injury; consistent harm signal by RIFLE (Risk, Injury, Failure, Loss, End stage) criteria from large randomized, controlled trials; increased bleeding risk in 6S for patients receiving HES; lack of demonstrable benefit; and the availability of a safe alternative (crystalloid) make continued use of starch solutions in a potentially at-risk population, such as cardiac surgical patients, untenable.

Although used for decades in cardiac surgical patients, albumin may also have legitimate safety concerns. An increase in adverse outcomes with albumin use among patients with traumatic brain injury[30] has been known for some time now. Impairment of the blood-brain barrier in cardiac surgical patients is also now well described.[31] Albumin is considerably more expensive[1] and as a human-derived product carries a small but definite risk for the transmission of prions. The costs of complications from inappropriate fluid use, however, are far more important than the costs of the actual fluids themselves. Furthermore, even when viewed as a possible choice during goal directed therapy (GDT), the optimal type of fluid for preemptive volume optimization is actually unclear because head-to-head trials with crystalloids and albumin for GDT have not been conducted. Given safe alternatives, it is also hard to defend the continued use of albumin.

CRYSTALLOIDS IN CARDIAC SURGERY

Crystalloid solutions are given to every patient who undergoes heart surgery, whatever their age, location, operation type, and urgency. In this section these issues are reviewed in the broad context of cardiac surgical practice and then the effects of some of the commonly available crystalloid solutions when they are administered to patients undergoing cardiac operations are described.

The Importance of Physiologically Balanced Solutions

Crystalloid solutions that contain unphysiologic concentrations of electrolytes have been used in surgical practice for more than 100 years. Perhaps the commonest (at least historically) has been 0.9% sodium chloride solution—normal saline. It is anything but normal. There are 9 g of salt in each bag, the equivalent of approximately 30 bags of regular potato chips, and the chloride concentration of 154 mEq/L is profoundly abnormal relative to plasma. As the amount of 0.9% saline administered increases, plasma chloride concentration tends to increase, as does the severity of the accompanying metabolic acidosis. This is caused by a progressive reduction in the plasma strong ion difference (SID) and is entirely dose related. Chowdhury and colleagues[32] have shown that administration of a mere 2 L of 0.9% saline is sufficient to reduce renal blood flow in human volunteers, an effect that has been seen consistently in animal models.[33,34] Fluid administration is an acid-base intervention, and the SID of an intravenous fluid directly determines the plasma acid-base effects of that fluid. The pH of the intravenous solution being administered has little effect on plasma pH. Thus, even though 0.9% saline solutions are slightly acidic, this acidity is not the reason for the metabolic acidosis that results from saline administration. Rather, metabolic acidosis results from lowering of plasma SID.

Physiologically balanced solutions are those in which the electrolyte content more closely resembles that of human plasma, and the SID is closer to the physiologic range (vs SID of 0 for normal saline). Examples are Ringer's lactate solution, Hartmann's solution, Plasma-Lyte 148, Accusol and Normasol. Such fluids generally contain slightly less sodium and significantly less chloride and have a SID significantly closer to that of plasma. The extra cations are generally potassium, calcium and/or magnesium while the anion deficit is accounted for by inclusion of buffers such as lactate and acetate. **Table 1** shows the electrolyte composition of several of the crystalloid solutions currently available in the United States compared with their distributions across several body fluid compartments.

Data supporting the use of physiologically balanced solutions have (until recently) been confined to animal studies. Infusion of saline causes progressive renal vasoconstriction in dogs,[33] and hyperchloremic metabolic acidosis in rodents,[34] particularly septic rodents. Recently, there have been volunteer human studies[32] and large observational studies[35–37] showing adverse effects associated with saline use that are not evident when balanced crystalloids are used. Furthermore, there are no published data describing a definite benefit from the use of 0.9% saline solution for resuscitation in unselected perioperative patients. There is mounting evidence of harm and little evidence of benefit from saline use. With the ready availability of inexpensive and familiar alternatives, it seems prudent to discontinue the routine use of saline for resuscitation in perioperative practice, including cardiac surgery. Use may be restricted to co-administration with citrated blood products.

The debate over whether colloid solutions should be used should also reflect that the net effect of a colloid solution is also affected by the carrier solution in which it is dissolved. This aspect of colloid therapy has not been studied sufficiently in either the observational or the interventional literature.

Hypertonic Solutions and Their Place in the Cardiac Operating Room

Hypertonic solutions are those that would draw water across a semipermeable membrane were plasma to be placed on its other side. As mentioned above, they tend to lead to cellular dehydration and have been used in an attempt to limit the total volume of fluid administered and to produce cellular dehydration in the setting of cerebral edema. In the cardiac surgery setting, the solutions used typically have been 7.2%–7.5% saline[38] with the goal of improving overall cardiovascular performance while maintaining effective tissue oxygen delivery. Benefits of hypertonic solutions include a dramatic reduction in positive fluid balance,[39,40] an increase in cardiac index,[39,40] and reduced systemic vascular resistance.[41,42] On the other hand, all these studies report a high incidence of hypernatremia and did not examine renal function closely. One can imagine that the effect of a high chloride load on the kidney is just the same whether it is delivered in a high or low volume. In the authors' practice, the use of hypertonic solutions is not common, particularly in the era of retrograde

Table 1
Electrolyte concentrations of commonly available crystalloid solutions

Fluid	Osmolarity mOsm/L	Na$^+$ mEq/L	Cl$^-$ mEq/L	K$^+$ mEq/L	Ca^{2+} mEq/L	Mg^{2+} mEq/L	Lactate mEq/L	Gluconate mEq/L	Acetate mEq/L	Glucose g/L
Plasma	290	142	103	4	5	3	2	—	—	1
NaCl 0.9% Dextrose 5%	230	154	154	—	—	—	—	—	—	50
NaCl 0.45% Dextrose 5%	203	77	77	—	—	—	—	—	—	50
NaCl 0.9%	308	154	154	—	—	—	—	—	—	—
Lactated Ringer's	273	130	109	4	3	—	28	—	—	—
Dextrose 5%	252	—	—	—	—	—	—	—	—	50
Plasmalyte 148	294	140	98	5	—	3	—	23	27	—
Normasol	294	140	98	5	—	3	—	23	27	—

autologous priming of the CPB circuit and aggressive on-pump ultrafiltration to minimize residual volume overload.

A Brief Note on Cardioplegia Solutions

To permit the surgeon to operate on a still, bloodless heart, some way of safely immobilizing it while minimizing damage is required. Once the patient has safely transferred on to CPB, cardioplegia solution is infused either antegrade into the aortic root proximal to an occlusive cross clamp itself applied proximal to the innominate artery or retrograde via the coronary sinus using a balloon-tipped catheter. Historically, this solution was infused under pressure at 4°C and comprised a crystalloid fluid containing 20–35 mEq/L potassium chloride and various other components (lidocaine, sodium bicarbonate, mannitol). The aim is to arrest the heart in diastole and to reduce myocardial oxygen consumption as much as possible during the period of aortic cross clamping and mandatory myocardial ischemia. It was found that mixing the cardioplegia solution with cold blood both reduced the myocardial enzyme leak during cross clamping and reduced the incidence of low output syndrome, which indicate improved myocardial protection. Cold blood cardioplegia is now the technique of choice in most centers performing cardiac surgery, with most centers using a combination of antegrade (aortic root or direct coronary injection) and retrograde (into the coronary sinus) delivery systems. The high potassium concentration does not persist into the postoperative period, where most patients (end-stage renal patients excepted) require potassium supplementation. This perhaps reflects the somewhat ubiquitous use of kaliuretic agents during and after cardiac surgery, furosemide being the most common.

Cardiac Surgery–associated Acute Kidney Injury and the Role of Crystalloids

Acute kidney injury (AKI) occurs commonly after cardiac surgery and is associated with increased morbidity and mortality.[43] This is one of the few situations in which there is a generally agreed-upon clinical risk prediction model,[43] although even this model does not perform well on an individual patient basis. There has been much work published recently on consensus definitions of AKI[44–46] and regarding novel diagnostic biomarkers of risk, diagnosis, and prognosis of AKI.[47,48] The electrolyte content of the intravenous fluids given to cardiac surgical patients has received little consideration as a causative agent in AKI pathophysiology, despite some convincing evidence from the noncardiac surgical literature that this may be important.

The authors analyzed a prospective claims database to study 31,000 noncardiac surgical patients and showed an increased incidence of dialysis in those who received 0.9% saline on the day of surgery instead of a balanced crystalloid solution.[35] In the nonelective patients, there was also a statistically significant increase in hospital mortality. Wilcox[33] showed a reduction in arterial vessel diameter as chloride concentration increased, and Lobo showed a reduction in both total renal blood flow and cortical perfusion when human volunteers received 2 L 0.9% saline that did not occur when the same subjects were given balanced fluids.[32] The authors suggest that increased serum chloride concentrations (even within the normal clinical range) lead to increased arteriolar vasoconstriction in the kidneys of patients who receive large volumes (and what volume constitutes large may be as little as 3 L) of chloride-rich IV solutions and that this, in turn, translates into worsened renal function, manifesting as increased rates of dialysis if severe. There are recent data published from Australia showing that when chloride-rich solutions are removed from the intensive care unit, the incidence of AKI and dialysis is reduced.[37]

Inflammation, Infection, and Immunity—Is There a Link with High Chloride Concentrations?

Kellum and colleagues[34] found an adverse effect of chloride on outcome in animal models of sepsis, and although cardiac surgical patients are not septic, they are certainly subject to a systemic inflammatory insult and share many of the clinical features of patients with sepsis. In the authors' study of noncardiac surgical patients,[35] there was a statistically significant increase in the composite endpoint of morbidity, and this was driven predominantly by an increased incidence of infection in those receiving 0.9% saline. It is conceivable, therefore, that high chloride concentrations may impair innate immunity and inhibit naturally occurring anti-inflammatory pathways, leading to increased postoperative infection rates. This hypothesis has not been proven (or disproven) in a randomized, controlled clinical trial, but when no data suggest a benefit, it may be wise to avoid chloride-rich intravenous solutions for cardiac surgical patients because alternatives are readily available.

Postoperative Atrial Fibrillation—Is There a Preventive Role for Electrolyte-Enhanced Crystalloid Solutions?

Postoperative atrial fibrillation (AF) is a common and troublesome complication of cardiac surgery. It occurs in approximately 20%–30% of patients and there is an association with new-onset AF and AKI.[49] Because it is common practice to administer magnesium supplements to cardiac surgical patients, we will briefly review the physiology of magnesium in the context of cardiac surgery. It is the second most prevalent intracellular cation (behind potassium), and, as such, serum levels do not reflect total body stores—the intracellular fluid to ECF ratio is about 15:1.[6] Although it is approximately 60% ionized, most laboratories do not report this fraction; thus, total

Table 2
Fluid types and their respective advantages and disadvantages

Fluid Type	Advantages	Disadvantages
Isotonic saline solution	Inexpensive, safe for co-administration with citrated blood products	Causes hyperchloremic metabolic acidosis Reduces plasma strong ion difference
Balanced solutions	Physiologic electrolyte concentrations Reduce renal, infectious, bleeding complications	Slightly more expensive than saline
Older starch solutions		Long elimination half-life Acute kidney injury Bleeding risks
Modern starch solutions		Acute kidney injury Bleeding risks
Albumin	Slightly greater volume efficacy than crystalloids with an intact EGL	Expensive Human-derived Prion disease
Hypertonic electrolyte solutions	Reduction of total volume needed Reduction of interstitial edema	Hyperchloremia
Hypertonic albumin solutions	Reduction of total fluid volume needed	

magnesium content is used for clinical decision making. It may be considered a physiologic calcium antagonist, and, when levels are low, patients are at increased risk for all tachyarryhthmias, especially torsades de pointes and atrial fibrillation. The latter is especially common when the patient is also hypokalemic. The first-line treatment (assuming hemodynamic stability) of new-onset AF is always potassium and magnesium supplementation. It is tempting to speculate, therefore, that the routine use of intravenous solutions that contain magnesium and potassium might be especially beneficial in cardiac surgical patients. The authors stress, however, that there are few clinical data showing a clear advantage of these fluids over their calcium-containing counterparts **Table 2**.

RECOMMENDATIONS

- Assessment of volume responsiveness should precede fluid resuscitation
- Starch solutions should be avoided during and after cardiac surgery
- Balanced crystalloids have several advantages, including maintenance of renal blood flow, avoidance of metabolic acidosis, and possibly the reduction of POAF

REFERENCES

1. Perel P, Roberts I. Colloids versus crystalloids for fluid resuscitation in critically ill patients. Cochrane Database Syst Rev 2012;(6):CD000567.
2. Raghunathan K, McGee WT, Higgins T. Importance of intravenous fluid dose and composition in surgical ICU patients. Curr Opin Crit Care 2012;18(4):350–7.
3. Finfer S, Liu B, Taylor C, et al. Resuscitation fluid use in critically ill adults: an international cross-sectional study in 391 intensive care units. Crit Care 2010;14(5): R185.
4. Chappell D, Jacob M, Hofmann-Kiefer K, et al. A rational approach to perioperative fluid management. Anesthesiology 2008;109(4):723–40.
5. Kehlet H, Bundgaard-Nielsen M. Goal-directed perioperative fluid management: why, when, and how? Anesthesiology 2009;110(3):453–5.
6. Neligan P. Monitoring and managing perioperative electrolyte abnormalities, acid base disorders and fluid replacement. In: Longnecker DE, editor. Anesthesiology. 2nd edition. McGraw Hill; 2012. p. 507–45.
7. Rhee P. Shock, electrolytes and fluids. In: Townsend CM, editor. Sabiston textbook of surgery: the biological basis of modern surgical practice. 17th edition. Philadelphia: Elsevier Saunders; 2012. p. 66–119.
8. Finfer S, Bellomo R, Boyce N, et al. A comparison of albumin and saline for fluid resuscitation in the intensive care unit. N Engl J Med 2004;350(22):2247–56.
9. Myburgh JA, Finfer S, Bellomo R, et al. Hydroxyethyl starch or saline for fluid resuscitation in intensive care. N Engl J Med 2012;367(20):1901–11.
10. Perner A, Haase N, Guttormsen AB, et al. Hydroxyethyl starch 130/0.42 versus Ringer's acetate in severe sepsis. N Engl J Med 2012;367(2):124–34.
11. Hahn RG. Volume kinetics for infusion fluids. Anesthesiology 2010;113(2):470–81.
12. Woodcock TE, Woodcock TM. Revised Starling equation and the glycocalyx model of transvascular fluid exchange: an improved paradigm for prescribing intravenous fluid therapy. Br J Anaesth 2012;108(3):384–94.
13. Kozar RA, Peng Z, Zhang R, et al. Plasma restoration of endothelial glycocalyx in a rodent model of hemorrhagic shock. Anesth Analg 2011;112(6):1289–95.
14. Bruegger D, Rehm M, Abicht J, et al. Shedding of the endothelial glycocalyx during cardiac surgery: on-pump versus off-pump coronary artery bypass graft surgery. J Thorac Cardiovasc Surg 2009;138(6):1445–7.

15. Marik PE, Baram M, Vahid B. Does central venous pressure predict fluid respon-siveness? A systematic review of the literature and the tale of seven mares. Chest 2008;134(1):172–8.
16. Lansdorp B, Lemson J, van Putten MJ, et al. Dynamic indices do not predict volume responsiveness in routine clinical practice. Br J Anaesth 2012;108(3):395–401.
17. Hatton KW. Do hemodynamic measures accurately predict volume responsive-ness when lung compliance is severely reduced by acute lung injury/acute respi-ratory distress syndrome? Crit Care Med 2012;40(1):327–8.
18. Cecconi M, Parsons AK, Rhodes A. What is a fluid challenge? Curr Opin Crit Care 2011;17(3):290–5.
19. Monnet X, Bleibtreu A, Ferre A, et al. Passive leg-raising and end-expiratory occlusion tests perform better than pulse pressure variation in patients with low respiratory system compliance. Crit Care Med 2012;40(1):152–7.
20. Smetkin AA, Kirov MY, Kuzkov VV, et al. Single transpulmonary thermodilution and continuous monitoring of central venous oxygen saturation during off-pump coronary surgery. Acta Anaesthesiol Scand 2009;53(4):505–14.
21. McKendry M, McGloin H, Saberi D, et al. Randomised controlled trial assessing the impact of a nurse delivered, flow monitored protocol for optimisation of circu-latory status after cardiac surgery. BMJ 2004;329(7460):258.
22. Goepfert MS, Reuter DA, Akyol D, et al. Goal-directed fluid management reduces vasopressor and catecholamine use in cardiac surgery patients. Intensive Care Med 2007;33(1):96–103.
23. Mizzi A, Tran T, Karlnoski R, et al. Voluven, a new colloid solution. Anesthesiol Clin 2011;29(3):547–55.
24. Jungheinrich C, Neff TA. Pharmacokinetics of hydroxyethyl starch. Clin Pharm 2005;44(7):681–99.
25. Lehmann GB, Asskali F, Boll M, et al. HES 130/0.42 shows less alteration of phar-macokinetics than HES 200/0.5 when dosed repeatedly. Br J Anaesth 2007;98(5): 635–44.
26. Cittanova ML, Leblanc I, Legendre C, et al. Effect of hydroxyethylstarch in brain-dead kidney donors on renal function in kidney-transplant recipients. Lancet 1996;348(9042):1620–2.
27. Bellmann R, Feistritzer C, Wiedermann CJ. Effect of molecular weight and substi-tution on tissue uptake of hydroxyethyl starch: a meta-analysis of clinical studies. Clin Pharm 2012;51(4):225–36.
28. Hartog CS, Reuter D, Loesche W, et al. Influence of hydroxyethyl starch (HES) 130/0.4 on hemostasis as measured by viscoelastic device analysis: a systematic review. Intensive Care Med 2011;37(11):1725–37.
29. Godier A, Durand M, Smadja D, et al. Maize- or potato-derived hydroxyethyl starches: is there any thromboelastometric difference? Acta Anaesthesiol Scand 2010;54(10):1241–7.
30. Myburgh J, Cooper D, Finfer S, et al. Saline or albumin for fluid resuscitation in patients with traumatic brain injury. N Engl J Med 2007;357(9):874–84.
31. Merino JG, Latour LL, Tso A, et al. Blood-brain barrier disruption after cardiac surgery. AJNR Am J Neuroradiol 2012. [Epub ahead of print].
32. Chowdhury A, Cox E, Francis S, et al. A randomized, controlled, double-blind crossover study on the effects of 2-L infusions of 0.9% saline and plasma-lyte(R) 148 on renal blood flow velocity and renal cortical tissue perfusion in healthy volunteers. Ann Surg 2012;256(1):18–24.
33. Wilcox C. Regulation of renal blood flow by plasma chloride. J Clin Invest 1983; 71(3):726–35.

34. Kellum J, Song M, Almasri E. Hyperchloremic acidosis increases circulating inflammatory molecules in experimental sepsis. Chest 2006;130(4):962–7.
35. Shaw AD, Bagshaw SM, Goldstein SL, et al. Major complications, mortality, and resource utilization after open abdominal surgery: 0.9% saline compared to Plasma-Lyte. Ann Surg 2012;255(5):821–9.
36. Yunos N, Bellomo R, Hegarty C, et al. Association between a chloride-liberal vs chloride-restrictive intravenous fluid administration strategy and kidney injury in critically ill adults. JAMA 2012;308(15):1566–72.
37. Yunos N, Kim I, Bellomo R, et al. The biochemical effects of restricting chloride-rich fluids in intensive care. Crit Care Med 2011;39(11):2419–24.
38. Azoubel G, Nascimento B, Ferri M, et al. Operating room use of hypertonic solutions: a clinical review. Clinics (Sao Paulo) 2008;63(6):833–40.
39. Oliveira R, Velasco I, Soriano F, et al. Clinical review: hypertonic saline resuscitation in sepsis. Crit Care 2002;6(5):418–23.
40. Tollofsrud S, Noddeland H. Hypertonic saline and dextran after coronary artery surgery mobilises fluid excess and improves cardiorespiratory functions. Acta Anaesthesiol Scand 1998;42(2):154–61.
41. Sirieix D, Hongnat J, Delayance S, et al. Comparison of the acute hemodynamic effects of hypertonic or colloid infusions immediately after mitral valve repair. Crit Care Med 1999;27(10):2159–65.
42. Bueno R, Resende A, Melo R, et al. Effects of hypertonic saline-dextran solution in cardiac valve surgery with cardiopulmonary bypass. Ann Thorac Surg 2004; 77(2):604–11 [discussion: 611].
43. Thakar C, Arrigain S, Worley S, et al. A clinical score to predict acute renal failure after cardiac surgery. J Am Soc Nephrol 2005;16(1):162–8.
44. Group KDIGOKAKIW. KDIGO clinical practice guideline for acute kidney injury. Kidney Int Suppl 2012;2(Suppl):1–138.
45. Mehta R, Kellum J, Shah S, et al. Acute Kidney Injury Network: report of an initiative to improve outcomes in acute kidney injury. Crit Care 2007;11(2):R31.
46. Bellomo R, Ronco C, Kellum JA, et al. Acute renal failure - definition, outcome measures, animal models, fluid therapy and information technology needs: the Second International Consensus Conference of the Acute Dialysis Quality Initiative (ADQI) Group. Crit Care 2004;8(4):R204–12.
47. Parikh C, Coca S, Thiessen-Philbrook H, et al. Postoperative biomarkers predict acute kidney injury and poor outcomes after adult cardiac surgery. J Am Soc Nephrol 2011;22(9):1748–57.
48. Alge J, Karakala N, Neely B, et al. Urinary angiotensinogen and risk of severe AKI. Clin J Am Soc Nephrol 2012. [Epub ahead of print].
49. Albahrani M, Swaminathan M, Phillips-Bute B, et al. Postcardiac surgery complications: association of acute renal dysfunction and atrial fibrillation. Anesth Analg 2003;96(3):637–43 Table of contents.

Ischemic Mitral Regurgitation
Mechanisms, Intraoperative Echocardiographic Evaluation, and Surgical Considerations

John M. Connell, MD, MPH[a], Andrea Worthington, BA[b],
Frederick Y. Chen, MD, PhD[a], Stanton K. Shernan, MA, FAHA, FASE[b],*

KEYWORDS

- Ischemic mitral regurgitation • Ventricular remodeling
- Intraoperative transesophageal echocardiography • Mitral valve repair

KEY POINTS

- Ischemic mitral regurgitation (IMR) is a subcategory of functional rather than organic, mitral valve (MV) disease.
- Whether reversible or permanent, left ventricular remodeling creates IMR that is complex and multifactorial.
- A comprehensive TEE examination in patients with IMR may have important implications for perioperative clinical decision making. Several TEE measures predictive of MV repair failure have been identified.
- Current practice among most surgeons is to typically repair the MV in patients with IMR. MV replacement is usually reserved for situations in which the valve cannot be reasonably repaired, or repair is unlikely to be tolerated clinically.

DEFINITION AND PRESENTATION

Ischemic mitral regurgitation (IMR) is a subcategory of functional rather than organic, mitral valve (MV) disease. By definition, IMR occurs directly as a result of coronary artery disease (CAD), and is therefore not an intrinsic pathologic process. As opposed to structural mitral regurgitation (MR), the valve leaflets in patients with IMR have normal architecture and are therefore neither myxomatous, rheumatic, endocarditic, congenitally malformed, nor otherwise diseased. The valve instead is adversely affected by abnormal, subvalvular support structures. Carpentier[1] described 3 general types of mechanisms of MR associated with abnormal leaflet motion (**Fig. 1**). Type I

[a] Division of Cardiac Surgery, Brigham and Women's Hospital, Harvard Medical School, 75 Francis Street, Boston, MA 02115, USA; [b] Department of Anesthesiology, Perioperative and Pain Medicine, Brigham and Women's Hospital, Harvard Medical School, 75 Francis Street, Boston, MA 02115, USA
* Corresponding author.
E-mail address: sshernan@partners.org

Anesthesiology Clin 31 (2013) 281–298
http://dx.doi.org/10.1016/j.anclin.2013.01.002
1932-2275/13/$ – see front matter © 2013 Elsevier Inc. All rights reserved.

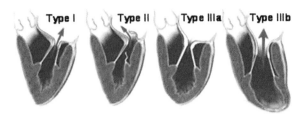

Fig. 1. Carpentier classification scheme for defining MR mechanisms based on leaflet motion abnormalities. Type I: normal leaflet motion (annular dilation; leaflet perforation); type II: increased leaflet motion (prolapse; flail); type III a: leaflet restriction during systole and diastole; type IIIb: leaflet restriction only during systole. (*Modified from* Carpentier A, Adams D, Filsoufi F. Carpentier's reconstructive valve surgery. From valve analysis to valve reconstruction. Philadelphia: Saunders Elsevier; 2010.)

describes pure annular dilation or leaflet perforation with otherwise normal leaflet architecture, usually resulting from left ventricular (LV) dilation and ventricular remodeling. Type II denotes excessive leaflet motion from leaflet prolapse or flail resulting from laxity or rupture of the chordae tendineae, or less commonly from acute papillary muscle rupture after myocardial infarction (MI). Type III describes 2 forms of valve leaflet restriction, occurring during both diastole and systole most commonly seen with rheumatic heart disease (type IIIa), or primarily only during systole (type IIIb).

Ischemic MR is divided into 2 broad categories: acute or chronic. The mechanism of each is different. In acute IMR, regurgitation is secondary to type II dysfunction with excessive leaflet motion caused by acute, postinfarction papillary muscle rupture or severe dysfunction. Although this condition represents a smaller percentage of IMR presentations, it is immediately life-threatening and requires more emergent decision making. Typically, the treatment of acute, ischemic MR is MV replacement (MVR).

Chronic IMR occurs as a consequence of ventricular dilatation secondary to ischemic ventricular remodeling, which results in papillary muscle displacement and a subsequent failure of leaflet coaptation. Regurgitation occurs secondary to annular dilation (type I) and leaflet restriction during systole (type IIIb). Chronic IMR requires regional or global ventricular dysfunction with chronic remodeling and subsequent apical displacement (eg, apical tethering or tenting), which prevents normal leaflet coaptation during systole. The cycle of long-standing CAD leading to negative ventricular remodeling with annular dilation and MR exacerbates cardiac ischemia, leads to worsened MR, and causes greater ventricular deterioration and heart failure.[2] Most patients with chronic IMR present with varying degrees of both coronary ischemia and congestive heart failure, with volume overload with poor exercise tolerance.

MECHANISMS

Specific mechanisms for the development of IMR may be reversible with revascularization and restoration of oxygen delivery or the MR may be fixed with irreversible LV remodeling. Whether reversible or permanent, remodeling creates MR that is complex and multifactorial (**Fig. 2**).[1] LV remodeling secondary to acute and chronic ischemia remains the fundamental, general mechanism for IMR and depends on apical tethering and an excessive tenting volume, which cause coaptation failure of the mitral leaflets (**Fig. 3**). Although both regional and general LV remodeling have been implicated as probable causes for IMR, the specific site of remodeling may be most relevant. Posterior MIs, especially when involving at least 30% of the LV, are more likely associated

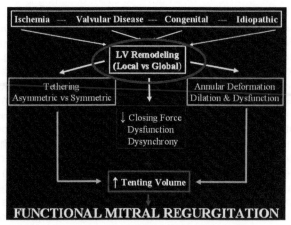

Fig. 2. Multiple causes and complex mechanisms of functional MR.

with annular dilation and excessive apical tethering compared with anterior MIs.[3] In addition, in a study of 128 patients with LV dysfunction defined as an ejection fraction (EF) less than 50%, Yiu and colleagues[4] reported a close correlation between the severity of tenting area and both apical displacement of the posterior papillary muscle (PPM) and posterior displacement of the anterior papillary muscle (APM). However, tenting area was only weakly correlated with LV end-diastolic volume index or wall stress, suggesting that local remodeling, although related to global LV deformation, is a stronger independent factor for IMR and functional MR (FMR) severity. LV dyssynchrony has also been proposed as a potential factor associated with MR severity. Hemodynamically significant MR occurs nearly twice as often in patients with a QRS greater than 130 milliseconds compared with normal duration.[5] Uncoordinated contraction of the LV basal musculature seems to impair sphincteric contraction of the

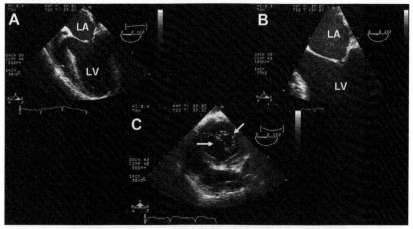

Fig. 3. Mitral leaflet apical tethering. (*A*) Transesophageal echocardiography (TEE) midesophageal 4-chamber view showed mild annular dilatation and apical displacement of both leaflets (ie, tethering). (*B*) High-resolution image showing tethering of both anterior and posterior leaflets. (*C*) TEE transgastric basal short-axis view showing posterior (*yellow arrow*) greater than anterior leaflet (*white arrow*) restriction. LA, left atrium; LV, left ventricle.

posterior MV annulus and interferes with leaflet coaptation.[6] Furthermore, delayed activation of the APM can cause uncoordinated contraction of the papillary muscles, resulting in malalignment of the MV leaflets.[5] Nonetheless, in a series of 74 patients with EF less than 40%, Agricola and colleagues[7] showed that local LV remodeling and global remodeling indices were the main determinants of systolic valvular tenting, which in turn was the primary independent predictor of effective regurgitant orifice (ERO). Regional dyssynchrony index was only a minor independent predictor in patients with nonischemic LV dysfunction in this study. Thus, although local remodeling in the vicinity of the papillary muscles is important for the development of FMR, regional dyssynchrony, which is more likely the result of ischemia or chronic scarring rather than an index of global remodeling, may have only a modifying role.[8]

Other variables related to the degree of apical tenting have also been considered in the mechanism of IMR. Controversy still exists over which force is more predominant for the development of IMR: increased tethering forces or decreased LV systolic closing force associated with impaired LV contraction. In a dog model of microembolization-induced heart failure, although increased end-systolic sphericity index (a surrogate for apical tethering) was associated with the development of FMR, there was no association between measures more consistent with closing force, including LVEF, chamber volume, or regional wall motion.[9] Yiu also showed in 128 patients with LV dysfunction (EF <50%) that the ERO correlated most closely with tenting area compared with MV annular contraction and end-diastolic volume index, whereas there was no correlation with LVEF or wall stress.[4] Therefore, increased tethering force seems to play a more important role than decreased closing forces in the development of IMR. The symmetry of the distribution of tethering along the MV leaflet coaptation line may also affect the location and degree of malcoaptation. Asymmetric tethering (**Fig. 4**) is often associated with isolated inferolateral MI with PPM involvement with leaflet coaptation that is displaced more posterior than apical. The echocardiographic appearance often shows anterior leaflet restriction by the strut chord from the PPM, which produces a hockey-stick deformity, with posterior leaflet override and posteriorly directed eccentric MR. Symmetric tethering often involves an MI with anterior and posterior distributions with significant LV remodeling associated with increased sphericity, decreased function (closing force), and bileaflet apical tethering (**Fig. 5**). Using

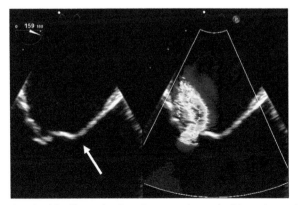

Fig. 4. Asymmetric mitral leaflet tethering. Transesophageal midesophageal long-axis view showing anterior mitral leaflet restriction by a strut chord, which produces a hockey-stick deformity (*arrow*), with posterior leaflet override and an eccentric, posteriorly directed, mitral regurgitant jet.

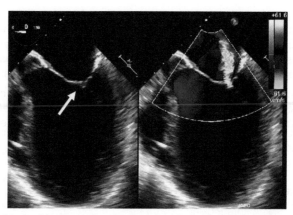

Fig. 5. Symmetric mitral leaflet tethering. Transesophageal midesophageal 5-chamber view showing bileaflet apical tethering (*arrow*), which results in a centrally directed, mitral regurgitant jet.

a three-dimensional (3D) transthoracic echocardiography, Watanabe and colleagues[10] also reported geometric differences of MV tenting between inferior MI and anterior MI. Percent of tethered leaflet area was significantly smaller, more regional, and less apically displaced in inferior MI compared with anterior MI. Concurrent mitral annular dilation and dysfunction may also play a role in IMR. Compared with the normal annulus, the FMR annulus tends to have a more relaxed, flatter saddle shape (larger nonplanimetry angle), reduced height, and larger area manifesting as a longer anteroposterior diameter.[11] However, annular dilation can occur without significant tethering when an MI is limited to the basal inferior-posterior segments, which can cause structural and functional changes in the posterior annulus without significant remodeling and LV dilation.[12] Thus, annular dilation in the context of IMR generally acts more as a modulating factor, increasing the degree of MR in the presence of leaflet tethering.[8] More recently, there has been increased interest in dynamic changes in mitral annular geometry, which has revealed that in IMR, the normal mitral annular area reduction during systole is delayed and smallest in late-systole, consistent with regional wall motion abnormalities.[13] Annular contraction in early systole is important for effective MV closure and is coupled with the synergistic, midsystolic to late-systolic LV contraction closing force. Delayed annular contraction might contribute to impaired leaflet coaptation seen in IMR. The recent introduction of commercially available software designed to investigate the dynamic nature of MV geometry has also revealed that compared with normal patients, those with IMR and FMR have larger mean mitral annular areas, larger anteroposterior and anterolateral-posteromedial diameters (4.3 cm vs 3.6 cm), as well as greater tenting volumes (6.2 mm³ vs 3.5 mm³), and nonplanarity angle at all points during systole compared with controls ($P<.01$).[14] Vertical mitral annular displacement (5.8 mm vs 8.3 mm) was also reduced in FMR compared with controls ($P<.01$).[14] Thus, although LV remodeling and apical tethering remain the fundamental geometric changes responsible for the development of IMR, the underlying mechanisms pertaining to MR severity remain complex and multifactorial.

INTRAOPERATIVE ECHOCARDIOGRAPHY EXAMINATION

A comprehensive intraoperative transesophageal echocardiography (TEE) examination in patients with IMR may have important implications for perioperative clinical decision making. The precardiopulmonary bypass (pre-CPB) echocardiographic inter-rogation of IMR begins with a thorough two-dimensional evaluation to discern the specific mechanism. The degree of leaflet motion restriction, annular dimensions, anterior and posterior leaflet heights, assessment of regional and global LV function, localization of regurgitant jet, and severity of MV incompetence should all be assessed along with potential involvement of collateral structures. Further delineation of MV disease and mechanisms, and the functional geometry associated with IMR may be obtained using 3D reconstruction or real-time 3D echocardiography (**Fig. 6**).[15–21]

The pre-CPB intraoperative echocardiographic evaluation of IMR must also take into consideration the effects of general anesthesia and positive pressure ventilation, which typically cause a reduction in the severity of MR compared with preoperative assessments.[22,23] Other hemodynamic factors, including alterations in preload, acute myocardial ischemia, as well as heart rate and rhythm, may also be responsible for the dynamic nature of IMR. Ideally, efforts should be made to optimize myocardial perfor-mance by administering volume, vasoconstrictors, or inotropes before a definitive diagnosis, which can affect surgical decision making, is ascertained.[24,25] Dobutamine stress echocardiography has also been used as a diagnostic technique to optimize cardiac performance conditions for the perioperative evaluation of MR.[26]

Although MV repair remains the ideal surgical treatment of choice for degenerative MV disease, controversy still exists regarding the optimal interventional approach for IMR. The fundamental concern is durability of MV repair and the subsequent recur-rence of clinically significant MR.[27] There is a relative paucity of data pertaining to prospective trials that have randomized patients to various interventional and nonin-terventional treatments. Nonetheless, several echocardiographic measures predictive of MV repair failure have been identified (**Fig. 7**).[8] Some of these predictors are related to LV remodeling and function, whereas others are related to MR jet characteristics and the extent of apical tethering and the preoperative geometry of the MV apparatus (**Table 1**).[8,27–34]

The initial postcardiopulmonary bypass (post-CPB) TEE examination is essential in helping to determine MV competency and begins with an understanding of the surgical procedure that was performed, which almost universally involves the use of an undersized annuloplasty ring or band. Whereas flatter prosthetics have an easily

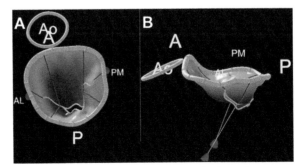

Fig. 6. 3D, parametric model of an MV with IMR created using a 3D transesophageal matrix array and software (Q-labs; MVQ; IE33;X7-2t; Philips Healthcare, Andover, MA). (*Left*) En-face view from left atrial perspective obtained during systole, demonstrating bileaflet tethering and central regurgitant orifice area. (*Right*). The same MV viewed in the lateral to medial perspective, showing significant tenting height and area associated with apical displacement of both leaflets. A, anterior; AL, anterolateral commissure; Ao, aortic valve; P, posterior; PM, posteromedial commissure.

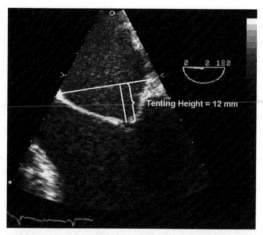

Fig. 7. Echocardiographic measures predictive of MV repair failure. A tenting height greater than 10 mm has been associated with decreased durability of MV repair for IMR. (*Data from* Magne J, Pibarot P, Dagenais F, et al. Preoperative posterior leaflet angle accurately predicts outcome after restrictive valve annuloplasty for ischemic mitral regurgitation. Circulation 2007;115:782–91; and Calafiore AM, Gallina S, DiMauro M, et al. Mitral valve procedure in dilated cardiomyopathy: repair or replacement? Ann Thorac Surg 2001;71:1146–53.)

Table 1
Echocardiographic predictors of MV repair failure

Variable	Value	Reference
LV Geometry		
ESV	≥145 mL	28
SSI	≥0.7	28
LVEDI	>3.5 cm/m²	29
Mitral annular dimension	≥3.7 cm²	30
LV Function		
WMSI	≥1.5	28
MPI	≥0.9	28
Diastolic filling pattern	Restrictive	31
MR Characteristics		
MR grade	>3.5	30
Jet location	Central or complex jet > isolated posterior jet	27
MV Apparatus Geometry		
Tenting height	≥1.0 cm	32,33
Tenting area	≥2.5 cm² ≥1.6 cm²	30,32
Distal anterior leaflet angle	>25°	34
Posterior leaflet angle	≥45°	32

Abbreviations: ESV, end-systolic volume; LVEDI, LV end-diastolic index; MPI, myocardial performance index; SSI, systolic sphericity index; WMSI, wall motion score index.

recognizable echocardiographic appearance, geometric rings that aim to restore the shape of the annulus may vary depending on the vendor (**Fig. 8**). In addition, the use of an edge-to-edge repair to induce coaptation between the anterior and posterior MV leaflets creates a characteristic double-barrel orifice (see **Fig. 8**).[35]

Although persistent MR in the immediate post-CPB period may be associated with perivalvular leaks or residual leaflet malcoaptation, the mechanism of recurrent and persistent functional IMR in the chronic phase after surgical annuloplasty is usually caused by progressive and recurrent posterior leaflet tethering[36] or anterior leaflet tethering.[34] Recurrent tethering is almost always secondary to continued LV remodeling,[37] as well as other mechanisms (**Fig. 9**).

Systolic anterior motion remains a concern for patients with degenerative MV disease undergoing repair, However, in patients with IMR, post-MV repair does not occur because the inherent apical tethering and LV remodeling prevent the abnormal dynamic geometry associated with the subvalvular MV apparatus and the subsequent obstruction of the LV outflow tract. Significant mitral stenosis after MV repair surgery is also less common than persistent MR and can be more challenging to diagnose.[38–40]

SURGICAL INDICATIONS/CONSIDERATIONS

For sudden-onset IMR after an acute MI, the recommendations for surgical intervention are relatively straightforward. MR resulting from an acute wall motion abnormality, chordal derangement, or papillary muscle rupture is unlikely to be resolved by medical management alone and usually requires operative intervention. The choice to repair or replace the valve is guided by the extent of the loss of normal architecture and the clinical stability of the patient, but frequently involves valve replacement. The decision to implant biological or mechanical prostheses is then based on their prognosis for longevity and potential contraindications to anticoagulation.

For chronic IMR, guidelines have been proposed from professional societies to assist with preoperative and intraoperative decision making. The American College of Cardiology (ACC) and the American Heart Association (AHA) recommend an MV intervention for patients undergoing coronary artery bypass graft (CABG) with moderate or severe MR, and in most instances, the ACC/AHA considers mitral ring annuloplasty alone sufficient.[41]

The European Society of Cardiology (ESC) and the European Association for Cardio-Thoracic Surgery (EACTS) also recommend an MV intervention for patients

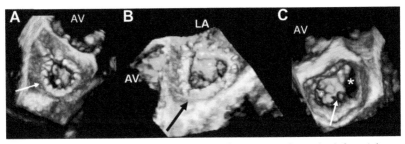

Fig. 8. 3D transesophageal echocardiographic en-face images from the left atrial perspective showing MV repair surgical approaches for patients with IMR. (*A*) Flat ring annuloplasty (*arrow*). (*B*) Saddle-shaped ring annuloplasty (*arrow*). (*C*) Edge-to edge repair with central suture between the anterior and posterior leaflets (*arrow*), producing a double-barrel orifice (*asterisks*). AV, aortic valve; LA, left atrium.

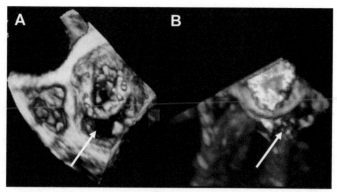

Fig. 9. 3D transesophageal echocardiographic en-face images showing (*A*) an MV annulo-plasty ring dehiscence (*arrow*) and (*B*) the corresponding large regurgitant jet (*arrow*).

undergoing CABG with moderate or severe MR and provide classes of recommenda-tions and levels of evidence for the following further indications.[42] Mitral intervention is indicated for patients with severe MR and LVEF greater than 30% undergoing CABG (class I, level C) (**Table 2**). Surgical intervention is also indicated for patients with moderate MR undergoing CABG if MV repair is feasible (class IIa, level C). For symp-tomatic patients with severe MR and LVEF less than 30%, mitral intervention is indi-cated if the patient can be revascularized (class IIa, level C), and mitral intervention is recommended for patients experiencing severe, symptomatic MR with LVEF greater than 30% who are not capable of being revascularized, who have failed medical management, and have few comorbidities (class IIb, level C).

Although intervention may be recommended, clinical practice is varied, and, in most cases, the type of intervention is left to surgeon discretion when deciding between repair and replacement. Typically, with moderate MR, the decision is to repair or not repair, whereas with severe MR, the decision is between replacement versus repair.[43] To assist with this decision-making process, the Cardiothoracic Surgical Trials Network (CSTN), with 10 core, 7 affiliate, and 15 satellite institutions in conjunc-tion with the National Institutes of Health National Heart Lung and Blood Institute and the Canadian Institute for Health Research has recently completed enrollment for

Table 2	
ESC recommendation classes and levels of evidence	
Class I	Evidence or general agreement that a given treatment or procedure is beneficial, useful, and effective
Class II	Conflicting evidence or a divergence of opinion about the usefulness/efficacy of a given treatment or procedure
Class IIa	Weight of evidence/opinion is in favor of usefulness/efficacy
Class IIb	Usefulness/efficacy is less well established by evidence/opinion
Level of evidence A	Data derived from multiple randomized clinical trials or meta-analyses
Level of evidence B	Data derived from a single randomized clinical trial or large nonrandomized studies
Level of evidence C	Consensus of opinion of the experts or small studies, retrospective studies, registries

a prospective, randomized trial comparing MV repair versus replacement for severe ischemic MR.[44] The CSTN is also conducting an ongoing trial for moderate MR.

The controversy again is centered on the possibility of recurrent MR. If not repaired, moderate MR may progress, and the patient becomes more symptomatic, with progressive heart failure over time. In severe MR that is repaired, the same recurrence is possible. Furthermore, patients with severe MR, poor ventricular function, and symptomatic heart failure engender more perioperative morbidity and mortality with replacement compared with repair. Informed consent at these decision points is critical, and choices are made in context with each patient's preoperative clinical status.

Current practice among most clinicians is to typically extend repair to all feasible patients with ischemic MR greater than mild severity (**Fig. 10**). In addition, for some patients with mild MR when CABG is being performed, an MV intervention may be considered when perioperative TEE shows significant annular dilation, leaflet tenting, or evidence of episodic increased MR, indicating the likelihood of significant progression of MR in the near future.

SURGICAL INTERVENTIONAL OPTIONS

The goals of surgical intervention are to reverse the pathophysiology of IMR. The key alterations sought are annular shape change, chordal repair, and favorable ventricular remodeling to restore the normal valvular supporting architecture. A median sternotomy is the most common surgical approach. Other, more minimally invasive approaches that enter through the right pleural space may offer less patient discomfort

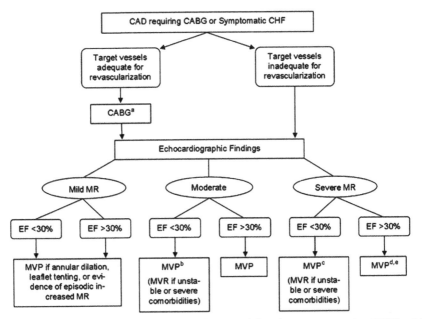

Fig. 10. Decision algorithm for chronic IMR. [a] CSTN trial under way comparing CABG + MV repair (MVP) versus CABG alone for moderate IMR (MR). [b] ESC and EACTS guidelines class IIa, level C if undergoing CABG and MVP is feasible. [c] ESC/EACTS guidelines class IIa, level C if target vessels are adequate for CABG. [d] ESC/EACTS guidelines class I, level C if undergoing CABG. [e] ESC/EACTS guidelines class IIb, level C, if target vessels are inadequate for CABG, symptoms are refractory to medical therapy, and the patient has low comorbidity.

but provide more limited exposure and more difficult cannulation for cardiopulmonary bypass. The 3 conventional surgical options are coronary revascularization alone, valve repair with or without revascularization, and valve replacement with or without revascularization.

For moderate MR, the argument in support of CABG alone assumes that revascularization may cause favorable ventricular remodeling, resulting in normalization of ventricular geometry and improvement in valve performance.[45] This hypothesis was supported by early evidence[46] that MV intervention showed no improvement in survival over CABG alone. However, Aklog and colleagues[22] reported that 40% of patients suffered persistent moderate to severe MR after CABG alone. More recent evidence from the STICH (Surgical Treatment for Ischemic Heart Failure) trial showed that CABG with MV repair was associated with a greater short-term and long-term survival benefit over CABG alone.[47] To definitively determine if revascularization alone is sufficient to treat IMR, the CSTN is enrolling patients for a prospective, randomized trial to compare MV repair with CABG versus CABG alone for moderate ischemic MR.[48]

Mitral repair, or valvuloplasty, is generally preferred whenever possible based on valve pathology and patient stability, because it avoids long-term anticoagulation, decreases infective endocarditis risk, and provides greater leaflet durability. Also, retrospective studies have shown lower perioperative mortality and, in 1 propensity-matched comparison, improved 5-year survival for repair versus replacement (58 vs 36%).[14,49] Among repairs, ring annuloplasty is considered the gold standard. Full-ring annuloplasty undersized by 1 to 2 sizes restores annular geometry, ensuring proper leaflet coaptation and providing proper annular reduction and minimal risk for stenosis.[50] Failure to downsize can result in a recurrence rate of 30% to 40%.[50] Saddle-shaped, full annuloplasty rings have also been advocated by some surgeons to improve restoration of annular geometry, decrease leaflet strain, and increase durability.[51,52] Partial-ring annuloplasty is believed to be inadequate for preventing progressive annular dilation.[27,53] Similarly, flexible rings also permit annular distortion and have been found to have a 4-fold greater recurrence of MR over rigid rings.[27,52] Annuloplasty ring size is determined by measuring the size of the anterior leaflet, and prolapsed posterior leaflet segments can be removed with quadrangular or triangular resection to better coapt with the anterior leaflet.[54] However, even with ring-induced annular reduction, concomitant prolapse or tethering of the valve leaflets may persist, requiring additional procedures. Tethered or elongated chordae of the anterior leaflet can be relocated by transposition of chordae or replacement with suture. Papillary muscles may also be relocated to a more favorable position on the ventricular wall.[55] Releasing strut chordae at the base of a tethered leaflet has also been proposed.[56,57] However, this release can cause greater tenting of leaflets and progression of regurgitation.

MVR is usually reserved for situations in which the valve cannot be reasonably repaired, or repair is unlikely to be tolerated clinically. MVR is more appropriate for complex valve disease with both structural and FMR, involving multiple or eccentric regurgitant jets. MVR is also usually faster than repair with a shorter CPB time, and therefore may be more appropriate for high-risk surgical candidates, because it obviates revising a repair or performing a salvage replacement after a failed repair. Biological prostheses are generally reserved for older patients, those with expected survival less than 10 years, and in patients unable to tolerate or maintain compliance with anticoagulation. Replacement can be performed without preservation of the mitral apparatus and chordal structures but is not recommended because preservation of the mitral apparatus has shown improved survival over nonpreservation, likely from

Table 3
Percutaneous MV technologies

	Device	Mechanism of Action		Recent Activity
Leaflet repair	MitraClip (Abbott Vascular, Abbott Park, IL)	Edge-to-edge leaflet repair, similar to Alfieri suture		EVEREST II trial complete: • 74% had MR reduced to less than 2+ • 1% mortality[70] Await COAPT trial in high-risk patients (NCT01626079)
	Percu-Pro (Cardiosolutions, West Bridgewater, MA)	Balloon spacer occupies gap between valve leaflets, anchored in place by tether to apical septum		Entering phase I trial stage
Valve replacement	Endovalve (Endovalve, Princeton, NJ)	Transcatheter replacement valve		Decreased MR in sheep, preclinical development
	CardiAQ (Cardiaq Valve Technologies, Irvine, CA)	Transcatheter replacement valve		First human implant 2012, Denmark
Chordal replacement	MitraFlex (Transcardiac Therapeutics, Atlanta, GA)	Apically tethered chordae[71]		Preclinical development
Annular shape change	Mitralign (Mitralign, Tewksbury, MA)	Mimics Paneth-Burr suture annuloplasty[72] Pledgeted sutures anchored through posterior annulus, then pulled together and locked to reduce annulus		European CE Mark trial, autumn, 2012

Accucinch (Guided Delivery Systems, Santa Clara, CA)	Subvalvular placement of anchors around the annulus, approximated by a tensioning cable		First human implant 2009, Germany Successful reduction of MR
QuantumCor (QuantumCor, Bothell, WA)	Radiofrequency energy at subablative temperatures to produce mitral annular contraction Transseptal or transapical delivery		Annular reduction and decreased MR in sheep[73]
Cardioband (Valtech Cardio, Or Yehuda, Israel)	Annuloplasty ring adhered with spiral tacks		Currently enrolling patients in phase I trial (NCT01533883)
Carillon XE (Cardiac Dimensions, Kirkland, WA)	External annular compression from within coronary sinus		TITAN trial showed significant reduction in MR and end-diastolic volume, but 30% had device removed for coronary artery compression CE mark obtained
Ventricular shape change iCoapsys (Edwards Lifesciences, Irvine, CA)	Transventricular suture restraint		RESTOR-MV trial: • Decreased LV end-diastolic dimension and MR at 2 y • Greater survival and complication-free survival than surgery[74]

Abbreviations: CE, Conformité Européene; COAPT, Clinical Outcomes Assessment of the MitraClip Percutaneous Therapy for High Surgical Risk Patients; RESTOR-MV, Randomized Evaluation of a Surgical Treatment for Off-Pump Repair of the Mitral Valve; TACT, Transapical Artificial Chordae Tendineae; TITAN, Transcatheter Implantation of Carillon Mitral Annuloplasty Device.

Modified from Chiam PT, Ruiz CE. Percutaneous transcatheter mitral valve repair: a classification of the technology. JACC Cardiovasc Interv 2011;4:1–3; Additional images printed with permission from Cardiac Dimensions and Valtech Cardio.

maintenance of overall ventricular geometry.[14,49,58] Removal of the valve and chordae should be performed only if the apparatus is severely deformed, such as if it is rheumatic or caused by a congenital malformation. The decision to repair or replace a valve still remains at the discretion of the surgeon. In the absence of definitive professional guidelines, the CSTN trial that is under way comparing repair and replacement for severe IMR should ideally elucidate more specific recommendations for the future.[48]

Surgical remodeling of the LV can also be performed. Infarction scars can be reduced by plication, whereas external ventricular restraint can be applied with mesh or adjustable balloons to restore adequate geometry.[59,60] Effective leaflet coaptation can be achieved with an edge-to edge repair (ie, Alfieri repair) to create a double-orifice valve.[35,44]

SURGICAL OUTCOMES

Operative mortality for MV surgery is favorable at approximately 3% to 4%.[14,49,58,61] Five-year survival has been traditionally low, at approximately 30% to 40%, because of the significance of this disease and the concurrent ischemic condition.[62–65] Braun and colleagues[66] observed minimal recurrence of MR at 18 months in 1 series with downsized annuloplasty rings. However, other studies have reported recurrence of MR of 28% to 30% at 6 months[27,67] and up to 72% at 4 years for annular reduction alone.[67] Ideal therapies most likely need to address a combination of interventional options, including revascularization, annular reduction, chordal integrity, and ventricular remodeling.

PERCUTANEOUS OPTIONS

A variety of percutaneous approaches have been devised for the minimally invasive treatment of MR, with the goal of serving the large demand for restoration of mitral function without the increased perioperative risk of traditional surgery. Each percutaneous system attempts to address a component of the pathophysiology associated with the mechanism of MR similar to those of open surgical intervention (**Table 3**).[68–74] These devices enable leaflet repair, chordal replacement, annular shape change, ventricular geometry change, or even complete valve replacement. Although the use of percutaneous approaches is often limited to patients who present as poor surgical candidates, their effectiveness and usefulness should continue to increase to engage a wider elective market. The usefulness and effectiveness of these devices will be compared with the gold standard of ring annuloplasty, yet clinical decisions with these devices will be tempered by patient valvular disease, overall prognosis, complicating comorbidities, and patient autonomy.

REFERENCES

1. Carpentier A. Cardiac valve surgery–the "French correction". J Thorac Cardiovasc Surg 1983;86:323–37.
2. Atluri P, GR, Gorman RC. Ischemic mitral regurgitation. In: Cohn LH, editor. Cardiac surgery in the adult. 4th edition. New York: McGraw-Hill; 2012. p. 629–46.
3. Gorman JH 3rd, Jackson BM, Gorman RC, et al. Papillary muscle discoordination rather than increased annular area facilitates mitral regurgitation after acute posterior myocardial infarction. Circulation 1997;96(Suppl 9):II-124–7.
4. Yiu S, Maurice Enriquez-Sarano M, Christophe Tribouilloy C, et al. Determinants of the degree of functional mitral regurgitation in patients with systolic left ventricular dysfunction: a quantitative clinical study. Circulation 2000;102:1400–6.

5. Erlebacher JA, Barbarash S. Intraventricular conduction delay and functional mitral regurgitation. Am J Cardiol 2001;88:83–6.
6. Kanzaki H, Bazaz R, Schwartzman D, et al. A mechanism for immediate reduction in mitral regurgitation after cardiac resynchronization. J Am Coll Cardiol 2004;44: 1619–25.
7. Agricola E, Oppizzi M, Galderisi M, et al. Role of regional mechanical dyssynchrony as a determinant of functional mitral regurgitation in patients with left ventricular systolic dysfunction. Heart 2006;10:1390–5.
8. Silbiger J. Mechanistic insights into ischemic mitral regurgitation: echocardiographic and surgical implications. J Am Soc Echocardiogr 2011;24:707–19.
9. Sabbah HN, Kono T, Rosman H, et al. Left ventricular shape: a factor in the etiology of functional mitral regurgitation in heart failure. Am Heart J 1992;123:961–6.
10. Watanabe N, Ogasawara Y, Yamaura Y, et al. Geometric differences of the mitral valve tenting between anterior and inferior myocardial infarctions with significant ischemic mitral regurgitation: quantification by novel software system with transthoracic real-time three-dimensional echocardiography. J Am Soc Echocardiogr 2006;1:71–5.
11. Kaplan S, Bashein G, Sheehan F, et al. Three-dimensional echocardiographic assessment of annular shape changes in the normal and regurgitant mitral valve. Am Heart J 2000;139:378–87.
12. Otsuji Y, Kumanohoso T, Yoshifuku S, et al. Isolated annular dilation does not usually cause important functional mitral regurgitation: comparison between patients with lone atrial fibrillation and those with idiopathic or ischemic cardiomyopathy. J Am Coll Cardiol 2002;39:1651–6.
13. Daimon M, Saracino G, Fukuda S, et al. Dynamic changes of mitral annular geometry and motion in ischemic mitral regurgitation assessed by a computerized 3D echo method. Echocardiography 2010;27:1069–77.
14. Khabbaz K, Mahmood F, Shakil O, et al. Dynamic 3-dimensional echocardiographic assessment of mitral annular geometry in patients with functional mitral regurgitation. Ann Thorac Surg 2013;95:105–10.
15. Abraham T, Warner J, Kon N, et al. Feasibility, accuracy, and incremental value of intraoperative three-dimensional transesophageal echocardiography in valve surgery. Am J Cardiol 1997;80:1577–82.
16. Jassar A, Brinster C, Vergnat M, et al. Quantitative mitral valve modeling using real-time three-dimensional echocardiography: technique and repeatability. Ann Thorac Surg 2011;91:165–71.
17. Vergnat M, Jassar A, Jackson B, et al. Ischemic mitral regurgitation: a quantitative three-dimensional echocardiographic analysis. Ann Thorac Surg 2011;1:157–64.
18. Watanabe N, Ogasawara Y, Yamaura Y, et al. Mitral annulus flattens in ischemic mitral regurgitation: geometric differences between inferior and anterior myocardial infarction: a real-time 3-dimensional echocardiographic study. Circulation 2005;112(Suppl 9):I458–62.
19. Salcedo E, Quaife R, Seres T, et al. A framework for systematic characterization of the mitral valve by real-time three-dimensional transesophageal echocardiography. J Am Soc Echocardiogr 2009;22:1087–99.
20. Sugeng L, Shernan S, Weinert L, et al. Real-time three-dimensional transesophageal echocardiography in valve disease: comparison with surgical findings and evaluation of prosthetic valves. J Am Soc Echocardiogr 2008;12:1347–54.
21. Lang R, Badano L, Tsang W, et al. Recommendations for image acquisition and display using three-dimensional echocardiography. J Am Soc Echocardiogr 2012;1:3–46.

22. Aklog L, Filsoufi F, Flores K, et al. Does coronary artery bypass grafting alone correct moderate ischemic mitral regurgitation? Circulation 2001;104:I-68–75.

23. Grewal K, Malkowski M, Piracha A, et al. Effect of general anesthesia on the severity of mitral regurgitation by transesophageal echocardiography. Am J Cardiol 2000;85:199–203.

24. Shiran A, Merdler A, Ismir E, et al. Intraoperative transesophageal echocardiography using a quantitative dynamic loading test for the evaluation of ischemic mitral regurgitation. J Am Soc Echocardiogr 2007;20:690–7.

25. Mihalatos D, Gopal A, Kates R, et al. Intraoperative assessment of mitral regurgitation: role of phenylephrine challenge. J Am Soc Echocardiogr 2006;19: 1158–64.

26. Roshanali F, Mandegar M, Yousefnia M, et al. Low-dose dobutamine stress echocardiography to predict reversibility of mitral regurgitation with CABG. Echocardiography 2006;23:31–7.

27. McGee E, Gillinov A, Blackstone E, et al. Recurrent mitral regurgitation after annuloplasty for functional ischemic mitral regurgitation. J Thorac Cardiovasc Surg 2004;128:916–24.

28. Gelsomino S, Lorusso R, De Cicco G, et al. Five-year echocardiographic results of combined undersized mitral ring annuloplasty and coronary artery bypass grafting for chronic ischaemic mitral regurgitation. Eur Heart J 2008;29:231–40.

29. Lee L, Kwon M, Cevasco M, et al. Postoperative recurrence of mitral regurgitation after annuloplasty for functional mitral regurgitation. Ann Thorac Surg 2012;94: 1211–7.

30. Kongsaerepong V, Shiota M, Gillinov A, et al. Echocardiographic predictors of successful versus unsuccessful mitral valve repair in ischemic mitral regurgitation. Am J Cardiol 2006;98:504–8.

31. Eremiene E, Vaskelyte J, Benetis R, et al. Ischemic mitral valve repair: predictive significance of restrictive left ventricular diastolic filling. Echocardiography 2005; 22:217–24.

32. Magne J, Pibarot P, Dagenais F, et al. Preoperative posterior leaflet angle accurately predicts outcome after restrictive valve annuloplasty for ischemic mitral regurgitation. Circulation 2007;115:782–91.

33. Calafiore AM, Gallina S, DiMauro M, et al. Mitral valve procedure in dilated cardiomyopathy: repair or replacement? Ann Thorac Surg 2001;71:1146–53.

34. Lee A, Acker M, Kubo S, et al. Mechanisms of recurrent functional mitral regurgitation after mitral valve repair in nonischemic dilated cardiomyopathy: importance of distal anterior leaflet tethering. Circulation 2009;119:2606–14.

35. Alfieri O, Maisano F, De Bonis M, et al. The double-orifice technique in mitral valve repair: a simple solution for complex problems. J Thorac Cardiovasc Surg 2001; 122:674–81.

36. Kuwahara E, Otsuji Y, Iguro Y, et al. Mechanism of recurrent/persistent ischemic/functional mitral regurgitation in the chronic phase after surgical annuloplasty: importance of augmented posterior leaflet tethering. Circulation 2006;114: I-529–34.

37. Magne J, Pibarot P, Dumensil J, et al. Continued global left ventricular remodeling is not the sole mechanism responsible for the late recurrence of ischemic mitral regurgitation after restrictive annuloplasty. J Am Soc Echocardiogr 2009;22: 1256–64.

38. Williams M, Daneshmand M, Jollis J, et al. Mitral gradients and frequency of recurrence of mitral regurgitation after ring annuloplasty for ischemic mitral regurgitation. Ann Thorac Surg 2009;88:1197–201.

39. Maslow A, Gemignani A, Singh A, et al. Intraoperative assessment of mitral valve area after mitral valve repair: comparison of different methods. J Cardiothorac Vasc Anesth 2011;25:221–8.

40. Riegel1 A, Busch R, Segal S, et al. Evaluation of transmitral pressure gradients in the intraoperative echocardiographic diagnosis of mitral stenosis after mitral valve repair. PLoS One 2011;6:1–8.

41. Bonow R, Carabello B, Chatterjee K, et al. Focused update incorporated into the ACC/AHA 2006 guidelines for the management of patients with valvular heart disease: a report of the American College of Cardiology/American Heart Association Task Force on Practice Guidelines. Circulation 2008;118:e523–661.

42. Vahanian A, Baumgartner H, Bax J, et al. Guidelines on the management of valvular heart disease: the Task Force on the Management of Valvular Heart Disease of the European Society of Cardiology. Eur Heart J 2007;28:230–68.

43. Kwon MH, Cevasco M, Chen FY. Functional, ischemic mitral regurgitation: to repair or not to repair? Circulation 2012;125:2563–5.

44. Perrault L, Moskowitz A, Kron I, et al. Optimal surgical management of severe ischemic mitral regurgitation: to repair or to replace? J Thorac Cardiovasc Surg 2012;143:1396–403.

45. Balu V, Hershowitz S, Zaki Masud A, et al. Mitral regurgitation in coronary artery disease. Chest 1982;81:550–5.

46. Wu A, Aaronson K, Bolling S, et al. Impact of mitral valve annuloplasty on mortality risk in patients with mitral regurgitation and left ventricular systolic dysfunction. J Am Coll Cardiol 2005;45:381–7.

47. Deja M, Grayburn P, Sun B, et al. Influence of mitral regurgitation repair on survival in the surgical treatment for ischemic heart failure trial. Circulation 2012;125:2639–48.

48. Cardiothoracic Surgical Trials Network (CSTN). Surgical interventions for moderate ischemic mitral regurgitation. 2012. Available at: http://www.ctsurgerynet.org/currenttrials.html. Accessed January 3, 2013.

49. Gillinov A, Wierup P, Blackstone E, et al. Is repair preferable to replacement for ischemic mitral regurgitation? J Thorac Cardiovasc Surg 2001;122:1125–41.

50. Acker M. Should moderate or greater mitral regurgitation be repaired in all patients with LVEF <30%? Mitral valve repair in patients with advanced heart failure and severe functional mitral insufficiency reverses left ventricular remodeling and improves symptoms. Circ Heart Fail 2008;1:281–4.

51. Jimenez J, Liou S, Padala M, et al. A saddle-shaped annulus reduces systolic strain on the central region of the mitral valve anterior leaflet. J Thorac Cardiovasc Surg 2007;134:1562–8.

52. Ryan L, Jackson B, Hamamoto H, et al. The influence of annuloplasty ring geometry on mitral leaflet curvature. Ann Thorac Surg 2008;86:749–60.

53. Mihaljevic T, Lam B, Rajeswaran J, et al. Impact of mitral valve annuloplasty combined with revascularization in patients with functional ischemic mitral regurgitation. J Am Coll Cardiol 2007;49:2191–201.

54. Gazoni L, Fedoruk L, Kern J, et al. A simplified approach to degenerative disease: triangular resections of the mitral valve. Ann Thorac Surg 2007;83:1658–64.

55. Kron I, Green G, Cope J. Surgical relocation of the posterior papillary muscle in chronic ischemic mitral regurgitation. Ann Thorac Surg 2002;74:600–1.

56. Messas E, Guerrero J, Handschumacher M, et al. Chordal cutting: a new therapeutic approach for ischemic mitral regurgitation. Circulation 2001;104:1958–63.

57. Messas E, Pouzet B, Touchot B, et al. Efficacy of chordal cutting to relieve chronic persistent ischemic mitral regurgitation. Circulation 2003;108(Suppl 1):II111–5.

58. Filsoufi F, Salzberg S, Adams D. Current management of ischemic mitral regurgitation. Mt Sinai J Med 2005;72:105–15.

59. Hung J, Guerrero J, Handschumacher M, et al. Reverse ventricular remodeling reduces ischemic mitral regurgitation: echo-guided device application in the beating heart. Circulation 2002;106:2594–600.

60. Kwon M, Cevasco M, Schmitto J, et al. Ventricular restraint therapy for heart failure: a review, summary of state of the art, and future directions. J Thorac Cardiovasc Surg 2012;144:771–777.e1.

61. Adams D, Filsoufi F, Aklog L. Surgical treatment of the ischemic mitral valve. J Heart Valve Dis 2002;11(Suppl 1):S21–5.

62. Connolly M, Gelbfish J, Jacobowitz I, et al. Surgical results for mitral regurgitation from coronary artery disease. J Thorac Cardiovasc Surg 1986;91:379–88.

63. Hendren W, Nemec J, Lytle B, et al. Mitral valve repair for ischemic mitral insufficiency. Ann Thorac Surg 1991;52:1246–51.

64. Hickey M, Smith L, Muhlbaier L, et al. Current prognosis of ischemic mitral regurgitation. Implications for future management. Circulation 1988;78:I51–9.

65. Pinson C, Cobanoglu A, Metzdorff M, et al. Late surgical results for ischemic mitral regurgitation. Role of wall motion score and severity of regurgitation. J Thorac Cardiovasc Surg 1984;88:663–72.

66. Braun J, van de Veire N, Klautz R, et al. Restrictive mitral annuloplasty cures ischemic mitral regurgitation and heart failure. Ann Thorac Surg 2008;85:430–6.

67. Hung J, Papakostas L, Tahta S, et al. Mechanism of recurrent ischemic mitral regurgitation after annuloplasty: continued LV remodeling as a moving target. Circulation 2004;110:II85–90.

68. Feldman T, Foster E, Glower D, et al, for the EVEREST II Investigators. Percutaneous repair or surgery for mitral regurgitation. N Engl J Med 2011;364: 1395–406.

69. Chiam P, Ruiz C. Percutaneous transcatheter mitral valve repair: a classification of the technology. JACC Cardiovasc Interv 2011;4:1–13.

70. Whitlow PL, Feldman T, Pedersen WR, et al. Acute and 12-month results with catheter-based mitral valve leaflet repair: the EVEREST II (Endovascular Valve Edge-to-Edge Repair) High Risk Study. J Am Coll Cardiol 2012;59:130–9.

71. Seeburger J, Leontjev S, Neumuth M, et al. Trans-apical beating-heart implantation of neo-chordae to mitral valve leaflets: results of an acute animal study. Eur J Cardiothorac Surg 2012;41:173–6.

72. Burr LH, Krayenbuhl C, Sutton MS. The mitral plication suture: a new technique of mitral valve repair. J Thorac Cardiovasc Surg 1977;73:589–95.

73. Heuser RR, Witzel T, Dickens D, et al. Percutaneous treatment for mitral regurgitation: the QuantumCor system. J Interv Cardiol 2008;21:178–82.

74. Grossi EA, Patel N, Woo YJ, et al. Outcomes of the RESTOR-MV trial (Randomized Evaluation of a Surgical Treatment for Off-Pump Repair of the Mitral Valve). J Am Coll Cardiol 2010;56:1984–93.

Robotic and Minimally Invasive Cardiac Surgery

William Vernick, MD[a],*, Pavan Atluri, MD[b]

KEYWORDS

- Robotic mitral valve surgery • Minimally invasive mitral valve surgery
- Cardiac anesthesia • Mitral valve repair • Transesophageal echocardiography

KEY POINTS

- Minimally invasive mitral valve surgery (MIMVS) and robotic-assisted MIMVS have become the approaches of choice among many surgeons throughout the world, and are providing patients with improved recovery without sacrificing safety or the quality of the surgical result.
- A significant learning curve exists for both surgeons and anesthesiologists when providing patients with minimally invasive surgical options, and not all patients are ideal candidates.
- In general, as surgery becomes less invasive the anesthesiologist's role in assessing the cardiovascular state and achieving access for cardiopulmonary bypass increases.

INTRODUCTION

The transition of mitral valve surgery away from the traditional sternotomy approach towards more minimally invasive strategies continues to evolve. This transition began during the 1990s with advancements in endoscopic instruments and visualization tools as well as peripheral cannulation circulatory systems for cardiopulmonary bypass (CPB).[1–9] By 2008, 20% of all mitral valve surgeries performed in the Unites States were done using minimally invasive techniques, with half being robotically assisted.[10]

The first minimally invasive mitral valve surgery (MIMVS) was performed by a surgical team from Stanford University in 1996.[5] The first robotic-assisted or telemanipulative mitral valve surgery was performed in France by Carpentier and colleagues[11] in 1997 using a prototype of the current da Vinci robotic system (Intuitive Surgical, Sunnyvale, CA). Chitwood and colleagues[12] from East Carolina followed in 2000 with the first robotic mitral valve case in the United States. In 2002 the Food and Drug Administration provided approval of the da Vinci system for use in cardiac surgery.[13]

[a] Department of Anesthesiology and Critical Care, The Perelman School of Medicine at the University Hosptial of Pennsylvania, 3400 Spruce Street, Philadelphia, PA 19104, USA;
[b] Division of Cardiovascular Surgery, Department of Surgery, University of Pennsylvania, 3400 Spruce Street, Philadelphia, PA 19104, USA
* Corresponding author.
E-mail address: william.vernick@uphs.upenn.edu

Anesthesiology Clin 31 (2013) 299–320
http://dx.doi.org/10.1016/j.anclin.2012.12.002
1932-2275/13/$ – see front matter © 2013 Elsevier Inc. All rights reserved.
anesthesiology.theclinics.com

Because the mitral valve lies in an annular plane that nearly approximates the sagittal plane of the body, the small right anterolateral incision generally associated with MIMVS is particularly well suited for exposure of the mitral valve during MIMVS. As the incision moves more laterally, this angle becomes even more direct, albeit at the cost of an increased distance to the valve. This distance however can easily be overcome with the use of robotic instruments.[14] Improved satisfaction and cosmesis have been important benefits for patients undergoing MIMVS,[15] particularly women, in whom the incision can be hidden in the right inframammary crease, and robotic-assisted surgery can be now be performed via an incision as small as 1.5 to 2 cm (**Fig. 1**).[16]

Nonrobotic MIMVS requires surgeons to use long endoscopic instruments through an access incision and then to visualize the valve as a 2-dimensional video image on a monitor (**Fig. 2**). By contrast, during robotic-assisted surgery the surgeon sits at a separate console (**Fig. 3**) and manipulates mechanical wrists (**Fig. 4**) that allow 7° of multidirectional motion.[17] The robotic system will transmit the scaled movements of the surgeon to the robotic arms and the computer will correct for any surgical tremors. Enhanced, near 3-dimensional visualization of the valve from the console is provided by 2 side-by-side camera arms that can also be controlled by the surgeon (**Fig. 5**). Moreover, the use of a dynamic atrial retractor with the robotic platform allows for rapid and continuous retractor repositioning to maximize valve exposure, providing an additional advantage over traditional endoscopic approaches. The lack of tactile sensation when telemanipulating the robotic arms during surgical repair is a limitation, leaving the surgeon to rely on visual cues to determine tissue strain. Potential difficulties with robotic knot-tying is a further negative aspect associated with robotic surgery.[13] In addition, there is a substantial fixed cost in purchasing the robotic system as well an increase in disposable costs with each use.

In addition to cosmetic benefits, case-control studies have consistently shown faster recovery times and less associated pain with MIMVS.[18–21] The Mayo Clinic

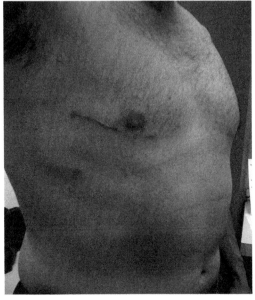

Fig. 1. Robotic-assisted incision along lateral inframammary crease as well as robotic port sites.

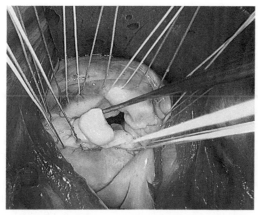

Fig. 2. Intraoperative videoscopic view of mitral valve during minimally invasive mitral valve surgery. Annuloplasty sutures have been placed to facilitate exposure of valve and inspection of leaflet pathology. Markedly redundant prolapsed posterior leaflet P2 segment is demonstrated.

described an improved early quality of life and return to work activities in patients undergoing robotic MIMVS compared with mitral valve surgery performed via sternotomy.[22] In a series by Murphy and colleagues,[23] more than 60% of robotically assisted MIMVS patients were discharged within 4 days of surgery. In the most recently published meta-analysis from Cheng and colleagues,[15] which is also the largest to date, a statistically significant improvement in bleeding, transfusion, incidence of atrial

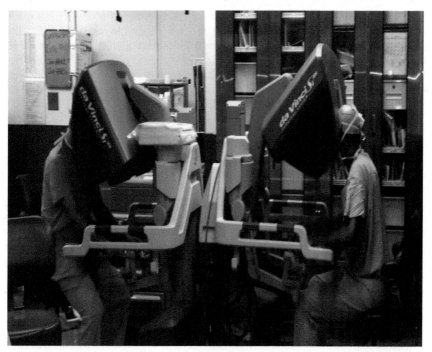

Fig. 3. Two surgeons seen sitting at a dual robotic console during robotic surgery.

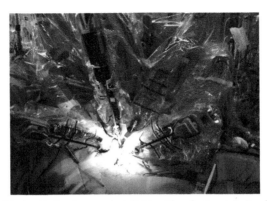

Fig. 4. Robotic-assisted mitral valve surgical field with robotic arms in place.

fibrillation, and time to resumption of normal activities was shown when comparing MIMVS with conventional mitral surgery.

Of course, these benefits would be of little consequence if the quality and durability of mitral surgery was limited by robotic MIMVS techniques or if MIMVS increased morbidity or mortality. In the available meta-analyses of MIMVS, perioperative and long-term mortality were equivalent between techniques for mitral valve surgery, as was long-term freedom from reoperation[15,18,24] These findings are supported by 2 recent large single-center outcomes studies. Eight-year freedom from reoperation was better with MIMVS[25] as was short-term and 1-year survival.[25,26] The largest single-center report of purely robotic MIMVS was from the East Carolina Heart Institute in 2012,[27] which showed a low short and long term mortality of 0.4% and 1.7% respectively in 540 consecutive patients with a 2.9% reoperation rate. These results of robotic surgery were comparable with, if not better than the results from Cheng's meta-analysis, in which 30-day mortality was 1.2% and reoperation rate was 2.3%.

However, a significant learning curve has been shown to exist with the use of both MIMVS and robotic-assisted MIMVS.[28] Both Cheng and colleagues[29] and Chitwood and colleagues[30] showed a decrease in failed mitral valve repair only after 74 and 100 robotic-assisted cases, respectively.[13] Operative times (4.5 vs 3.7 hours, 95%

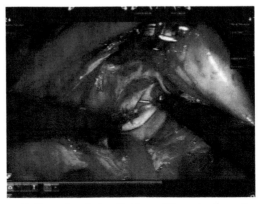

Fig. 5. Enhanced, near 3-dimensional visualization of the valve from the console is provided by 2 side-by-side camera arms, which can be controlled by the surgeon.

confidence interval [CI] 0.41–1.16) as well as CPB (144 vs 111 minutes, 95% CI 18.9–47.1) and aortic cross-clamp times (95 vs 74 minutes, 95% CI 10.14–32.69) have also been shown to be longer with MIMVS when compared with sternotomy approaches.[15] With more experience, operative times will decrease but will still remain longer than with standard approaches.[15,31] Perhaps more importantly, when comparing outcomes between MIMVS and conventional surgery, it should be considered that the data may be skewed. For example, patients with significant peripheral vascular disease may be excluded from consideration for MIMVS. In the meta-analysis of Cheng and colleagues, patients undergoing MIMVS were young and had a low incidence of baseline renal failure and pulmonary disease.

ANESTHESIA FOR ROBOTIC-ASSISTED MIMVS

Because most aspects are unchanged when comparing anesthesia for robotic-assisted MIMVS and non–robotic MIMVS, the conduct of anesthesia for both will be referred to interchangeably except when relevant differences exist.

Preoperative Preparation

The preoperative evaluation of patients for MIMVS and robotic MIMVS generally mimics the evaluation of patients undergoing standard mitral valve surgery. Because some degree of peripheral CPB cannulation is nearly universal with MIMVS, regardless of whether the surgery is to be performed completely endoscopically or if a large access incision is to be made, the most important difference in preoperative preparation relates to the feasibility and safety of accessing the vascular tree. Typically these concerns relate to a small-sized or diseased peripheral arterial system and/or descending aorta, although an abnormal venous system may pose problems as well. Although standard preoperative tests such as transesophageal echocardiography (TEE) and cardiac catheterization may identify significant abnormalities, many advocate for preoperative Doppler ultrasonography or computed tomography angiography (CTA) of the vascular tree before MIMVS. In a study of 141 patients scheduled for MIMVS from the Cleveland Clinic, 26 patients had their surgical approach changed because of CTA findings.[32]

Additional surgical concerns that might complicate MIMVS include previous right chest surgery or adhesions, as well as an abnormal orientation of the heart within the chest cavity. In addition to confirming surgical necessity, preoperative TEE may identify complex mitral valve abnormalities such as severe mitral annular calcifications that surgeons may consider will limit their ability to repair the valve via MIMVS. There is limited evidence to suggest that any preoperative pulmonary function testing should preclude MIMVS, although some consider the identification of severe pulmonary dysfunction to be a relative contraindication.

Type of Anesthesia and Patient Positioning

Although some centers use regional anesthesia techniques for minimally invasive direct coronary artery bypass surgery (MIDCAB), the need for CPB and intraoperative TEE (IOTEE) essentially eliminates this option for MIMVS and necessitates general anesthesia. The choice of anesthetic agents is practitioner and institutional dependent and is not dictated by MIMVS. Patient positioning is typically supine with the right upper trunk elevated in some manner. The right arm is positioned at the side to allow the shoulder to drop down to improve surgical exposure. This exaggerated position may potentially cause stress on the brachial plexus and the neck.

External defibrillator pads should be applied because limited surgical access makes use of internal defibrillator paddles more difficult, although not impossible through an access incision using pediatric paddles. One must remember that, depending on the exact location of the external pads, if defibrillation will be occurring across the right lung field, the empty right thoracic cavity during left single-lung ventilation may impair defibrillation success. The right lung can be reexpanded to attempt enhancement of defibrillation efficacy. Because direct skeletal muscle stimulation may occur during defibrillation, the robotic arms should be withdrawn beforehand to prevent iatrogenic injury.[13]

Airway Management

Because MIMVS utilizes a right thoracotomy, lung isolation has been a mainstay of anesthetic management. The right lung is typically deflated as the surgeon enters the chest cavity and opens the pericardium to expose the left atrium before the initiation of CPB. One-lung ventilation (OLV) is also typically used at certain points after separation from bypass: as surgical sites are checked, bleeding is controlled, and the chest closed.

Nonetheless, OLV is not mandatory for the conduct of MIMVS. Ventilation can be held or made intermittent when needed. CPB can also be initiated before exposing the left atrium at the beginning of the operation, although this approach will increase the total CPB time. The method of choice for achieving lung isolation is also debatable. The most common techniques for achieving lung isolation are with a left-sided double-lumen tube (DLT) or a right-sided bronchial blocker placed through a standard single-lumen endotracheal tube. Each technique has its own set of advantages and disadvantages. A DLT may be more challenging to place in certain patients, and may be associated with more airway trauma and bleeding. Another disadvantage of a DLT is that postoperative swelling may make the exchange to a single-lumen tube at the end of the case dangerous, even with the use of an airway-exchange catheter. Once properly positioned however, there are definite benefits to a DLT, as they are less likely to be dislodged than bronchial blockers and they allow for both the application of continuous positive airway pressure and suctioning to the deflated lung.

The institution of OLV may create significant management difficulties in patients presenting for cardiac surgery. Any hypoxemia and hypercarbia during OLV will increase pulmonary vascular resistance (PVR). Patients with mitral disease may already have elevated PVR, and the additional strain on the right ventricular may lead to dysfunction and an increase in any concomitant tricuspid regurgitation. Depressed cardiac function can further increase dead-space ventilation and limit pulmonary blood flow. Ventilation abnormalities may also lead to arrhythmias and increases in sympathetic tone, which may also be poorly tolerated, particularly in patients with marginal ventricular function. The degree of OLV ventilation/perfusion mismatch may significantly increase after CPB in MIMVS.[33] Although in general the time period when OLV is needed after CPB is relatively short when compared with lung surgery or MIDCAB, it may be protracted, particularly when intrathoracic bleeding requires persistent surgical attention.

Intraoperative TEE

The importance of IOTEE to help guide clinical decision making in cardiac surgery has been well established,[34,35] particularly in the setting of mitral valve repair.[36,37] Because IOTEE has become so intricately involved in guiding surgical cannulation, monitoring hemodynamics, and assessing the mitral valve before and after intervention in MIMVS,[38,39] it has become essentially mandatory for the operation. Therefore, the inability to obtain an intraoperative IOTEE often precludes the operation.

While it is common practice to confirm the presence of the surgical indication with IOTEE before incision, with MIMVS it is also useful for the anesthesiologist to use IOTEE to confirm the appropriateness of the patient for a minimally invasive technique before incision. Ideally this determination should also be completed before the placement of any specialized CPB cannulas. For example, the preincision finding of significant descending aortic atheroma will typically contraindicate retrograde arterial CPB flow, and requires alternative aortic cannulation strategies or a change in surgical approach. The presence of other significant concomitant disease that requires surgical intervention that cannot be addressed via a minimally invasive approach should also be excluded as soon as possible.

VASCULAR CANNULATION FOR MIMVS

For the anesthesiologist involved in MIMVS, a definite theme exists: the smaller the surgical incision, the more intimately involved the anesthesiologist becomes in the conduct of the operation and the more anesthesia preparation is required. In a small retrospective study of Port Access MIMVS, anesthesia preparation time was increased by 16 minutes on average when compared with conventional surgery.[33]

Venous Drainage

Venous return to the CPB circuit can be achieved in several ways (**Fig. 6**). There are various commercially available long percutaneous venous return cannulas (22F–28F) that may be introduced up to the right atrium or either vena cava via the femoral venous system. After accessing the femoral vein, a long wire is advanced toward, then visualized using TEE within, the right atrium or vena cava. The venous cannula

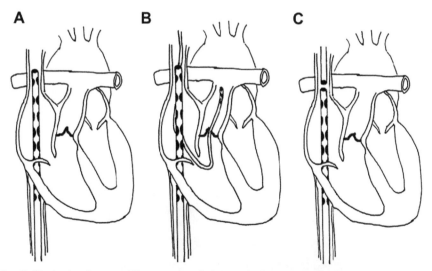

Fig. 6. Strategies for providing venous drainage during minimally invasive mitral valve surgery. (A) Single long femoral venous cannula advanced into the right atrium (RA). (B) Long femoral venous cannula advanced into RA in conjunction with endopulmonary vent catheter placed via right IJ introducer sheath. (C) Long femoral venous cannula advanced into RA in conjunction with venous drainage cannula advanced into superior vena cava from right IJ. (*Adapted from* Rehfeldt KH, Mauermann WJ, Burkhart H, et al. Robotic-assisted mitral valve repair. J Cardiothorac Vasc Anesth 2011;25(4):725; with permission.)

is then advanced over the wire into the right atrium or vena cava with TEE confirmation. As discussed later, the final position of this cannula depends on individual practice and the type of procedure being performed. If femoral venous access is not utilized, use of a larger access incision may allow for direct central venous cannulation.

Typically, adjunctive measures are used to assist venous drainage when using long percutaneous cannulas. Advances in perfusion techniques such as kinetic or vacuum-assisted venous drainage can increase flow dynamics by 20% to 40%.[40,41] In fact, adequate total body venous drainage may be achieved with a single femoral venous cannula as long as the cannula's multi-orificed side ports reside in the body of the right atrium with the tip in the proximal superior vena cava (SVC). However, additional measures to idealize surgical exposure for MIMVS are often critically important. In addition, drainage from the superior and inferior cava can effectively be separated by surgical retraction on the intra-atrial septum,[42] thereby complicating single-stage cannulation. Thus, in many practices it is standard to place an additional percutaneous venous drainage cannula that resides in the SVC from the neck (**Fig. 7**). This placement is best achieved via the right internal jugular (IJ) vein given the near direct path it takes to the SVC.

The placement of a large-bore drainage catheter in the neck is not without substantial risk of vascular injury. The risk likely increases with increasing size of the cannula, as more force must be generated to advance the catheter percutaneously. As with all upper extremity central venous cannulations, local traumatic injuries can occur as well as damage to more central structures, including the great vessels. Perforation of the right atrium, vena cava, or other vascular structure within the pericardium can lead to pericardial tamponade. Use of a strict Seldinger technique to minimize the chance of wire kinking during catheter advancement is a critical component to improving safety. Placement may be facilitated by sequential dilators of increasing size in advance of the cannula. Ideally an assistant with sterile gown and gloves should be present. Though not mandatory, the ability to visualize the wire in the right atrium on TEE may be useful.[43]

If the right IJ drainage cannula is placed well before the systemic heparinization for CPB, a small dose of heparin should be administered just before IJ cannula placement. The cannula should then be flushed vigorously after it is secured to prevent any clotting or thrombus formation within it. Sutures may be placed around the cannulation site at this point or later, to facilitate closure of the defect and provide hemostasis upon cannula removal.

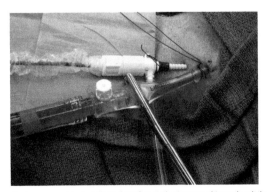

Fig. 7. A 16F venous drainage cannula placed in the right internal jugular (IJ) vein and connected to the bypass circuit. Note a boxed suture placed around the cannula site. A separate 9F introducer catheter with pulmonary artery catheter is seen more cephalad in the ipsilateral neck.

Some institutions use the Endopulmonary Vent Catheter (Edwards Lifesciences, Irvine, CA) in conjunction with a long femoral venous cannula to decompress the heart in lieu of the IJ drainage cannula. The Endopulmonary Vent Catheter has an appearance similar to that of a standard pulmonary artery catheter (PAC) and is placed in a similar fashion. However, because it is more flimsy, TEE or fluoroscopic guidance may be more necessary for proper positioning. It has a specialized design with multiple distal holes to allow vacuum-assisted venting of the pulmonary artery at approximately 50 mL/min.[41] Its tip should ideally reside within the main pulmonary artery.[13]

The use of a single long femoral venous cannula alone, or in conjunction with the Endopulmonary Vent Catheter, is generally acceptable for MIMVS because the surgical approach to the mitral valve is via a left atriotomy. However, when the right atrium must be opened during MIMVS (ie, concomitant closure of atrial septal defect or tricuspid valve repair), bicaval cannulation and occlusion are typically used to prevent associated air entrainment with an exposed right atrium. When the SVC is occluded, continuous monitoring of right IJ pressure is important to help ensure adequate SVC drainage from a percutaneous cannula. Many clinicians monitor right IJ pressure in all MIMVS for the same reason.

Arterial Outflow and Cross-Clamping

Regardless of whether arterial outflow from the CPB circuit is achieved via percutaneous peripheral, percutaneous central, or even direct central cannulation, the anesthesiologist is usually highly involved in assisting with placement. When Seldinger techniques are used by the surgeon, confirmation of correct wire position in either the ascending or descending aorta is usually made via TEE before advancement of the arterial cannula. In addition to the various techniques used for arterial cannulation, there are also several approaches to aortic cross-clamping, aortic venting, and cardioplegia administration. The anesthesiologist's role in these is discussed here.

The Port Access system (Edwards Lifesciences, Irvine, CA) was designed to facilitate MIMVS and was introduced into clinical practice in 1997. A similar product is also produced by Estech (Danville, CA). At the cornerstone of this new technology was the development of the EndoClamp Aortic Catheter (Edwards Lifesciences), which is an endoluminal aortic balloon. The EndoClamp is placed through a side port of a Y-shaped large (21F or 24F) arterial cannula (EndoReturn Arterial Cannula) and advanced into the ascending aorta (**Fig. 8**). This maneuver requires significant TEE guidance. The EndoClamp can also be advanced into the ascending aorta percutaneously from the right axillary artery[44] or the chest wall via the transthoracic Endo-Direct cannula. TEE examination should confirm that the size of the ascending aorta is appropriate. An ascending aorta greater than 3.5 cm in diameter may limit endo-occlusion, whereas a small-diameter aorta may increase the chance of catheter migration on balloon inflation as well as the risk of aortic injury.

The echocardiographer's role does not end with cannula placement. After the institution of CPB, the ascending aorta must be visualized on TEE (ascending aortic long-axis view) during inflation of the EndoClamp to confirm that it remains in place (**Fig. 9**). The flow of cardioplegia should also be noted using color flow Doppler. Proper position above the aortic root is essential to allow for adequate cardioprotection. At the same time, prevention of distal migration avoids malperfusion of the head vessels (**Fig. 10**). Motion of the balloon is a delicate balance between proximal flow from either residual cardiac contraction or infusion of antegrade cardioplegia versus distal flow from the aortic cannula.

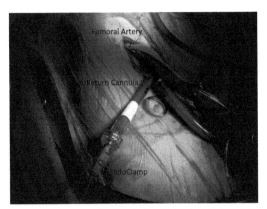

Fig. 8. EndoClamp aortic catheter advanced through the Y-shaped EndoReturn arterial cannula, which was placed into the right femoral artery.

Balloon migration may continue to occur throughout the procedure after initial inflation, but once the left atrium is opened, TEE visualization of the ascending aorta for TEE-guided balloon adjustment is limited by air interposition. The effects of air can be mitigated by filling the atrium with blood or another fluid when necessary. Monitoring for distal balloon migration can be achieved by continuously and simultaneously observing bilateral upper extremity arterial pressure (lower extremity pressure monitoring can be used in lieu of a left upper extremity arterial catheter). A precipitous, isolated drop in right upper extremity pressure indicates distal migration and occlusion of the innominate artery by the balloon, which is estimated to occur in 7% of cases.[33] Some centers use a single right-arm arterial catheter and watch for otherwise unexplained drops in blood pressure as a sign of migration. Proximal migration of the balloon may limit aortic occlusion, inhibit adequate myocardial protection, and possibly injure the aortic valve.

Many surgeons who use MIMVS have chosen to forgo Port Access. Use of the angled Chitwood Transthoracic Aortic Cross Clamp (Scanlan International Inc, Minneapolis, MN), which is inserted percutaneously and guided toward the ascending aorta under direct or endoscopic vision, is an alternative (**Figs. 11** and **12**). Use of this technique over Port Access for aortic cross-clamping is based on several factors, not the least of which are decreases in infrastructure demands and costs,[45] as well as shorter operative and cross-clamp times.[45] A disadvantage is the need to place a separate

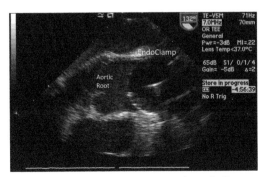

Fig. 9. Mid-esophageal aortic valve long-axis view with EndoClamp aortic catheter seen inflated in the ascending aorta just distal to the aortic root.

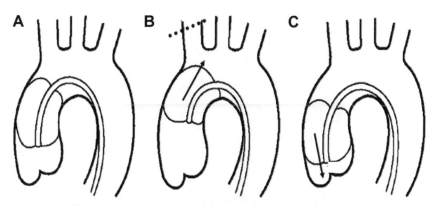

Fig. 10. (*A*) Well-positioned EndoClamp in the ascending aorta. (*B*) Distal migration (Shown by the *arrow*) of the EndoClamp and potentially obstructing flow to the innominate artery. (*C*) Proximal migration (shown by the *arrow*) of the EndoClamp, which may prevent adequate aortic occlusion or cardioplegia. (*Adapted from* Kottenberg-Assenmacher E, Kamler M, Peters J. Minimally invasive endoscopic port-access intracardiac surgery with one lung ventilation: impact on gas exchange and anesthesia resources. Anesthesia 2007;62:235; with permission.)

aortic root vent percutaneously onto the ascending aorta for cardiac venting and antegrade cardioplegia administration, as it can be surgically challenging to make repairs if needed after vent removal, particularly when more endoscopic surgical techniques are used. There is some circumstantial evidence that compared with the EndoClamp, use of an aortic root vent may provide more effective air venting of the aorta.[15,46,47]

Severe complications associated with vascular access and retrograde arterial perfusion have been reported by Mohr and colleagues[46] with Port Access surgery. By avoiding the endo-balloon with use of the transthoracic clamp, the larger Endo-Return arterial cannula becomes unnecessary and a smaller arterial perfusion cannula may be used. However, because this does not necessarily obviate peripheral arterial cannulation, peripheral vascular complications may still occur without the Port Access system, as can proximal embolization of descending aortic atheroma when retrograde

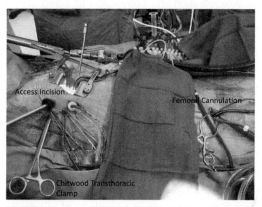

Fig. 11. Surgical field with access incision via small right anterior thoracotomy. The Chitwood clamp is placed percutaneously via an additional incision lateral to the access incision and is directed toward the ascending aorta under direct vision. The right femoral artery and vein are cannulated.

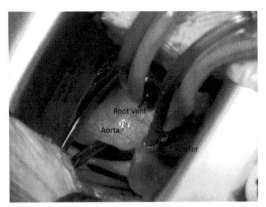

Fig. 12. Chitwood clamp seen via direct vision in surgical field during external occlusion of the ascending aorta. The aortic root vent is placed directly through the access incision and is proximal to the clamp in the aorta. The coronary sinus (CS) cannula is also seen passing through the access incision.

arterial flow is used. New York University Hospital describes an institutional drop in neurologic events from 4.7% to 1.2% during MIMVS, which they attribute to the avoidance of peripheral aortic cannulation.[48] Murphy and colleagues[23] report the use of a screening protocol to identify and avoid femoral cannulation in patients considered at higher risk for retrograde embolization.

Regardless of approach, as already discussed, during aortic cannulation with Seldinger technique, the wire should be clearly observed on TEE to be intraluminal in the aorta prior. The more wire and catheter manipulation occurs, the greater the potential for endothelial injury, which can predispose to dissection once CPB flow is initiated, although this is not the only cause of dissection. Although an elevation of arterial outflow-line pressure on the CPB circuit is often the first sign, early evaluation of the descending aorta after the initiation of retrograde CPB on TEE should be made to rule out dissection. Unlike with standard direct surgical cannulation, retrograde aortic dissection may not be apparent in the surgical field until it extends up to the ascending aorta. Early recognition and conversion to antegrade central arterial flow may limit the damage of this potentially devastating complication.

Despite an increased concern for iatrogenic dissection with Port Access, the most recent meta-analysis available found an extremely low dissection rate during MIMVS (8 in 5117 patients or 0.2%).[15] The report did not differentiate the dissection rate between Port Access and the use of a transthoracic clamp, even though this distinction was made for other outcomes and each group was equally represented in the cohort. When evaluating studies comparing the overall safety of the 2 approaches, it is important to consider the more significant learning curve associated with Port Access surgery. The steepness of the curve was exemplified by the findings of the first Port Access International Registry, in which the incidence of iatrogenic aortic dissection was 1.3% in the first half of the study followed by a decrease to 0.2% in the second half.[49]

Other alternatives to aortic cross-clamping exist, the simplest of which involves operating on a beating heart. The obvious advantage of this method is that it allows coronary flow to remain mostly uninterrupted. Disadvantages of this approach include a more disturbed surgical field and the possibility of systemic air embolization. Typically the empty or underfilled ventricle cannot generate enough pressure to open the aortic valve while on CPB. However, it remains important for the anesthesia and surgical team to monitor for this possibility. The occurrence of aortic valve opening can be signified by the appearance of "override" on the arterial waveform, or the valve can be visualized on IOTEE. The aortic vent should also be directly observed for the appearance of any air entrainment. These concerns can be limited by inducing ventricular fibrillation to create ventricular standstill. Fibrillation can be achieved either by a fibrillator applied directly to the heart or through the use of a pacing PAC.[50]

Cardioplegia

As discussed earlier, antegrade cardioplegia can be delivered via the EndoClamp or direct aortic root cannulation. Direct retrograde coronary sinus cannulation during MIMVS is more challenging but by adjusting the metal stylet to compensate for the more lateral surgical position, direct coronary sinus cannulation can be achieved through an access incision. With this approach, TEE guidance may be important. An additional option is the use of a percutaneous coronary sinus catheter.[51,52] The EndoPledge Coronary Sinus Catheter (Edwards Lifesciences) is advanced through an 11F introducer sheath, typically via the right IJ vein. The EndoPledge is a long triple-lumen catheter with a balloon on the end that allows for occlusion of the coronary sinus, measurement of distal pressure, and the infusion of cardioplegia. The obvious advantage of this approach is the ability to administer retrograde protection while remaining completely endoscopic.

EndoPledge cannulation can be guided by TEE, fluoroscopy, or both. TEE is most commonly used to help direct the cannula into the coronary sinus ostia (**Figs. 13 and 14**). Once in the coronary sinus, TEE is limited in its ability to exactly define the position of the tip, and provides limited functional information. The generation of a "ventricularized" distal pressure waveform during inflation of the occlusion balloon suggests adequate sinus occlusion. The cannula should be advanced until this ventricularized waveform is seen with balloon inflation. The cannula is deemed to be inserted too far if ventricularization occurs with less than 0.75 to 1 mL of balloon inflation and not far enough if more than 1 mL is required for occlusion.

Fluoroscopy can be used to better visualize the cannula in the coronary sinus. The cannula should be seen moving synchronously with each ventricular contraction to confirm its presence in the sinus. The appearance of the catheter "wrapped" too far behind the heart signifies distal displacement. Obstructive venography can also be performed, using diluted radiologic contrast agents to observe opacification of the entire coronary venous system, thus ensuring that the cannula is not misdirected

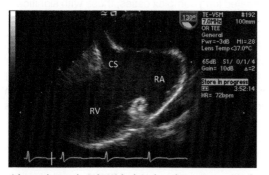

Fig. 13. Modified mid-esophageal right-sided 2-chamber view with focus on ostia of the coronary sinus. CS, coronary sinus; RA, right atrium; RV, right ventricle.

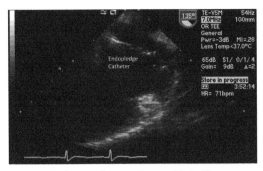

Fig. 14. EndoPledge coronary sinus catheter advanced into the coronary sinus.

into a cardiac vein or obstructing a major coronary vein. Thorough steps to ensure proper placement are important as, owing to its design, a careful balance exists between having the catheter distal enough in the sinus to prevent dislodgment and proximal enough to ensure adequate cardioplegia delivery to all myocardial segments. There is a single report suggesting that adequate cardioplegia distribution can occur irrespective of catheter depth because of the widespread network of collaterals within the cardiac venous system.[53]

Though conceptually appealing, the use of the EndoPledge cannula has not been widely adopted with MIMVS. Concerns about coronary sinus perforation risk, increased complexity of placement, and a high rate of dislodgment have limited its penetration. The overall incidence of coronary sinus disruption is unknown, but anecdotal reports clearly exist. Perforations of both the right atria and ventricle have also been reported.[54] A difficult and prolonged attempt at placement presumably increases the likelihood of trauma, particularly when there is difficulty with advancement after the coronary sinus ostia has been engaged.[55] In a recent retrospective study of 95 EndoPledge catheter insertions using a combined TEE and fluoroscopic approach with venography, the mean time for proper placement was 16.1 minutes (±14.1 minutes).[55] Successful positioning was achieved 87.5% of the time. Of the 13 failures, 9 were dislodged during surgery and not related to an inability to place the cannula.

Perhaps the most important reason for avoidance of the EndoPledge cannula is that many surgeons do not believe that retrograde cardioplegia is necessary for cardiac protection when adequate antegrade cardioplegia can be delivered; this has been demonstrated in several case series.[55–58] Suggested indications for retrograde cardioplegia include anticipated long complex cases; those with significant ventricular hypertrophy; patients with a history of prior coronary artery bypass grafting (CABG), particularly those with patent mammary grafts; and significant aortic insufficiency. However, none of these indications have been well established. Meyer and colleagues[59] reported successful results in 45 patients with previous CABG who underwent reoperative MIMVS without the use of retrograde cardioplegia. Even in the setting of moderate aortic insufficiency, adequate antegrade protection can still be achieved. However, increased vigilance regarding myocardial protection is required in this setting.

MIMVS AND PREVIOUS CARDIAC SURGERY

Previous cardiac surgery does not preclude MIMVS, and in fact MIMVS may provide some significant advantages in these patients. The right lateral thoracotomy incision limits exposure to chest-wall adhesions from previous sternotomy as well as most previous coronary bypass grafts. Multiple studies have shown an at least equal if not better mortality with redo MIMVS in comparison with redo sternotomy mitral valve surgery.[60–62] In addition, a decreased infection rate, transfusion requirement, and length of hospital stay were also consistently shown in these studies. However, Cleveland Clinic reported a higher incidence of repair failure as well as stroke in 80 MIMVS patients after previous sternotomy compared with a similar group of 2444 reoperative mitral repair sternotomies. Mortality was similar, however, at 6.7% and 6.3%.[63] Chitwood and colleagues[27] reported a 3% 30-day mortality in 167 previous sternotomy MIMVS patients over 15 years (19 robotically). During the last 5 years examined, their 30-day mortality dropped to 0% in 85 patients with a low stroke rate. They did note a higher than expected incidence of pneumonia, with 28% isolated to the right lung.

Management of patients with patent left internal mammary (LIMA) coronary bypass grafts requires some mention, although in practice it differs little from patients undergoing sternotomy. The ability to clamp the LIMA and prevent myocardial warming is limited, thus management strategies revolve around more aggressive systemic cooling or "beating-heart" surgical strategies.[27,64] The need for retrograde cardioplegia in patients with a patent LIMA graft is suggested by some but is not necessarily required, as discussed earlier.

The presence of anterior chest-wall adhesions from previous sternotomy may limit exposure to the right ventricle, preventing the ability to apply temporary epicardial pacing wires, and this may be particularly true when performing true endoscopic surgery. The preoperative placement of a pacing PAC can alleviate this problem. Similarly, the combination of previous cardiac surgery and endoscopic MIMVS may also create difficulties in achieving caval occlusion if the right side of the heart must be entered. The placement of an EndoReturn arterial cannula in the right IJ and of another interpositioned EndoReturn cannula distal to the femoral venous return cannula can allow for occlusion balloons to be placed into each respective cava. On opening of the right atrium, these balloons can be inflated percutaneously under direct vision to proximally occlude each cava while still draining the body. Placement of endoscopic bulldog clips on each cava during robotic MIMVS has also been reported.[65]

CARDIOPULMONARY BYPASS MANAGEMENT

Although most aspects of the conduct of CPB are unchanged relative to conventional mitral surgery, there are some additional considerations during MIMVS. Limitations to flow may occur through smaller peripheral arterial cannulas or when the EndoClamp limits the effective cannula orifice. An additional arterial cannula may need to be placed and added to the circuit if high arterial-line resistance occurs when attempting to achieve appropriate CPB flow. Similarly, even with assisted venous drainage, total heart decompression may not occur during normal systemic flows, requiring a permissive low-flow state.

Systemic blood pressure may also need to be lowered to prevent proximal migration of the balloon when the EndoClamp is used. It may also be more difficult to achieve a bloodless surgical field when the systemic blood pressure is elevated. Although these alterations in systemic flow and blood pressure are often out of the anesthesiologist's control, it is important to remain informed and involved in the management process. Normothermic or even tepid bypass may not be appropriate when low CPB flow is required.

MITRAL VALVE EXPOSURE AND REPAIR

Exposure and visualization of the mitral valve during robotic surgery varies from the standard sternotomy approach. Specialized left atrial retractors have been developed to expose the mitral valve. Placing the mitral valve repair ring annuloplasty sutures first and retracting under tension enhances exposure of the mitral valve. This tactic is often performed with the increased confidence of valve reparability provided by a detailed IOTEE. The robotic video imaging system greatly enhances field lighting and visualization of the mitral valve (see **Fig. 5**). The additional monitors in the operating room allow all members of the operative team to observe and even participate in the mitral valve repair. The immediate visual confirmation of the abnormality detected on IOTEE greatly strengthens the diagnostic skills of the anesthesiologist. Direct observation of the repair can also alert the anesthesiologist to specific concerns when evaluating the postrepair IOTEE.

SEPARATION FROM CPB AND IMMEDIATE POSTBYPASS MANAGEMENT

During separation from CPB, in principle there are no dramatic differences from open operations. However, if increased cross-clamp and CPB times occur, this may need to be factored into decision making regarding post-CPB pharmacologic, ventilatory, fluid, and blood-product management. After a period of reperfusion, preparations are made and any requirements for pacing and hemodynamic support are adjusted. If a pacing PAC is being used, adjustments in position may need to be made because once the heart fills, the wire may migrate away from the ventricular wall. The amplitude may also need to be increased if the ventricular pacing threshold has increased. Initial ventilation of both lungs should be instituted when possible. Attempts to de-air the heart are made in the usual fashion. The ability to dislodge retained left atrial air is typically not hampered by the incision, but exposure to the left ventricular apex may be.

With less surgical access to the heart and great vessels, the anesthesiologist plays an even greater role in monitoring all aspects of cardiac function. For example, with sternotomy, but not with MIMVS, the right ventricle can be observed in the surgical field for signs of dysfunction. As replacement of the components of CPB after their initial removal in MIMVS can be time consuming and technically involved, early and accurate TEE diagnoses before decannulation are important. Given the close proximity of the noncoronary leaflet of the aortic valve to the anterior mitral valve annulus, a directed TEE examination of the aortic valve after CPB is also important. Similarly, the proximity of the circumflex coronary artery to the posterior and lateral annulus requires assessment of ventricular wall motion. For the same reason, ensuring adequate de-airing is also important, as emergent reinstitution of CPB could be delayed if coronary air embolism leads to significant cardiac dysfunction after surgical decannulation.

During the initiation of surgical chest closure, OLV is typically needed. Superimposing this additional strain on the right ventricle in patients with preexisting dysfunction or residual myocardial stunning may lead to decompensation. Achieving control of surgical bleeding may prolong this period and further complicate hemodynamic management. Measures such as positive end-expiratory pressure to the ventilated lung or intermittent lung inflation may be necessary. It may be helpful to temporarily ventilate the deflated right lung in isolation on resolution of normal ventilation in order to fully reexpand it without having to generate excessive positive pressure.

PREPARING FOR TRANSFER AND THE INTENSIVE CARE UNIT

At the conclusion of surgery there are several preparations the anesthesia team must make before transport that are not usually necessary following sternotomy. First, if a double-lumen endotracheal tube has been used, it should be switched to a single-lumen tube, unless immediate extubation is planned or oropharyngeal swelling or trauma poses a significant risk for loss of airway during tube exchange. The use of an airway-exchange catheter may be helpful. In patients with significant upper body swelling or airway trauma, the double-lumen tube may need to be left in place. If a second arterial catheter or an IJ return venous catheter was used, they should be removed at the conclusion of surgery. Some technique to achieve hemostasis must be employed on removal of the IJ return catheter. A boxed purse-string or a U-stitch closure is commonly used. If cosmesis is a significant concern, after hemostasis is achieved, the closure stitch can be removed and a subcuticular closure made.

POSTOPERATIVE PAIN MANAGEMENT

There are numerous options available for pain control after MIMVS beyond the traditional use of parenteral opioids. The use of these adjunctive measures is widespread. Excitement for their use in MIMVS is enhanced by the desire for and possibility of a quicker extubation in many of these patients. Successful fast-track anesthesia has been well described in the setting of MIMVS.[66] Although many of the patients for MIMVS are excellent candidates for early extubation, caution must still be exercised because of the potential occurrence of significant postoperative chest-wall bleeding given the multiple chest-wall puncture sites.

The simplest adjunctive pain-management technique involves the use of limited intercostal injections of local anesthetic during surgical closure. The desire for a longer duration of local anesthesia has led many to use continuous infusions via temporary catheters and specialized pumps. Catheters may simply be left under the subcutaneous tissue before closure and then tunneled out through the skin.[67,68] An extrapleural intercostal catheter can also be placed under direct vision, and may also provide improvements in pain control and, possibly, pulmonary function.[69] The inability to adequately strip the parietal pleura posteriorly beyond the incision may limit optimal positioning of the catheter tip. Because of the high vascularity of the chest-wall cavity, caution must be exercised when injecting local anesthetics in this region because the possibility for systemic toxicity is quite real.

Whereas thoracic epidural use has been reported during MIDCAB surgery, both for postoperative pain and as the anesthetic technique,[70–73] epidural anesthesia has rarely been used with MIMVS. Paramount among the concerns with epidural catheters is the risk of epidural hematoma formation and consequent spinal cord injury. Additional concerns relate to bilateral sympathectomy leading to hypotension. Finally, the successful use of unilateral continuous paravertebral blocks has been described with MIMVS for postoperative pain control. Investigators have shown a high level of safety, with equally effective pain control in comparison with epidural anesthesia.[72,74] Advantages of a paravertebral block over a thoracic epidural include a higher safety margin for neurologic complications and avoidance of bilateral sympathectomy.

SUMMARY

Traditional mitral valve surgery is rapidly being supplanted as the primary surgical approach to the mitral valve by innovative minimally invasive techniques. Patients are experiencing a decrease in pain and faster recoveries without sacrificing the durability of their surgical repair. Most importantly, these results can be achieved with an equivalent morbidity and mortality in comparison with standard mitral valve surgery. At the forefront of innovation is the use of robotically assisted surgery. At present, the majority of robotic MIMVS cases are performed at only a small number of centers.[13] Although definitive advantages of robotic surgery over non–robotic-assisted MIMVS have yet to be shown, expansion of robotic MIMVS seems inevitable, fueled by continued technological advancements and patient demands. Despite the impressive results reported in the literature with robotic-assisted MIMVS, it is important to acknowledge that successful outcomes require a significant investment in training and experience as well as an increase in the cost of infrastructure and time.

REFERENCES

1. Coddens J, Deloof T, Hendrickx J, et al. Transesophageal echocardiography for port-access surgery. J Cardiothorac Vasc Anesth 1999;13(5):614–22.
2. Siegel LC, St Goar FG, Stevens JH, et al. Monitoring considerations for port-access cardiac surgery. Circulation 1997;96(2):562–8.
3. Arom KV, Emery RW. Minimally invasive mitral operations. Ann Thorac Surg 1997; 63(4):1219–20.
4. Chitwood WR Jr, Wixon CL, Elbeery JR, et al. Video-assisted minimally invasive mitral valve surgery. J Thorac Cardiovasc Surg 1997;114(5):773–80 [discussion: 780–2].
5. Chitwood WR Jr, Elbeery JR, Moran JF. Minimally invasive mitral valve repair using transthoracic aortic occlusion. Ann Thorac Surg 1997;63(5):1477–9.
6. Mohr FW, Falk V, Diegeler A, et al. Minimally invasive Port-Access mitral valve surgery. J Thorac Cardiovasc Surg 1998;115(3):567–74 [discussion: 574–6].
7. Navia JL, Cosgrove DM 3rd. Minimally invasive mitral valve operations. Ann Thorac Surg 1996;62(5):1542–4.
8. Schwartz DS, Ribakove GH, Grossi EA, et al. Minimally invasive cardiopulmonary bypass with cardioplegic arrest: a closed chest technique with equivalent myocardial protection. J Thorac Cardiovasc Surg 1996;111(3):556–66.
9. Glower DD, Siegel LC, Frischmeyer KJ, et al. Predictors of outcome in a multi-center port-access valve registry. Ann Thorac Surg 2000;70(3):1054–9.
10. Gammie JS, Zhao Y, Peterson ED, et al. J. Maxwell Chamberlain Memorial Paper for adult cardiac surgery. Less-invasive mitral valve operations: trends and outcomes from the Society of Thoracic Surgeons Adult Cardiac Surgery Database. Ann Thorac Surg 2010;90(5):1401–8, 1410.e1; [discussion: 1408–10].
11. Carpentier A, Loulmet D, Aupecle B, et al. Computer assisted open heart surgery. First case operated on with success. C R Acad Sci III 1998;321(5):437–42 [in French].
12. Chitwood WR Jr, Nifong LW, Elbeery JE, et al. Robotic mitral valve repair: trapezoidal resection and prosthetic annuloplasty with the Da Vinci Surgical System. J Thorac Cardiovasc Surg 2000;120(6):1171–2.
13. Rehfeldt KH, Mauermann WJ, Burkhart HM, et al. Robot-assisted mitral valve repair. J Cardiothorac Vasc Anesth 2011;25(4):721–30.
14. Anderson CA, Kypson AP, Chitwood WR Jr. Robotic mitral surgery: current and future roles. Curr Opin Cardiol 2008;23(2):117–20.
15. Cheng DC, Martin J, Avtar L, et al. Minimally invasive versus conventional open mitral valve surgery: a meta-analysis and systematic review. Innovations 2011; 6(2):84–103.

16. Smith JM, Stein H, Engel AM, et al. Totally endoscopic mitral valve repair using a robotic-controlled atrial retractor. Ann Thorac Surg 2007;84(2):633–7.
17. Atluri P, Woo YJ. Minimally invasive robotic mitral valve surgery. Expert Rev Med Devices 2011;8(1):115–20.
18. Modi P, Hassan A, Chitwood WR Jr. Minimally invasive mitral valve surgery: a systematic review and meta-analysis. Eur J Cardiothorac Surg 2008;34(5): 943–52.
19. Yamada T, Ochiai R, Takeda J, et al. Comparison of early postoperative quality of life in minimally invasive versus conventional valve surgery. J Anesth 2003;17(3): 171–6.
20. Walther T, Falk V, Metz S, et al. Pain and quality of life after minimally invasive versus conventional cardiac surgery. Ann Thorac Surg 1999;67(6):1643–7.
21. Vleissis AA, Bolling SF. Mini-reoperative mitral valve surgery. J Card Surg 1998; 13(6):468–70.
22. Suri RM, Antiel RM, Burkhart HM, et al. Quality of life after early mitral valve repair using conventional and robotic approaches. Ann Thorac Surg 2012;93(3):761–9.
23. Murphy DA, Miller JS, Langford, et al. Endoscopic robotic mitral valve surgery. J Thorac Cardiovasc Surg 2006;132(4):776–81.
24. Suri RM, Schaff HV, Dearani JA, et al. Survival advantage and improved durability of mitral repair for leaflet prolapse subsets in the current era. Ann Thorac Surg 2006;82(3):819–26.
25. Galloway AC, Schwartz CF, Ribakove GH, et al. A decade of minimally invasive mitral repair: long-term outcomes. Ann Thorac Surg 2009;88(4):1180–4.
26. Iribarne A, Karpenko A, Russo MJ, et al. Eight-year experience with minimally invasive cardiothoracic surgery. World J Surg 2010;34(4):611–5.
27. Arcidi JM Jr, Rodriguez E, Elbeery JR, et al. Fifteen-year experience with minimally invasive approach for reoperations involving the mitral valve. J Thorac Cardiovasc Surg 2012;143(5):1062–8.
28. Charland PJ, Robbins T, Rodriguez E, et al. Learning curve analysis of mitral valve repair using telemanipulative technology. J Thorac Cardiovasc Surg 2011;142(2):404–10.
29. Cheng W, Fontana GP, De Robertis MA, et al. Is robotic mitral valve repair a reproducible approach? J Thorac Cardiovasc Surg 2010;139(3):628–33.
30. Chitwood WR Jr, Rodriguez E, Chu MW, et al. Robotic mitral valve repairs in 300 patients: a single-center experience. J Thorac Cardiovasc Surg 2008;136(2):436–41.
31. Reich DL, Galati M. An American view. American and European anesthesia reimbursement policies' effects on the adoption of novel techniques. J Cardiothorac Vasc Anesth 2009;23(2):140–1.
32. Moodley S, Schoenhagen P, Gillinov AM, et al. Preoperative multidetector computed tomography angiography for planning of minimally invasive robotic mitral valve surgery: impact on decision making. J Thorac Cardiovasc Surg 2012. [Epub ahead of print].
33. Kottenberg-Assenmacher E, Kamler M, Peters J. Minimally invasive endoscopic port-access intracardiac surgery with one lung ventilation: impact on gas exchange and anaesthesia resources. Anaesthesia 2007;62(3):231–8.
34. Eltzschig HK, Rossenberger P, Loffler M, et al. Impact of intraoperative transesophageal echocardiography on surgical decisions in 12,566 patients undergoing cardiac surgery. Ann Thorac Surg 2008;85(3):845–52.
35. Minhaj M, Patel K, Muzic D, et al. The effect of routine intraoperative transesophageal echocardiography on surgical management. J Cardiothorac Vasc Anesth 2007;21(6):800–4.

36. Quigley RL. The role of echocardiography in mitral valve dysfunction after repair. Minerva Cardioangiol 2007;55(2):239–46.
37. Freeman WK, Schaff HV, Khandheria BK, et al. Intraoperative evaluation of mitral valve regurgitation and repair by transesophageal echocardiography: incidence and significance of systolic anterior motion. J Am Coll Cardiol 1992;20(3):599–609.
38. Wang Y, Gao CQ, Wang JL, et al. The role of intraoperative transesophageal echocardiography in robotic mitral valve repair. Echocardiography 2011;28(1): 85–91.
39. Applebaum RM, Cutler WM, Bhardwaj SB, et al. Utility of transesophageal echocardiography during port-access minimally invasive cardiac surgery. Am J Cardiol 1998;82(2):183–8.
40. Toomasian JM, McCarthy JP. Total extrathoracic cardiopulmonary support with kinetic assisted venous drainage: experience in 50 patients. Perfusion 1998; 13(2):137–43.
41. Chauhan S, Sukesan S. Anesthesia for robotic cardiac surgery: an amalgam of technology and skill. Ann Card Anaesth 2010;13(2):169–75.
42. Woo YJ. Minimally invasive valve surgery. Surg Clin North Am 2009;89(4): 923–49, x.
43. Chaney MA, Minhaj MM, Patel K, et al. Transoesophageal echocardiography and central line insertion. Ann Card Anaesth 2007;10(2):127–31.
44. Farivar RS, Lowy S, Fernandez J. Axillary cannulation for endo-occlusion and antegrade flow during complex reoperative mitral valve surgery. J Thorac Cardiovasc Surg 2011;142(2):462–4.
45. Reichenspurner H, Detter C, Deuse T, et al. Video and robotic-assisted minimally invasive mitral valve surgery: a comparison of the Port-Access and transthoracic clamp techniques. Ann Thorac Surg 2005;79(2):485–90 [discussion: 490–1].
46. Mohr FW, Onnasch JF, Falk V, et al. The evolution of minimally invasive valve surgery—2 year experience. Eur J Cardiothorac Surg 1999;15(3):233–8 [discussion: 238–9].
47. Onnasch JF, Schneider F, Falk V, et al. Five years of less invasive mitral valve surgery: from experimental to routine approach. Heart Surg Forum 2002;5(2): 132–5.
48. Grossi EA, Loulmet DF, Schwartz CF, et al. Evolution of operative techniques and perfusion strategies for minimally invasive mitral valve repair. J Thorac Cardiovasc Surg 2012;143(4 Suppl):S68–70.
49. Galloway AC, Shemin RJ, Glower DD, et al. First report of the Port Access International Registry. Ann Thorac Surg 1999;67(1):51–6 [discussion: 57–8].
50. Levin R, Leacche M, Petracek MR, et al. Extending the use of the pacing pulmonary artery catheter for safe minimally invasive cardiac surgery. J Cardiothorac Vasc Anesth 2010;24(4):568–73.
51. Siegel LC. Coronary sinus catheterization for minimally invasive cardiac surgery. Anesthesiology 1999;90(4):1232–3.
52. Plotkin IM, Collard CD, Aranki SF, et al. Percutaneous coronary sinus cannulation guided by transesophageal echocardiography. Ann Thorac Surg 1998;66(6): 2085–7.
53. Clements F, Wright SJ, de Bruijn N. Coronary sinus catheterization made easy for Port-Access minimally invasive cardiac surgery. J Cardiothorac Vasc Anesth 1998;12(1):96–101.
54. Abramson DC, Giannoti AG. Perforation of the right ventricle with a coronary sinus catheter during preparation for minimally invasive cardiac surgery. Anesthesiology 1998;89(2):519–21.

55. Lebon JS, Coutre P, Rochon AG, et al. The endovascular coronary sinus catheter in minimally invasive mitral and tricuspid valve surgery: a case series. J Cardiothorac Vasc Anesth 2010;24(5):746–51.

56. Casselman FP, Van Slycke S, Dom H, et al. Endoscopic mitral valve repair: feasible, reproducible, and durable. J Thorac Cardiovasc Surg 2003;125(2):273–82.

57. Casselman FP, La Meir M, Jeanmart H, et al. Endoscopic mitral and tricuspid valve surgery after previous cardiac surgery. Circulation 2007;116(11 Suppl): I270–5.

58. Vanermen H, Farhart F, Wellens F, et al. Minimally invasive video-assisted mitral valve surgery: from Port-Access towards a totally endoscopic procedure. J Card Surg 2000;15(1):51–60.

59. Meyer SR, Szeto WY, Augoustides JG, et al. Reoperative mitral valve surgery by the port access minithoracotomy approach is safe and effective. Ann Thorac Surg 2009;87(5):1426–30.

60. Sharony R, Grossi EA, Saunders PC, et al. Minimally invasive reoperative isolated valve surgery: early and mid-term results. J Card Surg 2006;21(3):240–4.

61. Bolotin G, Kypson AP, Reade CC, et al. Should a video-assisted mini-thoracotomy be the approach of choice for reoperative mitral valve surgery? J Heart Valve Dis 2004;13(2):155–8 [discussion: 158].

62. Burfeind WR, Glower DD, Davis RD, et al. Mitral surgery after prior cardiac operation: port-access versus sternotomy or thoracotomy. Ann Thorac Surg 2002; 74(4):S1323–5.

63. Svensson LG, Gillinov AM, Blackstone EH, et al. Does right thoracotomy increase the risk of mitral valve reoperation? J Thorac Cardiovasc Surg 2007;134(3):677–82.

64. Umakanthan R, Petracek MR, Leacche M, et al. Minimally invasive right lateral thoracotomy without aortic cross-clamping: an attractive alternative to repeat sternotomy for reoperative mitral valve surgery. J Heart Valve Dis 2010;19(2): 236–43.

65. Gullu AU, Senay S, Kocyigit M, et al. A simple method for occlusion of both venae cavae in total cardiopulmonary bypass for robotic surgery. Interact Cardiovasc Thorac Surg 2012;14(2):138–9.

66. Sostaric M, Gersak B, Novak-Jankovic V. Early extubation and fast-track anesthetic technique for endoscopic cardiac surgery. Heart Surg Forum 2010;13(3): E190–4.

67. Sostaric M, Gersak B, Novak-Jankovic V. The analgesic efficacy of local anesthetics for the incisional administration following port access heart surgery: bupivacaine versus ropivacaine. Heart Surg Forum 2010;13(2):E96–100.

68. Sostaric M. Incisional administration of local anesthetic provides satisfactory analgesia following port access heart surgery. Heart Surg Forum 2005;8(6): E406–8.

69. Ganapathy S. Anaesthesia for minimally invasive cardiac surgery. Best Pract Res Clin Anaesthesiol 2002;16(1):63–80.

70. Anderson MB, Kwong KF, Furst AJ, et al. Thoracic epidural anesthesia for cardiac surgery via left anterior thoracotomy in the conscious patient. Heart Surg Forum 2002;5(2):105–8.

71. Aybek T, Dogan S, Neidhart G, et al. Coronary artery bypass grafting through complete sternotomy in conscious patients. Heart Surg Forum 2002;5(1):17–20 [discussion: 20–1].

72. Mehta Y, Arora D, Sharma KK, et al. Comparison of continuous thoracic epidural and paravertebral block for postoperative analgesia after robotic-assisted coronary artery bypass surgery. Ann Card Anaesth 2008;11(2):91–6.

73. Ho AM, Chung DC, Joynt GM. Neuraxial blockade and hematoma in cardiac surgery: estimating the risk of a rare adverse event that has not (yet) occurred. Chest 2000;117(2):551–5.
74. Carmona P, Llagunes J, Canovas S, et al. The role of continuous thoracic paravertebral block for fast-track anesthesia after cardiac surgery via thoracotomy. J Cardiothorac Vasc Anesth 2011;25(1):205–6.

Advances and Future Directions for Mechanical Circulatory Support

Michelle Capdeville, MD[a],*, Nicholas G. Smedira, MD[b]

KEYWORDS

- Mechanical circulatory support • Ventricular assist device • Axial flow • HeartMate II
- HeartWare

KEY POINTS

- Second-generation axial flow ventricular assist devices (VADs) have demonstrated increased durability relative to first-generation devices.
- Advantages of second-generation and third-generation VADs include fewer moving parts, smaller size, lower infection rates, and silent operation.
- With the ongoing shortage of donor organs, current generations of VADs show promise as alternatives to transplant in select patients.
- Appropriate risk assessment can assist in the proper selection of VAD candidates.
- Echocardiography is indispensable in the perioperative management of VAD patients.

INTRODUCTION

Although cardiac transplant remains the gold standard for the treatment of end-stage heart failure, limited donor organ availability and growing numbers of eligible recipients have increased the demand for alternative therapies. This is in spite of the use of older and more high-risk donor hearts, DCD (donors after circulatory determination of death) hearts,[1,2] and the use of the newer Organ Care System (TransMedics Inc, Andover, MA, USA) "heart-in-a-box" technique, in which the donor heart is perfused at the time of harvest to allow for prolongation of the ischemic time and for acceptance of organs from longer geographic distances. At present, the number of heart transplant operations performed in the United States has remained constant at approximately 2200 per year, and there has been a steady decline in the number of these procedures over the past 15 years.[3]

Following the 2001 landmark publication of the REMATCH trial (Randomized Evaluation of Mechanical Assistance for the Treatment of Congestive Heart Failure),

[a] Department of Cardiothoracic Anesthesia, Cleveland Clinic, 9500 Euclid Avenue, J4-331, Cleveland, OH 44195, USA; [b] Department of Cardiovascular Surgery, Cleveland Clinic, 9500 Euclid Avenue, J4-1, Cleveland, OH 44195, USA
* Corresponding author.
E-mail address: capdevm@ccf.org

Anesthesiology Clin 31 (2013) 321–353
http://dx.doi.org/10.1016/j.anclin.2012.12.003   anesthesiology.theclinics.com
1932-2275/13/$ – see front matter © 2013 Elsevier Inc. All rights reserved.

which compared optimal medical management to device therapy in nontransplant candidates with end-stage heart failure, it became apparent that mechanical cardiac assist would become a viable alternative in properly selected patients.[4] The results of the REMATCH trial ultimately led to United States Food and Drug Administration (FDA) approval of the HeartMate XVE (Thoratec Corporation, Pleasanton, CA, USA) for destination therapy in November 2002, followed by approval for Medicare coverage for the same indication in October 2003.

The following sections discuss 2 rotary devices in current use: the HeartMate II (Thoratec Corporation, Pleasanton, CA, USA) and the newer investigational Heart-Ware HVAD (HeartWare, Inc, Miami Lakes, FL, USA).

SECOND-GENERATION VENTRICULAR ASSIST DEVICES

The first generation implantable VADs were pulsatile volume displacement pumps. Despite being successful as bridges to transplant, they were limited by several adverse events, including infection, thromboembolism, and mechanical failure.

The introduction of axial flow pumps, which include the HeartMate II, the Jarvik 2000 Flowmaker (Jarvik Heart, Inc, New York, NY, USA), and the MicroMed DeBakey (MicroMed Cardiovascular, Inc, Houston, TX, USA), eliminated several problems encountered with earlier-generation devices. The HeartMate II has been the most successful of these pumps[5] and received FDA approval for destination therapy in January 2010. The following are its advantages over first-generation devices:

- Fewer moving parts (the rotor is the only moving part)
- Wear-resistant bearings
- Small size and weight, allowing for implantation in smaller patients
- Silent operation
- Decreased power consumption
- More comfortable
- Smaller driveline, resulting in lower infection rates
- Relatively low rate of thromboembolism
- Lack of valves and reservoir chamber, with potentially increased durability

INDICATIONS
Bridge to Transplant

VAD support as a bridge to transplant has increased significantly in recent years. Patients awaiting cardiac transplant and who are managed medically may require VAD rescue if their condition deteriorates. In a US study of 3711 United Network for Organ Sharing status 1A patients between January 2000 and December 2006, of whom 2208 were initially medically managed and 1503 were supported with a VAD as a bridge to transplant, 20% of the medically treated patients went on to require VAD support. VAD support in medically managed status 1A patients was associated with a significantly greater probability of survival and/or transplant at 3 months (66.5%–87.1% increased probability). This observation has led to the suggestion that earlier/elective institution of VAD support in medically managed status 1A patients should be considered in those at greater risk of death or with long expected waiting times for organ availability.[6] In our center, nearly 40% of patients are supported with a left ventricular assist device (LVAD) at the time of transplant.

In patients who are not candidates for cardiac transplant because of pulmonary hypertension, some studies have demonstrated a reduction in pulmonary vascular resistance (PVR) after an extended period of support with a VAD, thereby allowing eventual transplant eligibility.[7]

Bridge to Recovery

A limited number of patients with idiopathic cardiomyopathy have demonstrated myocardial recovery after VAD support and were successfully weaned from device therapy.[8–10] Although the reported incidence of myocardial recovery from reverse remodeling in LVAD-supported patients has been variably low,[11] there has been ongoing interest in trying to identify some of the mechanisms involved in this process. Unfortunately, prediction of which patients are likely to recover has been elusive because there is no reliable marker of myocardial recovery with VAD support.[12] Myocardial samples taken at the time of LVAD implant and after explant have demonstrated several changes, including increased expression and responsiveness of myocyte β-adrenergic receptors and favorable changes in the enzymes that modify the extracellular matrix, as well as calcium cycling proteins.[13]

In a single-center prospective study of 15 patients with end-stage heart failure with nonischemic cardiomyopathy receiving a pulsatile HeartMate I (Thoratec Corporation, Pleasanton, California, USA) LVAD, pharmacologic interventions (lisinopril, carvedilol, spironolactone, and losartan) were initiated during device support with the goal of reversing pathologic hypertrophy, initiating reverse remodeling, and normalizing cellular metabolic function.[14] Echocardiography was used to determine whether maximal reverse remodeling had occurred, as evidenced by measurements of left ventricular (LV) dimensions with the pump turned off. At this point, the β_2-adrenergic agonist clenbuterol was administered. This protocol allowed for pump removal in approximately two-thirds of patients, with lasting recovery and favorable quality of life.[15] A similar study was conducted by the same investigators in 20 patients who received an axial flow LVAD for nonischemic cardiomyopathy.[16] The investigators also demonstrated reversal of end-stage heart failure in 12 of these patients, of whom 10 were alive and well at follow-up. Experimentally, clenbuterol has been shown to induce physiologic myocardial hypertrophy in several models of heart failure.[17,18]

The Harefield Recovery Study (HARP) is a multicenter trial that is currently underway in the United States and is examining whether patients with nonischemic cardiomyopathy on LVAD support can recover sufficient myocardial function to allow for pump explantation using clenbuterol.

Bridge to Decision

Patients with multisystem organ failure and refractory acute cardiogenic shock who undergo permanent LVAD implantation tend to have worse outcomes than patients who have been optimized before implant.[19] In many of these patients, neurologic status may be in question. Placement of an expensive long-term or permanent device may not be cost-effective. In these situations, placement of a short-term device, such as the Impella Recover (ABIOMED Inc, Danvers, MA, USA),[20] TandemHeart (Cardiac Assist Inc, Pittsburgh, PA, USA),[21] or extracorporeal membrane oxygenation,[22] can stabilize the patient clinically and allow one a greater window of time to decide on the more appropriate course of action, and at a lower cost.

When 1-year survival was assessed in 280 destination therapy HeartMate XVE LVAD patients who were divided into low-, medium-, high-, and very high risk groups based on a composite risk score, the higher-risk groups had significantly worse survival outcomes (81%, 62%, 28%, and 11%, respectively).[19] This led to the recommendation that very-high-risk patients be bridged to decision with a short-term device.

Destination Therapy

Following the favorable results of the REMATCH trial and with the ongoing shortage of donor hearts, destination therapy is becoming a viable option for a large number of patients with end-stage heart failure. The REMATCH trial set the stage for the future of destination therapy. In this study, 1-year survival was 52% in the LVAD group compared with 25% in the medically treated group, and 2-year survival was 28% in the LVAD group compared with 8% in medically managed patients.[4] LVAD patients who were recruited in the second half of the study had significantly better survival than patients recruited in the earlier study period, likely because of improved experience and management, as well as device modifications.[23]

The INTrEPID study (Investigation of Nontransplant-Eligible Patients who are Inotrope Dependent), which was a US-Canadian destination therapy trial that compared patients receiving the Novacor LVAS (World Heart Corporation, Oakland, CA, USA) to optimal medical management, showed 6-month survival rates of 46% and 22% (P = .03), respectively, and 12-month survival rates of 27% and 11% (P = .02). There was, however, a significant rate of neurologic events in the VAD cohort (62%) compared with medically managed patients (11%).[24]

CONTRAINDICATIONS

With the increasing experience and success of destination therapy, many of the contraindications that were once considered absolute are now relative. The contraindications to VAD implantation are outlined in **Table 1**.

RISK ASSESSMENT

Operative mortality is greatly influenced by severity of functional impairment, end-organ dysfunction, nutritional status, and global markers of cardiac dysfunction (low pulmonary artery pressures (PAP) and elevated levels of liver enzymes from hepatic congestion).[19] Risk assessment is an important tool in the appropriate selection of candidates for VAD therapy and enables clinicians to provide patients and families with realistic expectations, particularly with regard to decisions about destination therapy.

INTERMACS

INTERMACS, the Interagency Registry for Mechanical Assisted Circulatory Support, is an elective registry that follows-up patients with long-term FDA-approved mechanical

Table 1
Contraindications to VAD implantation

Relative	Absolute
Mechanical AVR	Irreversible end-organ damage
Active malignancy	Poor neurologic status
Morbid obesity	Ongoing coagulopathy
—	Sepsis
—	Social issues
—	Substance abuse
—	Noncompliance

Abbreviation: AVR, aortic valve replacement.

circulatory support devices in the United States, and has identified patient profiles and defined appropriate timelines for initiating VAD support.[25–27] Using data from the INTERMACS registry[28] patients have been risk stratified into 7 categories (**Table 2**) based on their condition at presentation for VAD implantation.

Data from INTERMACS has shown that preimplantation condition has a significant impact on patient survival and highlights the importance of early referral before cardiogenic shock and irreversible end-organ damage occur.[29] Patients in the higher-risk categories have been shown to have increased short-term morbidity and mortality, whereas data for outcomes of patients in INTERMACS levels 4 to 7 are still lacking.

LIETZ-MILLER RISK SCORE

Surgical risk has been estimated in pulsatile pumps using the Lietz-Miller Destination Therapy Risk Score (DTRS), which uses a point system assigned to clinical and laboratory variables, and bases mortality risk after VAD implantation on point totals. Patients with the highest point scores were shown to have estimated 1-year survival rates of only 11% post-LVAD implant, highlighting the importance of proper patient selection to maintain acceptable outcomes.[19] Significant prognosticators for in-hospital mortality included hematologic abnormalities, poor nutritional status, markers of end-organ dysfunction and right ventricular (RV) dysfunction, and lack of inotropic support.

When the DTRS was studied in patients receiving a continuous flow LVAD, the score was able to discriminate between patients with high and low 3-month in-hospital mortality but failed to discriminate between low- and medium-risk groups.[30] In bridge-to-transplant patients, the DTRS was a poor predictor of 2-year mortality, whereas in destination therapy patients, the score was able to stratify outcomes over 2 years but was unable to distinguish patients with a futile outcome.

Table 2 INTERMACS risk stratification			
Profile#	Description	Definition	Time to MCS
1	Crashing and burning	Critical cardiogenic shock	Within hours
2	Progressive decline	Inotrope dependence with continuing deterioration	Within a few days
3	Stable but inotrope dependent	Clinically stable on mild-to-moderate doses of intravenous inotropes (includes stable patients on temporary circulatory support without inotropes)	Within a few weeks
4	Recurrent advanced heart failure	"Recurrent" rather than "refractory" decompensation	Within weeks to months
5	Exertion intolerant	Comfortable at rest	Variable
6	Exertion limited	Able to do some mild activity; fatigued within a few minutes of any meaningful physical exertion	Variable
7	Advanced NYHA III	Clinically stable with a reasonable level of comfortable activity, despite nonrecent history of previous decompensation	Not a candidate for MCS

Abbreviations: MCS, mechanical circulatory support; NYHA, New York Heart Association.

MATTHEWS RISK SCORE

Matthews and colleagues[31] developed a right ventricular risk score (RVRS) to determine short-term risk of RV failure and postoperative mortality in destination therapy patients. The investigators found that independent predictors of RV failure included vasopressor requirement (4 points), aspartate aminotransferase levels of 80 IU/L or more (2 points), bilirubin levels greater than 2.0 mg/dL (2.5 points), and creatinine levels of 2.3 mg/dL or more (3 points). Odds ratios for RV failure were as follows: RVRS ≤ 3.0, 4.0–5.0, and ≥ 5.5; 0.49 (95% confidence interval [CI] 0.37–0.64), 2.8 (95% CI 1.4–5.9), and 7.6 (95% CI 3.4–17.1), respectively. The 180-day survival was $90 \pm 3\%$, $80 \pm 8\%$, and $66 \pm 9\%$, respectively.

PHYSIOLOGY OF AXIAL FLOW

With axial flow pumps, there is continuous unloading throughout the cardiac cycle. Concerns over the effects of reduced or absent pulsatility on organs such as the brain, gastrointestinal (GI) tract, and kidneys as well as endocrine effects have been raised with the use of rotary cardiac assist devices. Much of our current understanding comes from animal data, although increasing information from human patients with heart failure is slowly emerging.

Rotary pumps are capable of generating a full cardiac output; however, even small amounts of ventricular recovery result in a certain degree of pulsatility.[32] With increasing myocardial recovery, pulsatility increases and can be seen on the arterial waveform. A flat arterial trace is only seen when the pump is run at maximal speeds, which is not recommended (see below).[33] In most patients, pulsatility ranges between 5 and 25 mm Hg.[34]

Reduced pulsatility from continuous flow LVADs was shown in a calf model to induce severe periarteritis in the kidneys, because of upregulation of the local renin-angiotensin system in inflammatory cells.[35] Angiotensin II type 1 receptors, which play a role in cell growth and proinflammatory and profibrogenic activity, and angiotensin-converting enzyme were upregulated in renal mononuclear inflammatory cells.

Changes in aortic and arterial wall structure, including the renal artery have been described with continuous flow.[36,37] In the kidney, renal cortical hypertrophy and infiltration of inflammatory cells into the renal cortex were reported. The aortic wall in goats showed thinning and atrophic changes, with a reduced volume ratio of smooth muscle cells.

There has been some concern that low pulsatility might create areas of stasis distal to an existing stenosis, potentially leading to thrombosis. Frazier and colleagues[38] described thrombosis of a major branch artery in the presence of a 30% stenosis and full anticoagulation in patients in whom the LVAD outflow conduit was placed in the descending aorta.

Thrombosis of the aortic root has been rarely reported and is believed to be due to blood stasis and prolonged closure of the aortic valve. Laminated thrombus has been observed more frequently in the area of the noncoronary cusp, perhaps because of the lack of coronary flow relative to the other cusp areas.

Commissural fusion of the aortic valve has been noted with both pulsatile and axial flow devices.[39] In the case of axial flow pumps, commissural fusion has been thought to be related to mild-to-moderate degrees of continuous aortic insufficiency (AI).

It is generally believed that long-term nonpulsatile flow does not affect cerebral autoregulation.[40] At least in clinical practice, no major adverse effects have been observed.

Hemolysis has not been shown to be a clinically relevant event in patients supported with axial flow devices unless it is associated with pump thrombosis.

Bleeding from intestinal arteriovenous malformations (AVMs) is a complication that has been recognized with axial flow pumps. These AVMs are typically incidental findings in normal adults, but bleeding from these sites may be worsened by anticoagulation.[41] In a retrospective review of 33 patients receiving a long-term LVAD between June 1, 2006, and July 31, 2008, 40% of HeartMate II recipients ($n = 20$), experienced at least 1 episode of GI bleeding, whereas the remaining patients who had received pulsatile pumps had no reported episodes of GI bleeding.[42] In 65% of the bleeding episodes observed, no definite source could be identified. The investigators suggested that this bleeding might be due to angiodysplasias in the small bowel, as has been described in patients with aortic stenosis (AS).[43] This phenomenon is often referred to as Heyde syndrome, after the original description by Heyde in 1958.[44] This type of bleeding has been shown to resolve in patients with AS after valve replacement.[45] An association between shear-stress-induced acquired von Willebrand disease type 2A and bleeding from GI angiodysplasias in patients with AS has been suggested.[46,47] In one report, HeartMate II recipients were shown to be lacking the large von Willebrand factor (vWF) multimers, suggesting that the device might induce acquired von Willebrand disease.[48,49] Blood exposure to high sheer stress seems to be the common denominator in acquired von Willebrand disease in patients with AS and LVAD patients. Removal of the source of high shear stress has relieved the bleeding problems in both groups of patients.[50]

In a study of 26 patients who had received a HeartMate II device, vWF multimer assays were performed both with the device in place and postexplant for transplant. The investigators found that while on device support, all patients showed severely impaired platelet aggregation and loss of large vWF multimers. After device removal, normal platelet aggregation patterns and normal multimer analysis were noted, confirming that this hematologic abnormality is reversible.[51]

Despite the recognition of acquired von Willebrand disease in assist device patients, the importance of this condition remains uncertain.

HEARTMATE II

The HeartMate II has been the most successful of the second-generation axial flow rotary devices, and is approved both as a bridge to transplant and destination therapy (**Figs. 1–3**).[5] HeartMate II is a valveless axial flow pump with a titanium-coated rotor. This device has an implant volume of 63 mL, weighs 350 gm, and can generate flows between 3 and 10 L/min at pump speeds of 6000 to 15,000 rpm. As with first-generation devices, the inflow cannula is located at the LV apex and the outflow cannula is anastomosed to the ascending aorta. Both inflow and outflow cannulas are made of woven Dacron and require preclotting. The actual pump is implanted preperitoneally (most commonly) or intraabdominally. The pump's internal rotor has helical blades that curve around a central shaft. As the rotor spins, kinetic energy causes the blood to be drawn from the LV apex in a continuous manner. The motor is located within the pump housing and generates a spinning magnetic field that causes the rotor to spin. A tunneled percutaneous lead that is attached to a controller supplies power and control to the device. The percutaneous lead can be connected to a pair of rechargeable batteries worn by the patient or to an external power module. The absence of a blood sac has eliminated the need for venting, with a resultant reduction in the size of the driveline relative to first-generation devices. The HeartMate II received FDA approval as a bridge to transplant in April 2008.

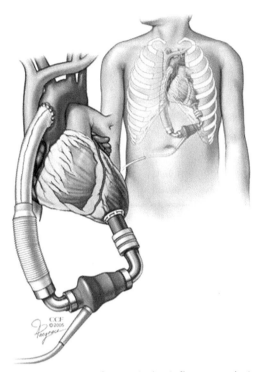

Fig. 1. HeartMate II LVAD in situ. Left ventricular inflow cannula is located at LV apex; outflow cannula is anastomosed to the ascending aorta.

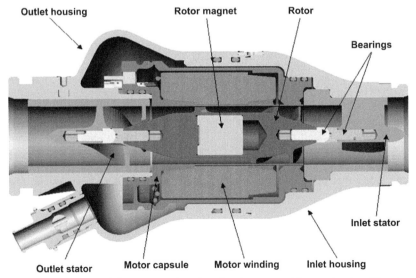

Fig. 2. HeartMate II axial flow pump showing titanium-coated internal rotor. (*Courtesy of* Thoratec Corporation, Pleasanton, CA, USA.)

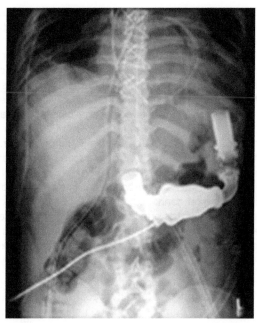

Fig. 3. Chest radiograph showing HeartMate II LVAD in situ. (*Courtesy of* Thoratec Corporation, Pleasanton, CA, USA.)

Anticoagulation consists of heparin initially, followed by transition to warfarin, with a targeted international normalized ratio (INR) between 1.5 and 2.5, and aspirin (early on, patients were more vigorously anticoagulated with a target INR 2.5–3.5). Dipyridamole has been removed from the original standard regimen. This anticoagulation regimen is in contrast to the HeartMate I, for which only aspirin was required.[52]

In a prospective US multicenter study of 133 transplant candidates who underwent implantation of the HeartMate II LVAD, the 6-month survival was 75% and the 12-month survival was 68%.[53] New York Heart Association (NYHA) functional classification and 6-minute walk test performance were significantly improved at 3 months, as were quality of life measures using the Minnesota Living with Heart Failure and Kansas City Cardiomyopathy measures. The most common complication was bleeding. Device-related infection occurred in 14% of patients and was limited to the driveline. The incidence of stroke was 8% (6% ischemic and 2% hemorrhagic). Hemolysis occurred in 3% of patients. About 4% required device replacement.

The HeartMate II Destination Therapy Trial compared the HeartMate II to the older HeartMate XVE.[5] In this study, the primary end point was survival without disabling stroke and without the need to repair or replace the device. About 46% of patients in the HeartMate II group reached the primary end point, compared with 11% (P<.001) in the HeartMate XVE group. These results were primarily due to improved durability of the axial flow pump, with only 10% of patients requiring pump replacement.

Pump Function and Settings

The speed of the rotor and the pressure gradient across the pump determine the pump performance. Simply stated, flow and pressure are inversely related. This pressure-flow relationship has been measured at different rotor speeds as illustrated in **Fig. 4**. As resistance is increased, there comes a critical point at which the pump will shut off and flow equals 0.

Throughout the cardiac cycle, the pressure differential between inlet and outlet cannulas is equal to the aortic pressure minus the LV pressure, plus a combined pressure loss across the inlet and outlet cannulas.[54] Because this system is devoid of valves, sufficient pump speeds must be generated to prevent reverse flow that could potentially result from pressure differentials that are lower than the expected aortic pressures.

These pumps are capable of generating relatively high negative pressures at the inlet conduit, which can lead to ventricular collapse (see below). Generation of negative pressure can occur when LV preload is less than that needed for the pump at any set speed or when there is inflow obstruction, as can occur with thrombosis or improper positioning of the inlet cannula.

There are 4 pump parameters that provide important information about LVAD function. Each parameter depends on the patient's clinical condition, and changes in baseline values and trends tend to be more important than the actual numbers themselves.

- *Pump speed:* In general, pump speed is set to maintain a degree of pulsatility during the cardiac cycle. The greatest flow occurs during systole, when the pressure differential across the pump is least, and minimum flow occurs during diastole, when inlet pressures are lowest and the pressure difference is greater. At specific pump speeds, there is an inverse relationship between flow and the pressure differential (aortic pressure minus LV pressure) across the pump.[55] At maximum pump speed, the LV volume is at its lowest and the LV does not contribute to the cardiac output. At lower pump speeds, there is more blood in the ventricle and systemic flow becomes pulsatile (LV systolic pressure exceeds aortic pressure, allowing the valve to open). The optimum speed is assessed with echocardiography and the following are established: no septal shift, normal LV size, adequate cardiac index, and intermittent opening of the aortic valve. A typical speed range is on the order of 8600 to 9800 rpm.
- *Pulsatility index (PI):* The PI is defined as the difference between maximum and minimum flow divided by the average flow during the cardiac cycle: $PI = (Q_{max} - Q_{min})/Q_{avg}$. PI is a dimensionless number with values ranging between

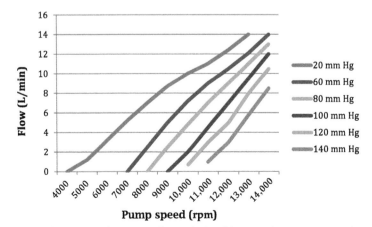

Fig. 4. Graphic illustration of pressure-flow relationship at various pump speeds.

1 and 10 (typical ranges seen clinically are between 3 and 4). PI is inversely related to the amount of pump support. With severely reduced LV contractility, minimal pulsatility (low PI) is observed. A low PI can also be seen in patients with better contractility, but in the presence of excessive pump speeds resulting in ventricular collapse. With hypovolemia, there is a fall in PI without a corresponding increase in pump speed. An increase in PI can be seen with increased contractility and ventricular pressure (ie, myocardial recovery, inotrope support, increased volume status).

- *Power:* Pump power, measured in Watts, reflects the motor's voltage and current. The power range with this device is between 0 and 25.5 W. The system controller measures power directly. Power at a specified speed and estimated flow are related. Increased power can be due to increases in pump flow, pump speed, or physiologic demand. When there is an increase in power that is unrelated to increased flow, as can be seen in the presence of pump thrombus, falsely elevated flow readings will be seen. There is an expected range of power for each set speed under normal operating conditions. Power values that fall outside of this range are displayed as +++ or --- instead of numerically when the estimated flow is above or below the expected limits at a specific set speed.

- *Estimated flow:* Flow rate, as seen on the system module, is an estimate and not a precise measurement. The flow rate is determined by power and pump speed. At a given pump speed, the relationship between power and flow tends to be linear, with the exception of very high or very low pump speeds. As LVAD preload and LV pressure increase, flow increases. As LVAD afterload and aortic pressure decrease, flow also increases. Flows should be maintained at greater than 3.0 L/min. Because this is a calculated value, at higher and lower ends of the power-flow relationship, this number becomes less reliable. Pump flows may overestimate and underestimate true flow by 500 mL. Increases in power that are not matched by an increase in flow are suspicious for pump thrombus. Decreases in power and estimated flow can be due to inflow cannula obstruction or suction.

SURGICAL CONSIDERATIONS
Patient Selection

Proper patient selection has a significant impact on surgical outcomes. Several scoring systems described above have been developed to better predict which patients will survive with medical management and which patients are more likely to have a favorable outcome after LVAD implant. Earlier implementation of mechanical support can prevent or lessen progressive end-organ dysfunction, particularly when prolonged waiting times are anticipated for a donor organ, and is an important part of the selection process. Specific considerations include:

- *Nutritional status:* Cachexia with a body mass index (BMI), calculated as the weight in kilograms divided by height in meters square, less than 22 kg/m^2 has a high associated perioperative mortality that is frequently related to infection.[56] This risk factor is potentially modifiable, and aggressive nutritional support should be instituted with specialty care providers.[57]

- *Infection:* Active infection must be controlled before device implant because this is a primary cause of morbidity and mortality.

- *Right ventricular dysfunction:* The increased venous return to the right side of the heart that occurs with LVAD support may worsen preexisting RV dysfunction. Leftward shift of the interventricular septum may also alter RV geometry, leading to tricuspid regurgitation.[58–60] Optimization of RV function may include central venous pressure (CVP) reduction (to 15 mm Hg or less) with diuresis to reduce RV workload, which helps reduce hepatic congestion and associated coagulation abnormalities. Elevated PVR should be managed pharmacologically with vasodilators (eg, sildenafil, prostaglandins) and inotropes (milrinone, dobutamine) as deemed appropriate.

- *Ventilatory support:* Preoperative ventilator support has been shown to be an independent predictor of RV failure.[61] Diuresis or hemofiltration may improve pulmonary function that is secondary to fluid overload.
- *Coagulation status:* Clotting abnormalities may be due to use of anticoagulants and antiplatelet agents or may be secondary to hepatic dysfunction. These medications should be discontinued preoperatively whenever possible. Patients on coumadin should be transitioned to heparin and can be treated with vitamin K and/or fresh frozen plasma.
- *Hematologic abnormalities:* Patients with low platelet counts should be tested for heparin-induced thrombocytopenia. If they test positive for this abnormality, alternative anticoagulation strategies will be required (ie, bivalirudin) for cardiopulmonary bypass. Sources of anemia should be investigated because this is a risk factor for poor outcomes.
- *End-organ dysfunction:* Renal, hepatic, pulmonary, and GI dysfunction should be optimized. A glomerular filtration rate less than 0.5 mL/kg/min is associated with poor outcomes.[62] Measures to help improve renal perfusion and reduce CVP should be instituted. Hepatic dysfunction that is secondary to RV dysfunction should be managed with preload and afterload reduction. In some instances, ultrafiltration may be beneficial. Pulmonary dysfunction in the presence of heart failure is difficult to assess with accuracy, and pulmonary function tests are not always helpful. Preoperative mechanical ventilation is a strong predictor of poor outcome.[63] Active GI bleeding should be thoroughly investigated and managed accordingly.

ANESTHETIC MANAGEMENT

Anesthetic management of the patient with end-stage heart failure undergoing LVAD implantation has been well described and is beyond the scope of this article.[64–68] General considerations before cardiopulmonary bypass are outlined in **Table 3**. Postbypass concerns include the following:

- *Right ventricular failure:* RV failure is one of the most challenging problems encountered postbypass. RV failure can be difficult to predict and is incompletely understood. Typically, it manifests as elevated CVP, poor LV filling, and reduced LVAD output. Perioperative RV failure is associated with a relatively high mortality in the LVAD recipient, ranging from 19% to 43%,[69–71] and posttransplant survival tends to be worse.[72,73] Postimplant, the pathophysiology of RV failure is complex and may include increased RV afterload, primary RV myocardial dysfunction, RV ischemia, and ventricular interdependence.

Low preoperative RV stroke work index (RVSWI), a correlate of RV contractility, plays a role in predicting RV dysfunction. RVSWI allows quantification of the ability of the RV to generate pressure and is given by [(mean PAP−mean CVP) × SVI]/BSA (SVI is the stroke volume index and BSA is the body surface area). In pulsatile LVADs, low RVSWI predicted the need for prolonged inotrope use.[74] An RVSWI less than 300 mm Hg/mL/m^{-2} is a strong predictor of the need for right ventricular assist device

Table 3
Prebypass anesthetic concerns

Overall Patient Stability	Elective vs Salvage Case
Monitoring	Standard ASA monitors, arterial line (cannulation strategy will determine proper placement site), pulmonary artery catheter, multiple large bore intravenous access, TEE
Ventilatory status	Intubated vs not intubated; ventilator settings
Reoperation status	Will require additional blood and blood products; check antibody status
Current symptoms	Can patient lay flat?
Anticoagulation status	Heparin (may require higher heparin doses, FFP or recombinant AT III if AT III deficient); Coumadin (may require FFP and vitamin K for reversal)
Current support	IABP, ECMO, short-term VAD, inotropes
Preoperative medications	Inotropes, vasodilators, diuretics, ACE inhibitors, anticoagulants, platelet inhibitors, antiarrhythmic medications
Cause of heart failure	Ischemic, idiopathic, viral (may affect degree of RV preservation)
Hematologic	Anemia (consider cause); thrombocytopenia (rule out heparin-induced thrombocytopenia); alternative anticoagulation strategy such as bivalirudin may be needed if patient tests positive for HIT
Systemic disease	Renal, hepatic, pulmonary function (may affect drug pharmacokinetics and drug dosing)
Right-sided heart failure	Hepatic engorgement and tricuspid regurgitation can lead to passive hepatic congestion and coagulopathy
Pulmonary hypertension	Can adversely affect right-sided heart function postbypass
Infection	Current antibiotic regimen should be continued per consultant recommendations
Pacemaker, AICD	When present, pacemakers should be interrogated and programed appropriately for the operating room; AICDs should be turned off and Zoll pads (Zoll Medical Corporation, Chelmsford, MA) applied to the patient

Abbreviations: ACE, angiotensin converting enzyme; AICD, automatic implantable cardioverter-defibrillator; ASA, American Society of Anesthesiologists; AT III, antithrombin III; ECMO; extracorporeal membrane oxygenation; FFP, fresh frozen plasma; HIT, heparin-induced thrombocytopenia; IABP, intra-aortic balloon pump; TEE, transesophageal echocardiography.

support.[72] In the presence of elevated preoperative PAP and normal CVP (ie, high RVSWI), the risk of postimplant RV failure is low. On the other hand, low PAP may reflect significant RV dysfunction and the inability to generate sufficient pressure across the pulmonary circuit.

A transpulmonary gradient greater than 16 mm Hg in the presence of a central venous pressure greater than or equal to 20 mm Hg has a relatively high sensitivity and specificity for predicting post-LVAD RV dysfunction.[75] Nonhemodynamic preoperative factors may be better predictors of RV failure than actual functional measurements.[73]

Intraoperative causes of RV failure include air embolism down the right coronary artery, which is seen as ST segment elevations in the inferior leads and ischemic changes in the right coronary territory, and is typically reversible with supportive management (increasing coronary perfusion pressure) with or without reinstituting cardiopulmonary bypass. Intracardiac air may or may not be evident on transesophageal echocardiography (TEE). If the right coronary artery is diseased, revascularization may be necessary.

When RV failure is due to preexisting RV dysfunction and does not improve with LV unloading, inotropic or mechanical support may be indicated. Inhaled nitric oxide and inhaled epoprostenol (Flolan) may reduce PAPs sufficiently to improve RV function.[76]

High pump speeds can have a negative effect on RV function by causing septal shift and altering RV geometry. Tricuspid regurgitation can also result.

The need to transfuse large volumes of blood and blood products to treat coagulopathy can lead to RV volume overload with resultant failure. The RV, being thin walled, is particularly vulnerable to volume overload and elevations in PVR. All volume administration should be done judiciously, and trends in CVP should be noted. Pulmonary hypertension can be related to hypoxemia, hypercarbia, elevated airway pressures, and acidosis. Interestingly, in the presence of normal PVR and decompression of the left side of the heart, moderate elevations in CVP may be adequate to generate blood flow across the pulmonary circuit, even in the presence of moderate-to-severe RV dysfunction.[77] In fact, patients in ventricular fibrillation have been reported to tolerate this arrhythmia with LVAD support.[78]

- *Vasoplegia:* Chronic vasodilator or inodilator use preoperatively, along with prolonged cardiopulmonary bypass times can result in profound vasoplegia postbypass. Agents such as norepinephrine, vasopressin,[79] and sometimes methylene blue[80] may be required to maintain adequate afterload conditions.
- *Hypothermia:* Hypothermia can worsen coagulopathy, increase metabolic rate with shivering, delay emergence from anesthesia, and lead to arrhythmias. Patients should be adequately rewarmed before separation from cardiopulmonary bypass, and warming measures should include fluid warmers, heated respiratory circuits, warm operating room ambient temperature, and forced air warming devices.
- *Coagulopathy:* Management of postpump coagulopathy can be challenging because administration of large volumes of blood and blood products can lead to volume overload and RV failure. First and foremost, prevention is essential and includes minimizing pump time, excellent surgical hemostasis, and maintenance of normothermia. Use of aminocaproic acid may help reduce bleeding. Early administration of platelets and fresh frozen plasma is encouraged when indicated. Clotting parameters should be checked at regular intervals. When available, thromboelastography can help to guide product administration. In instances of uncontrolled coagulopathy, there are reports of recombinant factor VII being used (off label) successfully.[81,82] There are, however, real concerns about the potential risk for thrombosis. In a retrospective study of 62 LVAD patients who received recombinant factor VII, patients were divided into low-dose (10–20 μg/kg) and high-dose (30–70 μg/kg) groups. Patients in the high-dose group had a significantly higher incidence of serious thromboembolic events (36.7% vs 9.4%, $P \leq .001$).[83] The risks and benefits of factor VII administration should be discussed with the surgical team, and strong consideration should be given to using lower doses.
- *Arrhythmias:* Arrhythmias may be related to suction events.
- *Target mean arterial pressure:* A target mean arterial pressure (MAP) of 70 to 80 mm Hg is desirable. A MAP greater than 90 mm Hg can lead to reduced pump output because this is an afterload-dependent system. Pump speed should therefore not be titrated to the desired blood pressure.

- *Target pulse pressure:* A pulse pressure of 10 to 20 mm Hg, with intermittent aortic valve opening (approximately every 3 beats), allows for a good balance between pump speed and LV pressure. It is unclear what the optimum frequency of aortic valve opening is. It is thought that aortic valve opening can reduce the risk of aortic valve thrombosis and aortic valve fusion over time.[84] The pulse pressure is determined by contractility, preload, and pump speed. At high pump speeds, diastolic pressure increases without much change in systolic pressure and pulse pressure decreases.
- *Volume status*
- *Pulse oximetry:* In the absence of pulsatility, pulse oximetry is unreliable, and frequent blood gas monitoring is recommended.

Separation from cardiopulmonary bypass is a coordinated exercise between the surgeon, perfusionist, anesthesiologist, and the individual who is adjusting the parameters on the pump module. The following events are essential for effective separation from cardiopulmonary bypass:

- Proper deairing of the heart and cannulas. TEE is used to guide deairing procedures as volume is added to the heart.
- The pump is activated at a fixed speed (generally 8000–9000 rpm) while still on partial bypass.
- Cardiopulmonary bypass flows are gradually reduced as volume is added to the heart, paying close attention to RV function, midline interventricular septal position, and LV volume status. Adequate preload is essential to providing adequate pump output. Ventricular collapse and septal shift may be due to inadequate preload or poor RV performance. LV dilatation can be due to improper inflow cannula position or very high afterload. Excessive afterload can result in reduced pump output because this is an afterload-dependent system. A MAP between 70 and 80 mm Hg is generally optimal.

ROLE OF TRANSESOPHAGEAL ECHOCARDIOGRAPHY

TEE is an indispensable tool in the LVAD patient. It provides real-time assessment of ventricular function, valvular pathology, and hemodynamics in a relatively noninvasive manner. Intraoperatively, TEE assists the surgeon in deciding whether the operation will extend beyond simple VAD placement, and postoperatively, it serves to monitor device function and myocardial recovery, and assists with weaning efforts and in the differential diagnosis of low-output states. The following should be included in the routine TEE assessment:

Prebypass

- *Tricuspid valve:* Tricuspid insufficiency is not uncommon in patients presenting for LVAD implant. Repair of significant tricuspid regurgitation, either with valvuloplasty or with bioprosthetic valve replacement, is indicated and important for preservation of RV function.
- *Mitral valve:* Mitral stenosis (MS) should be treated with valve replacement with a tissue prosthesis. MS impedes pump filling and results in elevated left atrial pressures, leading to RV dysfunction.

In general, mitral insufficiency does not require treatment. Decompression of the LV with pump activation usually leads to improvement in the degree of regurgitation by reducing filling pressures and reducing leaflet tethering that occurs with ventricular dilatation.

Preexisting mitral valve prostheses, whether mechanical or biologic, are generally left alone, keeping in mind that greater degrees of anticoagulation may be required postoperatively.

- *Aortic valve:* AS does not generally need to be addressed surgically unless there is associated AI. In the presence of hemodynamically significant AS, the LVAD generates most of the systemic output.

With rotary devices, AI may occur throughout the cardiac cycle, leading to high pump flows and an aorto-ventricular-LVAD circuit with wasted flow. Lowering the pump speed can decrease the transvalvular gradient and the amount of regurgitation, but at the expense of systemic perfusion.[85] Unloading of the LV with device placement can increase the gradient between the aorta and LV, leading to augmentation of the original degree of regurgitation. Moderate-to-severe AI must be surgically managed. This condition can be handled in several ways. Using the "Park stitch" technique, the edges of the aortic cusps can be sewn together to reduce or eliminate AI.[86] Another option is oversewing the aortic valve or outflow tract, keeping in mind that any device malfunction will certainly prove fatal, because the patient becomes totally device dependent.[87] Alternatively, the aortic valve can be replaced with a bioprosthesis.

In patients with a preexisting mechanical aortic prosthesis and anticipated long-term mechanical support, the valve should be replaced with a bioprosthesis or oversewn, because of the risk of thromboembolism.

- *Intracardiac shunt:* An intracardiac shunt (atrial septal defect, patent foramen ovale, ventricular septal defect) must be ruled out. A bubble study using agitated saline[88,89] and color flow Doppler should be used to interrogate the interatrial and interventricular septum. A negative bubble and color flow study may still fail to identify a patent foramen ovale because of elevated left-sided pressures, and these should be repeated postbypass. If a shunt is detected after left-sided decompression, it should be repaired. A Valsalva maneuver can enhance shunt detection, but should be used with caution, because it can provoke significant hemodynamic instability by altering venous return to the right side of the heart.
- *Right ventricular function:* RV size and function are assessed. This is only a semi-quantitative measure. More quantitative measures can be achieved preoperatively with transthoracic echocardiography (TTE) by calculating global right ventricular fractional area of change (RVFAC), which is equal to the difference between RV diastolic and systolic areas divided by the RV diastolic area.[90] If the RVFAC is less than 20%, patients may be more vulnerable to postoperative RV failure (normal RVFAC $\geq$40%). Because LV unloading increases RV preload and can cause a leftward shift of the interventricular septum, RV dysfunction can become unmasked or augmented postbypass.
- *Thrombus:* All chambers should be checked for the presence of thrombus, although this should never preclude visual inspection. Blood flow stasis can lead to thrombus formation in the left atrial appendage, left atrium, akinetic or aneurysmal ventricular segments, and on central monitoring catheters, pacing, or implantable defibrillator leads.
- *Ascending aorta:* The aorta should be assessed for the presence of atheromatous disease, particularly at the site of the outflow graft anastomosis.

Postbypass

- *Inflow cannula position:* The inflow cannula should be directed posteriorly, toward the mitral valve (**Fig. 5**). If it is directed toward the interventricular septum, inflow can be compromised, which can become a problem in the future because the LV size decreases over time. Flow into the inflow cannula should be laminar and unidirectional (**Fig. 6**). Any amount of turbulence or high Doppler velocities may indicate cannula obstruction by the septum or occlusion by thrombus. Normal peak Doppler velocities are between 0.7 and 2.0 m/sec (**Fig. 7**), depending on preload conditions and native heart function. The inflow cannula position should be rechecked after chest closure. A typical pulse wave Doppler flow trace shows a low-velocity phasic pattern.
- *Outflow cannula position:* The outflow cannula can be difficult to image (**Fig. 8**). Using pulse wave Doppler, the sample volume should be approximately 1 cm proximal to the aortic anastomosis. Normal velocities are approximately 0.5–2.0 m/sec (**Fig. 9**).[91] These flow velocities depend on pump speed and output, as well as the cannula's angle of insertion.[92]
- *Deairing:* This procedure should be accomplished before separation from bypass and at low LVAD speeds. Complete filling of the LV is necessary to prevent air aspiration around the inflow conduit.
- *Septal position:* Septal shift can occur at high pump speeds and with inadequate LV preload. Pump speed is adjusted and preload administered to maintain the septum in a midline position.
- *Aortic valve opening:* With full pump support, the aortic valve remains closed. Pump speed can be set based on the degree of valve opening.
- *Mitral valve:* Persistent significant mitral regurgitation may be related to inadequate LV decompression.
- *Tricuspid valve:* Increasing severity of tricuspid regurgitation can occur at increased pump speeds if there is septal shift with distortion of the tricuspid annulus. This condition can also occur in the presence of RV decompensation, as can occur with a right coronary air embolism. The severity of increasing

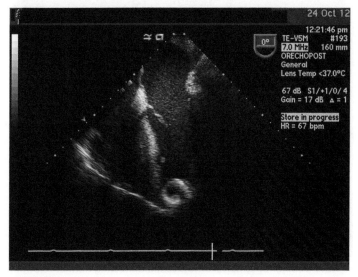

Fig. 5. TEE 4-chamber view showing proper positioning of LV apical inflow cannula.

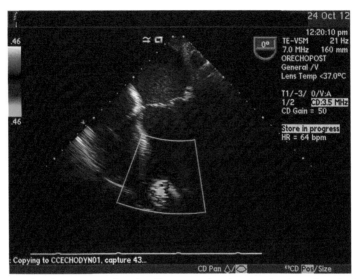

Fig. 6. TEE 4-chamber view with color flow Doppler showing laminar flow in the apical inflow cannula.

tricuspid regurgitation can sometimes be reduced by adjusting the pump speed.
- *Right ventricular function:* TEE can help determine the need for or response to inotropic support.
- *Intracardiac shunt:* The lack of intracardiac shunting should be reconfirmed postpump.

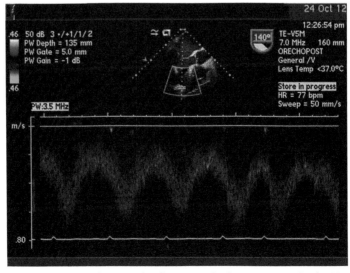

Fig. 7. Pulse wave Doppler of LV apical inflow cannula showing normal velocities (see text) and laminar flow.

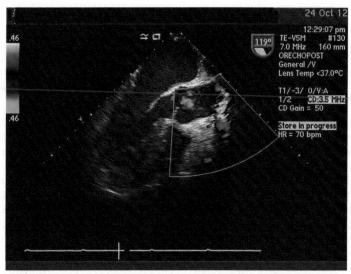

Fig. 8. TEE long-axis view with color flow Doppler showing laminar flow in the aortic outflow cannula.

- *Volume status:* Low LV volumes can be device or patient related. Hypovolemia and RV failure can lead to reduced LV preload, whereas too high pump speeds can cause LV collapse. High ventricular volumes, as can be seen with inflow cannula obstruction, can lead to rightward shift of the interventricular septum, tethering of the mitral valve leaflets, and functional mitral regurgitation.

Postchest closure, the patient should be reassessed with TEE. Chest closure can lead to deterioration of RV function. Increased peak airway pressures can adversely affect right-sided venous return, and resulting increased pulmonary artery pressures

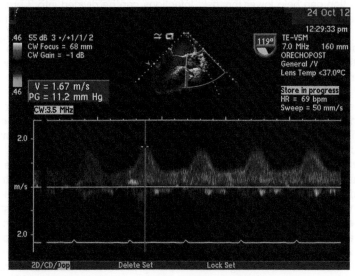

Fig. 9. Pulse wave Doppler of aortic outflow cannula showing normal velocities (see text).

can have detrimental effects. Inflow cannula position should also be reassessed post-chest closure.

Speed Ramp Study

When the patient is hemodynamically stable, a range of speed settings can be determined using the ramped speed test.[93] A ramped speed study[94] allows the operator to determine the range of safe operating pump speeds as follows:

- *Determine low-end range:* The pump speed is gradually reduced until the aortic valve opens with each beat and the patient shows no signs of cardiac failure. In the absence of aortic valve opening, with the use of a pulmonary artery catheter, the lowest speed setting should occur at a cardiac index of 2.5 L/min/m². Alternatively, TTE can be used to set the low speed cutoff when LV size increases and there is rightward septal shift. The speed should not be set below 8000 rpm.
- *Determine high-end range:* The pump speed is gradually increased until there is septal flattening, there is a decrease in LV end-diastolic dimension, the aortic valve remains closed, and the pulse pressure is 10 to 15 mm Hg. This speed is generally below 9600 rpm.

The proper speed setting will generally occur somewhere between the low and high-end speeds.

COMPLICATIONS

It should be emphasized that proper timing of device implant, along with meticulous patient selection, can help to lessen some of the complications encountered with these devices. Complications have included:

- *Bleeding/hemorrhage:* Bleeding can be secondary to anticoagulation or hepatic dysfunction or related to the operation itself (especially reoperations).
- *Infection and sepsis:* Infection remains a prevalent problem in LVAD patients. Device modifications have lowered this risk relative to first-generation LVADs; however, it remains a major cause of morbidity and mortality. Proper patient selection can help lower this risk. Infections can be divided into 3 broad categories: driveline, pump pocket, and LVAD-associated endocarditis.[95] The driveline is the most common infection site. In addition to device-related factors, pulsatile LVADs have been shown to induce alterations in the recipient's immune system that may contribute to the development of associated infections. These alterations include defects in T-cell function and cellular immunity.[96] At present, it is unclear if these same changes are seen in axial flow pumps. The newer-generation HeartWare device, which is implanted intrapericardially and has no pump pocket, has a lower device-related infection rate than historical controls, highlighting the contribution of device design to improved infectious outcomes.[97]
- *Pump thrombus:* Pump thrombus should be suspected when any of the 4 pump parameters are altered. In particular, power values greater than 10 to 12 W, gradual increases in power, or abrupt changes in power are worrisome for pump thrombus.[93] A developing thrombus can lead to pump flow obstruction. If the thrombus originated upstream and has embolized into the pump, the power increase will be more abrupt. Hemolysis can also be a sign of pump thrombosis.
- *Retrograde flow:* If the pump stops for any reason (eg, disconnection, power loss), blood can flow retrograde from the aorta to the LV because there are no valves in the circuit.

- *Suction:* If the pump speed is set too high in relation to the patient's volume status, LV suction occurs. Several factors can lead to inadequate LV filling, including hypovolemia, RV failure, tamponade, and elevated PVR. When suction is detected, the system is designed to automatically reduce pump speed to the lower set limit in the controller.
- *Stroke/Transient ischemic attack*
- *Hemolysis:* This is not a common problem, but can become clinically significant in the presence of pump thrombus.
- *Right-sided heart failure:* RV dysfunction remains a significant problem post-LVAD implant and can occur in up to one-third of patients.[71] The incidence does not seem to be much different between the HeartMate I and HeartMate II devices, although in a retrospective comparison, fewer patients receiving the HeartMate II required RV assist support or pure inotropic support for RV failure.[60]
- *GI bleeding*
- *Device failure*

TROUBLESHOOTING

In the postoperative period, several problems can occur, and their source must be identified promptly. Such complications can include:

- *Hypovolemia:* This can be due to surgical bleeding.
- *Tamponade:* Postoperatively, this can be due to localized clot formation compressing any or all cardiac chambers. A high index of suspicion is needed to make a prompt diagnosis.
- *RV failure:* This is seen as a dilated RV with functional tricuspid regurgitation, and low LV volumes with potential intermittent inflow cannula obstruction from suction events.
- *Arrhythmias:* These can occur as a result of suction events.
- *Hypoxemia:* An interatrial communication should be ruled out if no other source is identified.
- *Pulmonary embolism*
- *Device-related problems:* This includes inflow cannula malposition, outflow cannula kinking, and pump thrombosis.

Echocardiography is indispensable in the diagnosis and management of these types of problems.[93,98,99] The 4 pump parameters can provide a clue to the cause of pump- or patient-related problems as outlined in **Figs. 10** and **11**. It can be recalled that pump flow values are only estimates and are based on power. At low and high ends of the power-flow relationship, these estimates are imprecise. Increases in PI can result from increased LV filling and improved myocardial performance. Decreases in PI can be related to reduced LV filling and reduced contractility. Gradual or abrupt increases in power are highly suspect for pump thrombosis. Increases in pump power can be seen with increases in pump speed, with increases in pump flow, and during periods of increased physiologic demand. Close attention should be paid to the position of the interventricular septum, frequency of aortic valve opening, pulsatility, PAP estimates from tricuspid regurgitation Doppler velocities, LVAD output versus total output, and overall volume status. It must be remembered that power increases that are not matched by actual flow increases will lead to falsely elevated estimated flows.

- *Low flow, high power:* In the presence of low echocardiographically determined flow and high power, pump failure and increased afterload must be ruled out

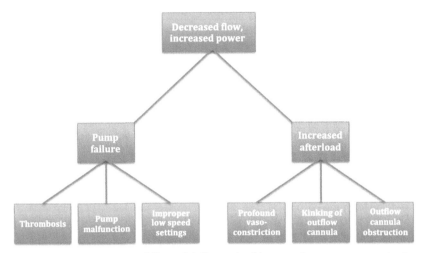

Fig. 10. Algorithm illustrating differential diagnosis of increased pump power and echocardiographically determined decreased flow (output).

(see **Fig. 10**). Pump failure can be due to thrombosis, malfunction, and improperly set low-speed settings. Echocardiography can show a rightward shift of the interventricular septum, an increase in functional mitral regurgitation, regular opening of the aortic valve, spontaneous echo contrast or "smoke" in the left atrium and/or ventricle, and regurgitation across the LVAD inflow and outflow cannulas. Pump thrombus can increase rotor drag leading to increased power requirement, and the PI decreases. The presence of hemolysis is also suspicious for pump thrombosis. LVAD thrombosis can be managed with anticoagulation or thrombolysis, whereas pump malfunction may require emergent pump exchange. Because the system contains no valves, any loss of power can potentially lead to retrograde flow. If the impeller fails to rotate, the pump becomes no

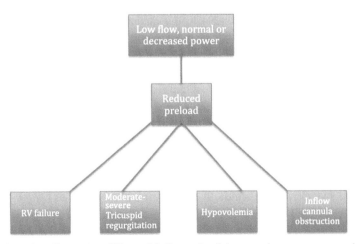

Fig. 11. Algorithm illustrating differential diagnosis of decreased pump power and echocardiographically determined low or normal flow (output).

more than a conduit between the ventricle and ascending aorta. If diastolic aortic pressure exceeds LV pressure, retrograde flow will ensue.

Elevated systemic vascular resistance will cause the aortic valve to remain closed. The PI is increased in this situation. The outflow cannula shows high-velocity flow (pressure in the LV is elevated) with a pulsatile contour despite reduced pump output. Aortic pressure is higher than ventricular pressure, which keeps the aortic valve closed. Continued rotation of the impeller augments the pressure wave generated by the LV. At low pump speeds and high afterload, retrograde flow can also occur. If there is obstruction of the outflow cannula from thrombus or kinking, LV systolic pressure will be greater than aortic pressure, leading to regular opening of the aortic valve.

Any of the following should alert the clinician to the possibility of pump thrombosis:

- Decreased pump flow
- Opening of the aortic valve with each beat because of increased LV preload
- Rightward septal bowing
- Increased mitral regurgitation from LV dilatation and leaflet tethering
- Hemolysis
- Altered pump parameters, especially increased power

- *Low flow, low/normal power*: In the presence of low echocardiographically detected flow and low or normal power, decreased preload should be suspected (see **Fig. 11**). This situation can be due to RV failure, moderate-to-severe tricuspid regurgitation, hypovolemia, and inflow cannula obstruction.
- In the presence of high echocardiographically detected flow with low estimated cardiac output as estimated by echocardiography, AI must be ruled out.

THIRD-GENERATION VENTRICULAR ASSIST DEVICES

Third-generation LVADs use magnetic and/or hydrodynamic levitation of the impeller, which has eliminated the need for contact bearings.[100] Third-generation devices include the HeartWare HVAD, which uses hydrodynamic levitation along with magnetic levitation for suspension; the HeartMate III (Thoratec Corporation, Pleasanton, CA, USA),[101] which uses full magnetic suspension; the Berlin Heart Incor (Berlin Heart AG, Berlin, Germany), and the DuraHeart (Terumo Heart, Inc, Ann Arbor, MI, USA),[102,103] which uses magnetic levitation. Advantages over previous-generation devices include:

- Smaller size
- Thinner driveline
- Lack of contact bearings
- Lack of pump pocket
- No mechanical wear-and-tear
- Potential for greater durability than previous-generation devices
- Ideal for small patients, including children
- Absence of friction and heat generation

HEARTWARE HVAD

The HeartWare VAD (HeartWare, Inc, Miami Lakes, FL, USA) is a 140 g miniaturized implantable centrifugal flow pump with a 50 mL displacement volume that is implanted in the pericardial space and was introduced clinically in 2006 (**Figs. 12–15**).[104,105] This device can generate flows up to 10 L/min. The wide-blade impeller of this device is

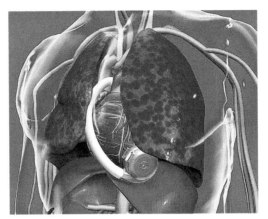

Fig. 12. HeartWare LVAD in situ. (*Courtesy of* Heartware, Inc, Miami Lakes, FL, USA.)

suspended by hybrid passive magnets and hydrodynamic forces.[106] Because there are no mechanical contact points within the pump, friction and heat generation have been eliminated and extended durability is expected. The integrated inflow cannula is inserted into the LV apex, and the pump itself is positioned in the pericardial space, eliminating the need for a pump pocket and thereby simplifying the surgical implant. The 10-mm outflow graft, made of zero porosity gelatin-impregnated

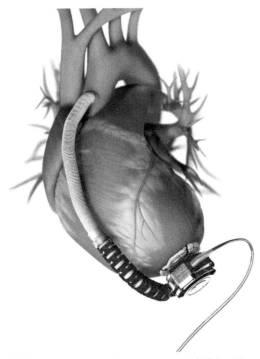

Fig. 13. HeartWare LVAD in situ showing LV apical (pericardial) location of pump. (*Courtesy of* Heartware, Inc, Miami Lakes, Florida.)

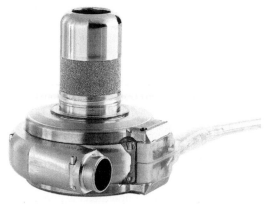

Fig. 14. Miniaturized HeartWare HVAD pump. (*Courtesy of* Heartware, Inc, Miami Lakes, FL, USA.)

material, is anastomosed to the ascending aorta.[107,108] Although it is intended for LV support, biventricular support has been reported.[109]

Components

- *Front housing:* The front housing includes the integrated 25-mm-long titanium inflow cannula.
- *Rear housing:* The rear housing includes a center post with a magnetic stack corresponding to a similar stack found within the impeller, which develops a strong repulsive force that helps to maintain the impeller's radial support. The center post's magnetic stack is vertically aligned and shifted downward relative to the impeller's magnetic stack. This position in turn creates an axial magnetic force that maintains the impeller position toward the front housing.

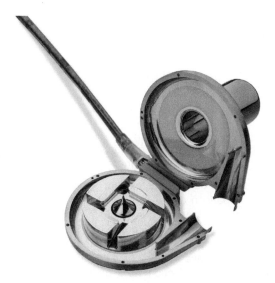

Fig. 15. Internal view of HeartWare HVAD showing impeller. (*Courtesy of* Heartware, Inc, Miami Lakes, FL, USA.)

- *Rotating impeller:* The rotating impeller has wide blades and accommodates 4 large rare-earth magnets, contributing to the pump's high efficiency. The impeller suspension system includes a separate stack of 3 rare earth magnets with like poles.
- *Outflow graft:* The 10-mm outflow graft is made of Vascutek Gelweave (Terumo Cardiovascular Systems Corp, Ann Arbor, MI, USA), which is a gelatin-impregnated graft material with zero porosity. Graft kinking is prevented by the inclusion of an articulating strain relief in the proximal portion. This strain relief consists of plastic interlocking vertebra links.
- *Driveline cable:* The driveline measures only 4.2 mm in diameter and is made up of 6 insulated fatigue-resistant cables. Woven Dacron polyester covers portions of the driveline cable to facilitate tissue ingrowth at the exit site.
- *Microprocessor-based controller:* The controller is connected to the pump via the percutaneous driveline. The controller operates the pump and monitors its function, provides diagnostic information, stores data, and manages the different available power sources (AC, DC, and battery power). Two separate power sources must be connected at all times.

Pump Operation

When the pump is activated, the impeller begins to rotate. The hydrodynamic thrust bearings push the impeller away from the front housing. The impeller is separated from the front housing by a blood barrier. Blood is forced through the pump by the rotating impeller using hydrodynamic and centrifugal forces. The electromagnetic coupling between motor magnets within the impeller and motor stators in the front and rear housings provide rotational energy to the impeller. Blood flow through the pump at a constant rotational speed (range 1800–4000 rpm) depends on the differential pressure across the pump. This system is a preload- and afterload-dependent one, and the difference between LV and aortic pressures is the most important determinant of flow through the pump. The lower the pressure differential, the higher is the flow rate generated. The highest flow rates occur under conditions of increased preload and decreased afterload, regardless of the impeller speed. Estimated flow is calculated from the pump speed, motor current, and blood viscosity (adjusted based on hematocrit), and baseline flow must exceed 1.8 L/min to prevent suction.

The ADVANCE Trial

The ADVANCE trial is a US nonrandomized multicenter study that enrolled 140 patients listed for transplant to receive the new HeartWare HVAD.[110] Results at 180 days were compared with data from 499 patients of the INTERMACS registry who had received an LVAD (mostly HeartMate II) as a bridge to transplant. Results from this study suggested that the HeartWare is at least as good as the currently available devices.

The primary outcome in this study was survival on the originally implanted HVAD, transplant, or explant (with 60-day postexplant survival) at 180 days. Secondary outcomes included comparison of survival between treatment groups and INTERMACS controls, functional outcomes, quality of life outcomes, and adverse events in the HVAD group. Patients in the HVAD group had 92% (compared with 90.1% in the control group, $P<.001$) success with regard to the primary outcome, the highest rate reported to date at 180 days with any type of VAD as a bridge to transplant.

Although less bleeding and infection were observed, stroke was a concerning adverse event. As with second-generation devices, GI bleeding from arteriovenous malformations was also seen.

Endurance Trial

The Endurance Trial is currently underway and is a randomized controlled unblinded multicenter comparison of the HeartWare HVAD with the HeartMate II as destination therapy in nontransplant candidates. This study will enroll 450 patients at 50 US hospitals.

SUMMARY

The evolution of mechanical circulatory support devices from large pulsatile pumps to smaller axial and centrifugal flow devices has dramatically altered the course of patients with advanced heart failure. Greater durability and lower complication rates have enhanced survival and quality of life. In select patients, destination therapy may result in survival rates comparable to transplant recipients.[111] At present, 2-year unadjusted survival after transplant is around 80%.[112] Using survival metrics based on this unadjusted survival in bridge-to-transplant transplant recipients, Kirklin and colleagues[111] have suggested that subsets of destination therapy patients might achieve comparable outcomes over this same time period. At present, nearly one-third of LVAD recipients are destination therapy patients. With little anticipated change in transplant donor availability, it can be expected that mechanical circulatory support will continue to be a viable alternative in transplant-eligible patients. Based on some of the promising results seen with the newer third-generation pumps, it is anticipated that they will receive FDA approval in the near future.

REFERENCES

1. Reich DJ, Mulligan DC, Abt PL, et al. ASTS recommended practice guidelines for controlled donation after cardiac death organ procurement and transplantation. Am J Transplant 2009;9:2004–11.
2. Ali AA, White P, Xiang B, et al. Hearts from DCD donors display acceptable biventricular function after heart transplantation in pigs. Am J Transplant 2011; 11:1621–32.
3. Stehlik J, Edwards LB, Kucheryavaya AY, et al. The Registry of the International Society for Heart and Lung Transplantation: twenty-seventh official adult heart transplant report—2010. J Heart Lung Transplant 2010;29:1089–103.
4. Rose EA, Gelijns AC, Moskowitz AJ, et al. Long-term use of a left ventricular assist device for end-stage heart failure. N Engl J Med 2001;345:1435–43.
5. Slaughter MS, Rogers JG, Milano CA, et al. Advanced heart failure treated with continuous-flow left ventricular assist device. N Engl J Med 2009;361: 2241–51.
6. Lietz K, Deng M, Morgan J, et al. Selection of UNOS status 1A candidates for mechanical circulatory support as bridge-to-transplantation (BTT)—Analysis of UNOS/OPTN 2000-2005. J Heart Lung Transplant 2008;27(2S):S244.
7. Zimpfer D, Zrunek P, Roethy W, et al. Left ventricular assist devices decrease fixed pulmonary hypertension in cardiac transplant candidates. J Thorac Cardiovasc Surg 2007;133:689–95.
8. Frazier OH, Benedict CR, Radovancevic B, et al. Improved left ventricular function after chronic ventricular unloading. Ann Thorac Surg 1996;62:675–81.
9. Dandel M, Weng Y, Siniawski H, et al. Long-term results in patients with idiopathic dilated cardiomyopathy after weaning from left ventricular assist devices. Circulation 2005;112(Suppl I):I37–45.

10. Simon MA, Kormos RL, Murali S, et al. Myocardial recovery using ventricular assist devices: prevalence, clinical characteristics, and outcomes. Circulation 2005;112:I32–6.

11. Mancini DM, Beniaminovitz A, Levin H, et al. Low incidence of myocardial recovery after left ventricular assist device implantation in patients with chronic heart failure. Circulation 1998;98:2383–9.

12. Klotz S, Danser AH, Burkhoff D. Impact of left ventricular assist device (LVAD) support on the cardiac reverse remodeling process. Prog Biophys Mol Biol 2008;97:479–96.

13. Maybaum S, Mancini D, Xydas S, et al. Cardiac improvement during mechanical circulatory support: a prospective multicenter study of the LVAD Working Group. Circulation 2007;115:2497–505.

14. Birks EJ, Tansley PD, Hardy J, et al. Left ventricular assist device and drug therapy for the reversal of heart failure. N Engl J Med 2006;355:1873–84.

15. George RS, Yacoub MH, Bowles CT, et al. Quality of life after removal of left ventricular assist device for myocardial recovery. J Heart Lung Transplant 2008;27:165–72.

16. Birks EJ, George RS, Hedger M, et al. Reversal of severe heart failure with a continuous-flow left ventricular assist device and pharmacological therapy: a prospective study. Circulation 2011;123:381–90.

17. Wong K, Boheler K, Petrou M, et al. Pharmacological modulation of pressure-overload cardiac hypertrophy: changes in ventricular function, extracellular matrix and gene expression. Circulation 1997;96:2239–46.

18. Wong K, Boheler KR, Bishop J, et al. Clenbuterol induces cardiac hypertrophy with normal functional, morphological, and molecular features. Cardiovasc Res 1998;37:115–22.

19. Lietz K, Long JW, Kfoury AG, et al. Outcomes of left ventricular assist device implantation as destination therapy in the post-REMATCH era: implications for patient selection. Circulation 2007;116:497–505.

20. Higgins J, Lamarche Y, Kaan A, et al. Microaxial devices for ventricular failure: a multicentre, population-based experience. Can J Cardiol 2011;27:725–30.

21. Bruckner BA, Jacob LP, Gregoric ID, et al. Clinical experience with the Tandem-Heart percutaneous ventricular assist device as a bridge to cardiac transplantation. Tex Heart Inst J 2008;35:447–50.

22. Marasco SF, Lukas G, McDonald M, et al. Review of ECMO (extra corporeal membrane oxygenation) support in critically ill adult patients. Heart Lung Circ 2008;17(Suppl 4):S41–7.

23. Park SJ, Tector A, Piccioni W, et al. Left ventricular assist devices as destination therapy: a new look at survival. J Thorac Cardiovasc Surg 2005;129:9–17.

24. Rogers JG, Butler J, Lansman SL, et al. Chronic mechanical circulatory support for inotrope-dependent heart failure patients who are not transplant candidates: results of the INTrEPID Trial. J Am Coll Cardiol 2007;50:741–7.

25. Holman WL, Pae WE, Teuteberg JJ, et al. INTERMACS: interval analysis of registry data. J Am Coll Surg 2009;208:755–61.

26. Kirklin JK, Naftel DC, Kormos RL, et al. The fourth INTERMACS annual report: 4000 implants and counting. J Heart Lung Transplant 2012;31:117–26.

27. Stevenson LW, Pagani FD, Young JB, et al. INTERMACS profiles of advanced heart failure: the current picture. J Heart Lung Transplant 2009;28:535–41.

28. Lietz K, Miller LW. Patient selection for left-ventricular assist devices. Curr Opin Cardiol 2009;24:246–51.

29. Alba AC, Rao V, Ivanov J, et al. Usefulness of the INTERMACS scale to predict outcomes after mechanical assist device implantation. J Heart Lung Transplant 2009;28:827–33.
30. Teuteberg JJ, Ewald GA, Adamson RM, et al. Risk assessment for continuous flow left ventricular assist devices: does the destination therapy risk score work? An analysis of over 1000 patients. J Am Coll Cardiol 2012;60:44–51.
31. Matthews JC, Koelling TM, Pagani FD, et al. The right ventricular failure risk score: a preoperative tool for assessing the risk of right ventricular failure in left ventricular assist device candidates. J Am Coll Cardiol 2008;51:2163–72.
32. Potapov EV, Loebe M, Nasseri BA, et al. Pulsatile flow in patients with a novel non-pulsatile implantable ventricular assist device. Circulation 2000;102(19 Suppl 3): III183–7.
33. John R. Current axial-flow devices: the HeartMate II and Jarvik 2000 left ventric-ular assist devices. Semin Thorac Cardiovasc Surg 2008;20:264–72.
34. Thalmann M, Schima H, Wieselthaler G, et al. Physiology of continuous blood flow in recipients of rotary cardiac assist devices. J Heart Lung Transplant 2005;24:237–45.
35. OOtaki C, Yamashita M, OOtaki Y, et al. Reduced pulsatility induces periarteritis in kidney: role of local renin-angiotensin system. J Thorac Cardiovasc Surg 2008;136:150–8.
36. Nishimura T, Tatsumi E, Takaichi S, et al. Prolonged nonpulsatile left heart bypass with reduced systemic pulse pressure causes morphological changes in the aortic wall. Artif Organs 1998;22:405–10.
37. Kihara S, Litwak KN, Nichols L, et al. Smooth muscle cell hypertrophy of renal cortex arteries with chronic continuous flow left ventricular assist. Ann Thorac Surg 2003;75:178–83.
38. Frazier OH, Myers TJ, Westaby S, et al. Use of the Jarvik 2000 left ventricular assist system as a bridge to heart transplantation or as destination therapy for patients with chronic heart failure. Ann Surg 2003;237:631–6.
39. Mudd JO, Cuda JD, Halushka M, et al. Fusion of aortic valve commissures in patients supported by a continuous axial flow left ventricular assist device. J Heart Lung Transplant 2008;27:1269–74.
40. Tominaga R, Smith WA, Massiello A, et al. Chronic non-pulsatile blood flow. I. Cerebral autoregulation in chronic nonpulsatile biventricular bypass: carotid blood flow response to hypercapnia. J Thorac Cardiovasc Surg 1994;108: 907–12.
41. Letsou GV, Shah N, Gregoric ID, et al. Gastrointestinal bleeding from arteriove-nous malformations in patients supported by the Jarvik 2000 axial flow left ventricular assist device. J Heart Lung Transplant 2005;24:105–9.
42. Stern DR, Kazam J, Edwards P, et al. Increased incidence of gastrointestinal bleeding following implantation of the HeartMate II LVAD. J Card Surg 2010; 25:352–6.
43. Pate GE, Mulligan A. An epidemiological study of Heyde's syndrome: an asso-ciation between aortic stenosis and gastrointestinal bleeding. J Heart Valve Dis 2004;13:713–6.
44. Heyde EC. Gastrointestinal bleeding in aortic stenosis [Letter to the editor]. N Engl J Med 1958;259:196.
45. Singh P, Scoyni R, Pooran N, et al. Aortic valve replacement: a last resort for aortic stenosis-associated refractory GI bleeding. Gastrointest Endosc 2002; 56:139–41.

46. Warkentin TE, Moore JC, Morgan DG. Aortic stenosis and bleeding gastrointes-tinal angiodysplasia: is acquired von Willebrand's disease the link? Lancet 1992; 340:35–7.
47. Vincentelli A, Susen S, Le Tourneau T, et al. Acquired von Willebrand syndrome in aortic stenosis. N Engl J Med 2003;349:343–9.
48. Geisen U, Heilmann C, Beyersdorf F, et al. Nonsurgical bleeding in patients with ventricular assist devices could be explained by acquired von Willebrand disease. Eur J Cardiothorac Surg 2008;33:679–84.
49. Klovaite J, Gustafsson F, Mortensen SA, et al. Severely impaired von Willebrand factor-dependent platelet aggregation in patients with a continuous-flow left ventricular assist device (HeartMate II). J Am Coll Cardiol 2009;53:2162–7.
50. Cappell MS, Lebwohl O. Cessation of recurrent bleeding from gastrointestinal angiodysplasias after aortic valve replacement. Ann Intern Med 1986;105:54–7.
51. Meyer AL, Malehsa D, Bara C, et al. Acquired von Willebrand syndrome in patients with an axial flow left ventricular assist device. Circ Heart Fail 2010;3: 675–81.
52. Boyle AJ, Russell SD, Teuteberg JJ, et al. Low thromboembolism and pump thrombosis with the HeartMate II left ventricular assist device: analysis of outpa-tient anti-coagulation. J Heart Lung Transplant 2009;28:881–7.
53. Miller LW, Pagani FD, Russell SD, et al. Use of a continuous-flow device in patients awaiting heart transplantation. N Engl J Med 2007;357:885–96.
54. Griffith BP, Kormos RL, Borovetz HS, et al. HeartMate II left ventricular assist system: from concept to first clinical use. Ann Thorac Surg 2001;71(Suppl 3): S116–20.
55. Khalil HA, Cohn WE, Metcalfe RW, et al. Preload sensitivity of the Jarvik 2000 and HeartMate II left ventricular assist devices. ASAIO J 2008;54:245–8.
56. Mano A, Fujita K, Uenomachi K, et al. Body mass index is a useful predictor of prognosis after left ventricular assist system implantation. J Heart Lung Trans-plant 2009;28:428–33.
57. Holdy K, Dembitsky W, Eaton LL, et al. Nutrition assessment and management of left ventricular assist device patients. J Heart Lung Transplant 2005;24:1690–6.
58. Farrar DJ, Compton PG, Hershon JJ, et al. Right heart interaction with the me-chanically assisted left heart. World J Surg 1985;9:89–102.
59. Santamore WP, Gray LA Jr. Left ventricular contributions to right ventricular systolic function during LVAD support. Ann Thorac Surg 1996;61:350–6.
60. Patel ND, Weiss ES, Schaffer J, et al. Right heart dysfunction after left ventricular assist device implantation: a comparison of the pulsatile HeartMate I and axial-flow HeartMate II devices. Ann Thorac Surg 2008;86:832–40.
61. Kormos RL, Teuteberg JJ, Pagani FD, et al. Right ventricular failure in patients with the HeartMate II continuous-flow left ventricular assist device: incidence, risk factors, and effect on outcomes. J Thorac Cardiovasc Surg 2010;139: 1316–24.
62. Sandner SE, Zimpfer D, Zrunek P, et al. Renal function and outcome after contin-uous flow left ventricular assist device implantation. Ann Thorac Surg 2009;87: 1072–8.
63. Kormos RL, Teuteberg JJ, Siegenthaler MP, et al. Pre-VAD implant risk factors influence the onset of adverse events (AEs) while on VAD [abstract]. J Heart Lung Transplant 2009;28:S153–4.
64. Feussner M, Mukherjee C, Garbade J, et al. Anaesthesia for patients under-going ventricular assist-device implantation. Best Pract Res Clin Anaesthesiol 2012;26:167–77.

65. Nussmeier NA, Probert CB, Hirsch D, et al. Anesthetic management for implantation of the Jarvik 2000 left ventricular assist system. Anesth Analg 2003;97:964–71.
66. Broussard D, Donaldson E, Falterman J, et al. Anesthesia for left ventricular assist device insertion: a case series and review. Ochsner J 2011;11:70–7.
67. Stone ME. Current status of mechanical circulatory assistance. Semin Cardiothorac Vasc Anesth 2007;11:185–204.
68. Thinberg CA, Gaitan BD, Arabia FA, et al. Ventricular assist devices today and tomorrow. J Cardiothorac Vasc Anesth 2010;24:656–80.
69. Kavarana MN, Pessin-Minsley MS, Urtecho J, et al. Right ventricular dysfunction and organ failure in left ventricular assist device recipients: a continuing problem. Ann Thorac Surg 2002;73:745–50.
70. Deng MC, Edwards LB, Hertz MI, et al. Mechanical circulatory support device database of the International Society for Heart and Lung Transplantation: Third Annual Report—2005. J Heart Lung Transplant 2005;24:1182–7.
71. Dang NC, Topkara VK, Mercando M, et al. Right heart failure after left ventricular assist device implantation in patients with chronic congestive heart failure. J Heart Lung Transplant 2006;25:1–6.
72. Fukamachi K, McCarthy PM, Smedira NG, et al. Preoperative risk factors for right ventricular failure after implantable left ventricular assist device insertion. Ann Thorac Surg 1999;68:2181–4.
73. Kormos RL, Gasior TA, Kawai A, et al. Transplant candidate's clinical status rather than right ventricular function defines need for univentricular versus biventricular support. J Thorac Cardiovasc Surg 1996;111:773–82.
74. Ochiai Y, McCarthy PM, Smedira NG, et al. Predictors of severe right ventricular failure after implantable left ventricular assist device insertion: analysis of 245 patients. Circulation 2002;106(12 Suppl I):I198–202.
75. Nakatani A, Thomas JD, Savage RM, et al. Prediction of right ventricular dysfunction after left ventricular assist device implantation. Circulation 1996;94(Suppl 9):II216–21.
76. De Wet CJ, Affleck DG, Jacobsohn E, et al. Inhaled prostacyclin is safe, effective, and affordable in patients with pulmonary hypertension, right heart dysfunction, and refractory hypoxemia after cardiothoracic surgery. J Thorac Cardiovasc Surg 2004;127:1058–67.
77. Oz MC, Argenziano M, Catanese KA, et al. Bridge experience with long-term implantable left ventricular assist devices: are they an alternative to transplantation? Circulation 1997;95:1844–52.
78. Salzberg SP, Lachat ML, Zund G, et al. Left ventricular assist device (LVAD) enables survival during 7 h of sustained ventricular fibrillation. Eur J Cardiothorac Surg 2004;26:444–6.
79. Argenziano M, Choudhri AF, Oz MC, et al. A prospective randomized trial of arginine vasopressin in the treatment of vasodilatory shock after left ventricular assist device placement. Circulation 1997;96(Suppl 9):II286–90.
80. Maslow AD, Stearns G, Butala P, et al. The hemodynamic effects of methylene blue when administered at the onset of cardiopulmonary bypass. Anesth Analg 2006;103:2–8.
81. Potapov EV, Pasic M, Bauer M, et al. Activated recombinant factor VII for control of diffuse bleeding after implantation of ventricular assist device. Ann Thorac Surg 2002;74:2182–3.
82. Heise D, Brauer A, Quintel M. Recombinant activated factor VII (Novo7) in patients with ventricular assist devices: case report and review of the current literature. J Cardiothorac Surg 2007;2:47.

83. Bruckner BA, DiBardino DJ, Ning Q, et al. High incidence of thromboembolic events in left ventricular assist device patients treated with recombinant activated factor VII. J Heart Lung Transplant 2009;28:785–90.

84. Banchis JE, Dawn B, Abdel-Latif A, et al. Acquired aortic cusp fusion after chronic left ventricular assist device support. J Am Soc Echocardiogr 2006; 19:1401.e1–3.

85. Haghi D, Suselbeck T, Saur J. Aortic regurgitation during left ventricular assist device support. J Heart Lung Transplant 2007;26:1220–1.

86. Park SJ, Liao KK, Segurola R, et al. Management of aortic insufficiency in patients with left ventricular assist devices: a simple coaptation stitch method (Park's stitch). J Thorac Cardiovasc Surg 2004;127:264–6.

87. Stringham JC, Bull DA, Karwande SV. Patch closure of the aortic anulus in a recipient of a ventricular assist device. J Thorac Cardiovasc Surg 2000;119: 1293–4.

88. Marriott K, Manins V, Forshaw A, et al. Detection of right-to-left atrial communication using agitated saline contrast imaging: experience with 1162 patients and recommendations for echocardiography. J Am Soc Echocardiogr. Available at: http://dx.doi.org/10.1016/j.echo.2012.09.007. Accessed October, 2012.

89. Lynch JJ, Schuchard GH, Gross CM, et al. Prevalence of right-to-left atrial shunting in a healthy population: detection by Valsalva maneuver contrast echocardiography. Am J Cardiol 1984;53:1478–80.

90. Scalia GM, McCarthy PM, Savage RM, et al. Clinical utility of echocardiography in the management of implantable ventricular assist devices. J Am Soc Echocardiogr 2000;13:754–63.

91. Catena E, Milazzo F, Merli M, et al. Echocardiographic evaluation of patients receiving a new left ventricular assist device: the Impella® Recover 100. Eur J Echocardiogr 2004;5:430–7.

92. May-Newman KD, Hillen BK, Sironda CS, et al. Effect of LVAD outflow conduit insertion angle on flow through the native aorta. J Med Eng Technol 2004;28: 105–9.

93. Topilsky Y, Maltais S, Oh JK, et al. Focused review on transthoracic echocardiographic assessment of patients with continuous axial flow left ventricular assist devices. Cardiol Res Pract 2011;2011:187434.

94. Slaughter MS, Pagani FD, Rogers JG, et al. Clinical management of continuous-flow left ventricular assist devices in advanced heart failure. J Heart Lung Transplant 2010;29(Suppl 4):S1–39.

95. Maniar S, Kondareddy S, Topkara VK. Left ventricular assist device-related infections: past, present, and future. Expert Rev Med Devices 2011;8: 627–34.

96. Ankersmit HJ, Edwards NM, Schuster M, et al. Quantitative changes in T-cell populations after left ventricular assist device implantation: relationship to T-cell apoptosis and soluble CD95. Circulation 1999;100(Suppl 19):II211–5.

97. Aaronson KD, Slaughter MS, Miller LW, et al. Use of an intrapericardial, continuous-flow, centrifugal pump in patients awaiting heart transplantation. Circulation 2012;125:3191–200.

98. Catena E, Milazzo F, Montorsi E, et al. Left ventricular support by axial flow pump: the echocardiographic approach to device malfunction. J Am Soc Echocardiogr 2005;18:1422.e7–e13.

99. Estep JD, Stainback RF, Little SH, et al. The role of echocardiography and other imaging modalities in patients with left ventricular assist devices. J Am Coll Cardiol 2010;3:1049–64.

100. Hoshi H, Shinshi T, Takatani S. Third-generation blood pumps with mechanical noncontact magnetic bearings. Artif Organs 2006;30:324–38.
101. Farrar DJ, Bourque K, Dague CP, et al. Design features, developmental status, and experimental results with the HeartMate III centrifugal left ventricular assist system with a magnetically levitated rotor. ASAIO J 2007;53:310–5.
102. Nojiri C, Kijima T, Maekawa J, et al. Development status of Terumo implantable left ventricular assist system. Artif Organs 2001;25:411–3.
103. Morshuis M, El-Banayosy A, Arusoglu L, et al. European experience with Dura-Heart magnetically levitated centrifugal left ventricular assist system. Eur J Cardiothorac Surg 2009;35:1020–7.
104. Slaughter MS, Sobieski MA II, Tamez D, et al. HeartWare miniature axial-flow ventricular assist device: design and initial feasibility test. Tex Heart Inst J 2009;36:12–6.
105. Tuzun E, Roberts K, Cohn WE, et al. In vivo evaluation of the HeartWare centrifugal ventricular assist device. Tex Heart Inst J 2007;34:406–11.
106. LaRose J, Tamez D, Ashenuga M, et al. Design concepts and principle of operation of the HeartWare ventricular assist system. ASAIO J 2010;56:285–9.
107. Strueber M, O'Driscoll G, Jansz P, et al. Multicenter evaluation of an intrapericardial left ventricular assist system. J Am Coll Cardiol 2011;57:1375–82.
108. Wieselthaler GM, O'Driscoll G, Jansz P, et al. Initial clinical experience with a novel left ventricular assist device with a magnetically levitated rotor in a multi-institutional trial. J Heart Lung Transplant 2010;29:1218–25.
109. Hetzer R, Krabatsch T, Stepanenko A, et al. Long-term biventricular support with the HeartWare implantable continuous flow pump. J Heart Lung Transplant 2010;29:822–4.
110. Aaronson KD, Slaughter MS, McGee E, et al. Evaluation of the HeartWare® HVAD left ventricular assist system for the treatment of advanced heart failure: results of the ADVANCE Bridge to Transplant Trial [abstract]. Circulation 2010;122:2215–26.
111. Kirklin JK, Naftel DC, Pagani FD, et al. Long-term mechanical circulatory support (destination therapy): on track to compete with heart transplantation? J Thorac Cardiovasc Surg 2012;144:584–603.
112. Stehlik J, Edwards LB, Kucheryavaya AY, et al. The Registry of the International Society for Heart and Lung Transplantation: Twenty-eighth Adult Heart Transplant Report—2011. J Heart Lung Transplant 2011;30:1078–94.

Transcatheter Aortic Valve Replacement

Andrej Alfirevic, MD*, Anand R. Mehta, MD, Lars G. Svensson, MD

KEYWORDS

- Rapid ventricular pacing • Paravalvular aortic insufficiency • Transfemoral approach
- Transapical approach • Balanced general anesthesia

KEY POINTS

- Percutaneous transcatheter aortic valve replacement was introduced in 2002, with a recent approval in inoperable surgical candidates.
- Balanced general anesthesia or monitored anesthesia care in addition to local anesthesia have been used during transfemoral and transapical approaches.
- The results of different registries and the PARTNER trial showed excellent success and survival rates, but stroke and paravalvular insufficiency represent major concerns.

EQUIPMENT

The first human percutaneous transcatheter aortic valve replacement (TAVR) procedure was performed by Dr Alain Cribier in Rouen, France in 2002.[1] This innovative technology used a stent-valve, delivered by the deployment device via the femoral antegrade venous pathway, puncturing the interatrial septum (**Fig. 1**). The procedure was successful but was soon realized to be associated with many technical risks, predominantly related to many anatomic turns that need to be made to properly position the stent-valve at the aortic valve (AV) annulus. The acquirement of the technology by Edwards Lifesciences in 2004 opened up the possibility for further evolution, resulting in the implementation of retrograde transfemoral arterial and anterograde transapical approaches that are currently used (**Fig. 1**). The initial results and success of the procedure in very high-risk octogenarians, reported by Webb and colleagues,[2] showed a 30-day mortality rate of 11%. The experience with the percutaneous stent-valve technology in the majority of United States medical centers has been limited, until recently, to the Edwards SAPIEN (Edwards Lifesciences, Irving, CA) valves. This review focuses predominantly on the use of this technology for transfemoral and transapical TAVR procedures because this is the only stent-valve technology that is approved by the

Cardiothoracic Anesthesiology, Cleveland Clinic Lerner College of Medicine of Case Western Reserve University, Cleveland Clinic, 9500 Euclid Avenue, Cleveland, OH 44195, USA
* Corresponding author.
E-mail address: alfirea@ccf.org

Anesthesiology Clin 31 (2013) 355–381
http://dx.doi.org/10.1016/j.anclin.2012.12.004
1932-2275/13/$ – see front matter Published by Elsevier Inc.
anesthesiology.theclinics.com

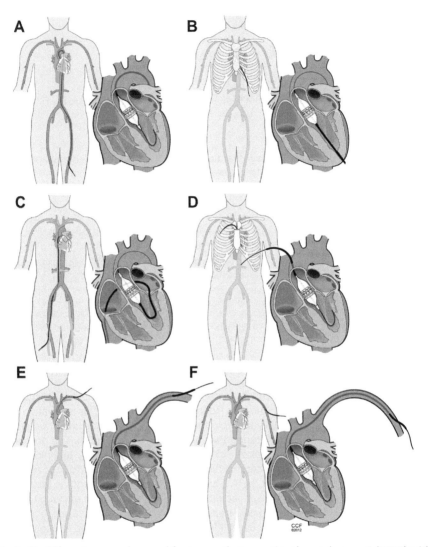

Fig. 1. Six different approaches used for transcatheter aortic valve replacement (TAVR) with a stent-valve. (*A*) Retrograde transfemoral arterial approach from femoro-iliac vessels. (*B*) Antegrade left ventricular transapical approach via anterolateral mini-thoracotomy. (*C*) Antegrade transfemoral venous approach, used during initial experience. (*D*) Retrograde trans-aortic approach via mini–anterior thoracotomy. (*E*) Retrograde trans-subclavian artery approach via surgical cut-down. (*F*) Retrograde trans-axillary artery approach via percutaneous Seldinger method.

Food and Drug Administration for the treatment of patients with symptomatic inoperable severe aortic stenosis (AS).

The current third-generation Edwards SAPIEN XT valve is made of bovine-pericardial tissue leaflets mounted inside a balloon-expandable cobalt chromium alloy tubular frame (**Fig. 2**).[3,4] Once the delivery device is introduced, the stent-valve is crimped on the balloon catheter by the technician. At present there are 2 stent-valve

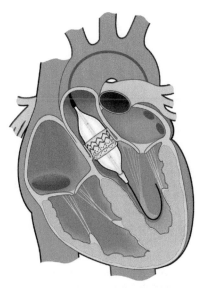

Fig. 2. Edwards SAPIEN aortic valve prosthesis. The prosthesis is crimped onto the expandable balloon and positioned via the retrograde arterial approach at the level of the aortic valve annulus.

sizes available, 23 and 26 mm, with 20- and 29-mm stent-valves awaiting clinical application in the United States. The stent-valve is sized according to the measurement of the AV annulus diameter. The 23-mm valve is reserved for an annular diameter of 18 to 21 mm and the 26-mm valve for annular diameter of 22 to 25 mm. The length of the stent-valve is 14 and 16 mm for the 23- and 26-mm stent-valve, respectively. The stent-valve is delivered via the RetroFlex transfemoral delivery system (Edwards Lifesciences) that includes an introducer sheath set and dilator kits measuring 22F for the 23-mm and 24F for the 26-mm stent-valve, respectively. The newer SAPIEN XT technology uses 16F to 19F SAPIEN XT/NovaFlex delivery sheaths, enabling its use in patients with smaller vessels and also potentially decreasing the incidence of major vascular complications.[4] The delivery sheath used in transapical implantation procedures is 26F in size.

The CoreValve ReValving System (Medtronic CoreValve, Irving, CA) was initially introduced in 2006 for TAVR.[3] This self-expandable system consists of 3 porcine pericardial leaflets (**Fig. 3**). The CoreValve is mounted and sutured into a self-expandable nitinol stent, which deforms under cold temperatures and regains its undeformed shape at warmer body temperatures. The intraprocedural preparation of the valve involves crimping of the valve in ice water onto the delivery catheter. After proper positioning, at body temperature the stent will self-expand and assume the contours of the AV apparatus, namely AV annulus and sinotubular junction. The CoreValve system is available in 22- and 26-mm diameters with a stent frame that is 50 mm in length. The proximal part of the valve expands against the AV annulus and native leaflet tissue, while the middle part holds the leaflets and the distal part anchors the valve at the sinotubular junction of the proximal ascending aorta. The initial delivery system included sizes 22F to 25F, but the current system uses delivery systems (Accutrak delivery catheter [Medtronic]) that are 18F or 19F in diameter.[4,5] The potential advantage of the CoreValve system over the Edwards SAPIEN system includes absence of rapid

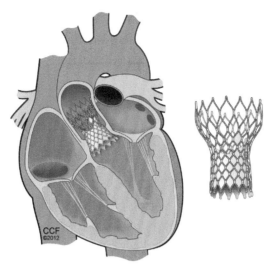

Fig. 3. CoreValve aortic valve prosthesis. This valve is self-expandable, with 2 anchoring points at the annulus and the sinotubular junction.

ventricular pacing (RVP) during deployment potentially related to less hemodynamic instability, ability for retrieval if positioned incorrectly, and 2, instead of 1, anchoring points.[5] However, the increased valve length may lead to a relatively high rate of acute and delayed heart block and potentially delayed occlusion of the coronary ostia.[3,5] The CoreValve can also be used for patients with predominant AV insufficiency. Because the literature is lacking as regards randomized comparative trials between the two stent-valve systems, it is hard to speculate about their potential clinical benefits.[5] The recent meta-analysis of high-risk patients scheduled for surgical aortic valve replacement (SAVR) and TAVR reported an increased incidence of pacemaker insertion in patients who received the CoreValve compared with those who received the Edwards SAPIEN valve (24.5% vs 5.9%; $P<.0001$), with a comparable rate of procedural success.[6] A variety of different manufacturers are battling for supremacy in the field, with designs more likely involving self-expandable features rather than balloon-expandable features.[5]

INDICATIONS AND CONTRAINDICATIONS

Patients with symptomatic severe AS have an increased risk of dying if treated medically alone.[7–9] Without SAVR about 75% of patients will die in 3 years after the onset of symptoms.[10] Therefore, SAVR is a treatment of choice for improving survival and quality of life in symptomatic patients with severe AS.[10] However, at least one-third of symptomatic patients may not undergo SAVR owing to refusal, comorbidities, or advanced age and frailty.[11,12] As with any other surgical procedure, risks associated with SAVR exist and are related to the patient's comorbidities and the expertise of the surgical team. Patients younger than 70 years undergoing isolated SAVR have a fairly low overall operative mortality of less than 3%.[13] Nevertheless, 30-day postprocedural mortality after SAVR in octogenarians with decreased left ventricular (LV) function is reported to be 12% and increases to 17% in nonagenerians.[14,15] In addition, a rate of stroke of 1.4% to 4.8% has been reported after SAVR in high-risk patients,[16,17] and of 8% in patients older than 80 years.[18] Therefore the minimally invasive TAVR was specifically developed with the hope of decreasing morbidity and mortality in the highest-risk patient population. TAVR registries from different centers worldwide are reporting a procedural success rate of more than 93%.[19–22] The 30-day mortality rate of patients at very high or prohibitive surgical risk is reported to be 9% to 11%, which is comparable with the estimated Society of Thoracic Surgeons (STS) risk scores for each patient.[19–21] Recently 2 randomized, prospective controlled trials describing the use of TAVR technology have been completed. The Placement of Aortic Transcatheter Valves (PARTNER) trial showed a 30-day mortality rate of 6.4% and 20% absolute improvement in survival at 1 year, compared with medically managed patients who were not suitable surgical candidates (Cohort B).[9,23] One year following the publication of these results, the analysis of the Cohort A arm of the PARTNER trial was published, showing a noninferior 1-year survival rate in the high-risk patient population undergoing TAVR in comparison with the SAVR procedure.[23,24] Even though the initial short-term and intermediate-term results show comparability with a more invasive surgical procedure, the trade-off, at least for now, is related to the increased incidence of neurologic events including major stroke and peripheral vascular injury. The PARTNER trial also demonstrated improvements in patients' quality of life demonstrated as a reduction in rehospitalization when compared with medically managed patients.[9,25] In comparison with surgically managed patients, patients with transfemoral TAVR had a significantly shorter length of stay as well as earlier improvement in functional status.[24] Recently, a 2-year outcomes analysis of patients from Cohorts A and B were published, sustaining the positive findings.[26,27] Current literature therefore shows positive results in the very high-risk or inoperable patient population whereby benefits associated with TAVR outweigh the risks. In March 2012 an expert consensus document reported: "TAVR is appropriate currently only for a highly select population and the valve team should systematically identify the characteristics that define that population with the most benefit and acceptable risk."[28] Furthermore, recent literature describes a shift of indications for TAVR procedure in patients to below the high-risk level.[29,30] Major contributors of the success and improved outcomes that may apply to the lower-risk patient population are related to the growing operator experience and evolution of technology.[21,29,31,32] The transfemoral or transapical approach has not been predicated as a risk factor for late mortality in lower-risk patients, given the caveat of selection bias that is present in most of the current literature.[32–34]

The advantage of using the transapical rather than the transfemoral approach includes avoidance of manipulation of the iliofemoral vessels, aorta, and aortic arch, particularly if atherosclerotic disease is present. In addition, the alignment of the stent-valve within the AV annulus is more coaxial. The disadvantage is related to the need for a thoracotomy incision, which is more painful. Moreover, injury to the myocardium resulting from access of the LV apex may result in catastrophic bleeding. The initial Feasibility study reported a 17.5% 30-day mortality rate in patients undergoing the transapical approach.[35] Initial studies reported higher rates of neurologic events in patients undergoing a transfemoral[36,37] (4%–10%) compared with a transapical[38,39] (0%–3%) approach. Contrary to these reports, recent large studies comparing transfemoral versus transapical approaches found similar postprocedural rates of cerebral ischemic events and no direct association with the burden of aortic atheroma.[20,21,33,34] In addition, no direct correlation was found with the severity of valvular calcification or amount of RVP.[34] The mechanical stress of AV valvuloplasty, stent-valve deployment, and gaseous embolism is more likely derived from mechanisms linking both transapical and transfemoral approaches with cerebral ischemic events.[34] Even though the patients presenting for the transapical approach may exhibit more significant risk factors before the procedure, the 30-day and 1-year mortality are comparable between the two approaches.[40] Newer approaches including transaortic and left subclavian techniques are being used, which are better tolerated by patients without inflicting direct myocardial injury.[41]

Although no strict exclusion criteria exist, patients with significant cognitive dysfunction due to Alzheimer dementia, concomitant severe mitral disease, Child B hepatic cirrhosis, and very poor physical condition may not be suitable candidates for TAVR.[28,42] Presence of LV dysfunction and nonrevascularized coronary disease, mitral valve regurgitation greater than 3+, tricuspid valve regurgitation greater than 3+, coagulopathy, uncontrolled atrial fibrillation, severe chronic obstructive pulmonary disease, and pulmonary hypertension all represent relative contraindications and predict a higher chance of intraprocedural instability.[28,36,37,43] In addition, strictly procedure-related contraindications to TAVR include an AV annulus that is too small (<18 mm) or too large (>25 mm) to accommodate currently available prostheses, and severe peripheral vascular disease (atherosclerosis, arterial aneurysm).[28,36,37,43] A recent case report highlights the presence of idiopathic hypertrophic subaortic stenosis as well as prominent septal hypertrophy as a contraindication for TAVR because of the increased risk of valve embolization.[44] The predictors of late mortality after TAVR include body mass index, periprocedural sepsis, the need for hemodynamic support, pulmonary hypertension, preexisting chronic kidney disease, chronic obstructive pulmonary disease, logistic EuroSCORE, STS score, age, liver disease, severe mitral regurgitation, and anemia.[9,20,45] In addition, the short-term or long-term risks and benefits of the TAVR procedure in asymptomatic patients with severe AS are currently unknown. Therefore, given the current risks associated with the TAVR procedure, this subgroup of AS patients are not optimal candidates for this technology.[46,47]

PATIENT PREPARATION

During the preprocedural evaluation, the multidisciplinary team is confronted with the elderly patient exhibiting multiple comorbidities. The intention of TAVR is to decrease the invasiveness of the open surgical procedure while maintaining the same rate of success. The current literature supports the use of TAVR in the inoperable patient population.[9,24] Predicting the risk of morbidity and mortality using the EuroSCORE and STS score overestimates the true risk of SAVR in older patients with comorbidities.[48] Furthermore, no scoring system exists that is able to risk-stratify patients who are being evaluated for TAVR procedure. It is interesting that none of the traditional scoring systems include specific evaluation for the presence of "porcelain aorta," frailty, "hostile chest," or coronary grafts crossing the midline or adherent to sternum. Thus the preoperative decision process strongly relies on the multidisciplinary team approach, evaluating factors such as frailty, functional status, availability, experience, technical skills, local results, referral patterns, and patient preference.[28,49,50] Preoperative evaluation does not significantly differ from the usual preoperative assessment of the patient scheduled for aortic valve replacement, although some additional procedure-specific details need attention. The patient criteria for TAVR eligibility are derived from the existent trials and include a high operative risk score (EuroSCORE and STS PROME score), advanced lung disease, surgery denied by at least 2 cardiac surgeons, and previous sternotomy with functional coronary bypass grafts.[28] Similarly, an estimated 30-day mortality risk is assessed by incorporating a thorough clinical evaluation with one of the traditional scoring systems.[50] In addition to a thorough history and physical examination, different diagnostic modalities such as echocardiography, angiography, and computed tomography (CT) are used for assessment of patient eligibility.

Preoperative transthoracic echocardiography (TTE) and transesophageal echocardiography (TEE) provide assessment of the AS severity, structural and functional assessment of the other valves, and assessment of left and right ventricular function and regional wall motion abnormalities.[51] The size of the AV annulus is measured with TTE, TEE, CT, and angiography, with the final decision made from careful evaluation of measurements derived from all modalities. Accurate measurement of the AV annulus is critical to assure adequate sizing of Edwards SAPIEN stent-valve, which was shown to minimize risks of paravalvular leaks, valve malposition, aortic root rupture, and heart block.[52,53] In addition, the degree and distribution of AV calcification were shown to be directly related to the severity of the paravalvular leak after TAVR.[54,55] The accurate measurement of the ascending aortic diameter is important for sizing during CoreValve TAVR. Although sizing has been primarily obtained by either TTE or TEE and has shown a good procedural success rate, more recent studies showed an underestimation of the AV diameters obtained by 2-dimensional (2D) echocardiography in comparison with multidetector CT (MDCT) or 3-dimensional (3D) echocardiography.[56–61] Furthermore, intraprocedural TEE evaluation assists with balloon valvuloplasty and confirms the accurate position of the stent-valve, and is important for timely diagnosis of the paravalvular or central leaks as well as procedural complications such as cardiac tamponade, aortic dissection, or myocardial ischemia.[51] Invasive angiography and CT scan of the chest and pelvis are important to assess the location, severity, and tortuosity of the atherosclerotic disease in the aorta and peripheral arteries, determining the eligibility for the transfemoral approach. Compliant arteries can accommodate sheaths that are 1 to 2 mm larger than their internal diameters, though not in cases of severe atheromatous disease, calcification, or tortuosity. Coronary angiography evaluates for the presence and severity of coronary artery lesions and patency of previous coronary grafts. In patients with previous open heart surgery, CT scan of the chest with angiographic contrast evaluates the proximity of the coronary grafts to the undersurface of the sternum, which may change the vascular cannulation strategy should the need for rescue cardiopulmonary bypass (CPB) arise. Laboratory workup should include assessment of the baseline kidney function because many patients present with some degree of chronic insufficiency. The assessment of liver function is focused on the coagulation profile with additional blood workup including hemoglobin, glucose, and type and crossmatch for packed red blood cells. The pulmonary function test, chest radiograph, and arterial blood gas analysis should be performed in patients with respiratory problems to assess the pattern and severity of the disease. Careful airway evaluation is important, not only to avoid possible unexpected difficulty but also to select patients who may benefit from general anesthesia by securing the airway in a more controlled nonemergent fashion. The list of preoperative medications should be reviewed, and the patient instructed to continue medications as they would for any other surgical procedure. Aspirin and clopidogrel may be already part of a patient's list of medications, or they may be newly administered before the procedure. Aspirin in a dose of 75 to 300 mg is usually started before the procedure and is continued indefinitely afterward.[36,62–65] No clear guidelines exist about the need and duration of an antiplatelet medication regimen. Thus, different regimens vary regarding the use of clopidogrel, which is given as a bolus of 75 to 300 mg preoperatively and is continued for 3 to 6 months after the procedure.[36,62–65] Prophylactic antibiotics are continued for 3 to 7 days following the procedure, though without substantial support in the literature.

TECHNIQUE, BEST PRACTICES, AND PROCEDURE STEPS

The transfemoral approach is the first choice in the majority of patients who are considered for TAVR. The eligibility for the transfemoral approach is driven by the size of the iliofemoral arterial vessels, lack of the tortuosity, and significant atherosclerotic disease. The alternative options, such as transapical, transaortic, and subclavian/axillary approaches, are available for patients ineligible for a transfemoral approach.[66] It is important for the success of the procedure that each team member is familiar with the key procedural details.[49] The key elements of the TAVR procedure are guided by the fluoroscopic and echocardiographic imaging. The procedure itself is performed in a catheterization suite or a hybrid operating room (**Figs. 4** and **5**). In either situation, anesthesiologists are working in remote locations where they have to possess flexibility and adaptability to perform the task. Communication between the team members is of utmost importance for the success of the procedure.

Transfemoral Approach

The transfemoral approach requires access to both femoral arteries and at least 1 femoral vein.[3] Initially the access was obtained via surgical cut-down but currently the sheaths are placed via the percutaneous approach, rendering the procedure less painful. A temporary pacemaker wire is introduced via the femoral vein to enable RVP. The same pacemaker wire can be used at the end of the procedure should the need for pacemaking arise owing to the development of heart block. Intraprocedural anticoagulation is achieved by administration of 70 to 100 U/kg of heparin and is titrated to an activated clotting time of longer than 300 seconds.[28] Heparin is given after the wire and small sheaths are in place, before the introduction of larger sheaths carrying the deployment device. In most instances following a successful procedure, protamine is used for the anticoagulation reversal in a 1:1 ratio, although at times reversal may not be needed if the risk of surgical bleeding is low and the risk of thromboembolic events is increased. After the retrograde introduction of the balloon catheter, AV valvuloplasty is performed to dilate and enable introduction of the stent-valve (**Fig. 6**). The AV valvuloplasty may be associated with the displacement of small calcium particles, resulting in stroke or coronary occlusion, sustained ventricular fibrillation, or hemodynamically significant aortic insufficiency.[3] Following AV valvuloplasty the stent-valve, crimped on a 20-mL deflated balloon, is introduced toward the AV annulus. Adequate positioning of the stent-valve at the level of the AV annulus is confirmed by echocardiography and fluoroscopy (**Fig. 7**). The recommended location for the deployed Edwards SAPIEN valve is 50% ventricular from the native leaflets' hinge point.[51] RVP is used to temporarily decrease the forward stroke volume ejection and therefore decrease the chance of stent-valve migration during the deployment.[3,28,66] The rate of RVP is most commonly within 160 to 220 beats/min, which decreases the systolic blood pressure to less than 70 mm Hg and the pulse pressure to less than 20 mm Hg.[28] Temporary suspension of breathing is used to prevent heart translocation during the deployment. The success of the deployment is assessed with echocardiography and angiography, and by obtaining invasive and noninvasive hemodynamic parameters.[28,67,68]

The CoreValve is placed in a similar fashion via the arterial retrograde approach. There are several differences relative to the SAPIEN valve as regards the deployment of the prosthesis. The valve has to be anchored 5 to 10 mm proximally from the AV annulus and distally at the sinotubular junction.[51] The valve's nitinol frame self-expands at body temperature, and RVP is not necessary for the deployment. The delivery sheath is positioned at the AV annulus, and angiography is performed to

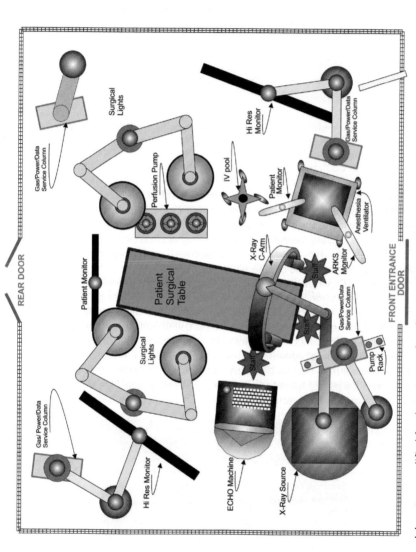

Fig. 4. Catheterization laboratory modified for the purpose of performing the TAVR procedure. Note the location of the anesthesia equipment and its relationship with the patient's table, floor-mounted biplane fluoroscopy machine, and positioning of the rest of the multidisciplinary team members. ARKS, Anesthesia Record-Keeping System; IV, intravenous.

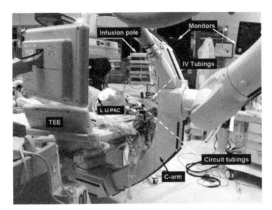

Fig. 5. Hybrid operating room and location of the anesthesia equipment, and its relationship with the patient's table and single-plane fluoroscopy machine coming in from the patient's right-hand side. LIJ, left internal jugular; PAC, pulmonary artery catheter; TEE, transesophageal echocardiography.

evaluate and locate coronary ostia. The crimped valve is deployed by withdrawal of the delivery sheath. The temporary pacemaker wire is still placed, because the AV valvuloplasty is performed under RVP.

Transapical Approach

This approach, which enables direct axial alignment of the stent-valve from the LV apex to the AV annulus, is the only antegrade approach currently in use,[69] and is only possible with the SAPIEN valve. The procedure is performed via mini left anterolateral thoracotomy incision (5–6 cm), usually in the fifth intercostal space. The pericardium is incised and retained with stay sutures. Reinforced purse-string sutures are applied to the LV apex, which is located by TEE visualization.[28] The apex is then punctured and a 14-gauge sheath inserted followed by the guide wire, then a Berman catheter (Arrow International Inc, Reading, PA) and, finally, extra-stiff wire. The balloon valvuloplasty catheter is introduced and valvuloplasty performed under RVP. After

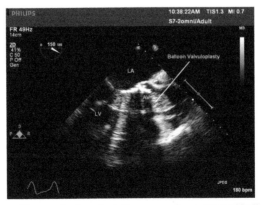

Fig. 6. Mid-esophageal long-axis view depicting properly positioned balloon (*arrow*) during the act of valvuloplasty. Note the electrocardiogram tracing during the rapid ventricular pacing. LA, left atrium; LV, left ventricle; AV, aortic valve.

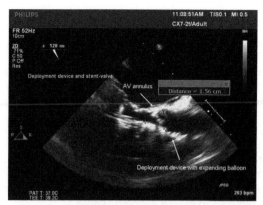

Fig. 7. Mid-esophageal long-axis view depicting properly positioned Edwards SAPIEN stent-valve before deployment. The stent-valve is positioned approximately 50/50 at the annulus. The measurement represents the length of the stent-valve ($\approx$16 mm for the 26-mm size valve). Note the difficulty of 2-dimensional echocardiography in depicting accurate coaxial alignment between the axis of crimped stent-valve and left ventricular outflow tract axis/aortic valve axis. Also note the shadowing of the anterior aortic valve annulus by the deployment device and stent-valve, representing potential difficulty in positioning of the stent-valve perpendicular to the annulus.

withdrawing the balloon catheter, the stent-valve system is introduced. Proper positioning of the stent-valve at the annulus is performed similarly to the transfemoral approach. Following successful deployment the transapical sheath is withdrawn, using RVP once again, and the LV apex closed with purse-string sutures. This approach also enables placement of the temporary or permanent epicardial pacemaker leads.[3,28,41,66]

Other Approaches

Recently a transaortic approach has been successfully used for both types of prosthesis.[28,66] This approach uses either an upper partial sternotomy J-incision or an anterior right mini-thoracotomy incision in the first or second intercostal space.[28,66] A guide wire is placed in retrograde fashion across the AV followed by balloon valvuloplasty and valve deployment. The approach gives the advantage of short distance from the AV, with more control and familiarity for the cardiac surgeon. It also avoids puncture of the LV apex and introduction of a large deployment device through peripheral vessels. Another alternative is the left subclavian approach via surgical cut-down, which may lead to better control during deployment of the prosthesis but is associated with the risk of major intrathoracic bleeding.[22,66] To avoid catastrophic bleeding associated with the left subclavian approach a left axillary approach may be used, which provides an easily reparable access site should injury occur.[66]

Anesthetic Concerns for TAVR

Patients presenting for the TAVR procedure are at the highest risk for encountering hemodynamic instability. The success of the procedure relies on meticulous preparation, vigilance, experience, and communication between the whole team involved in the patient's care. All of these competencies have been highlighted and impressed upon the operators and institutions involved in the care of the patients undergoing TAVR procedures.[49] Procedural requirements for the multidisciplinary team and specific equipment (fluoroscopy, 2D/3D echocardiographic imaging, cardiopulmonary bypass) mandates specific room size (>800 square feet [244 m²]).[28,49] Hybrid operating rooms or modified catheterization suites are used with appropriate air handling and air exchange.[28,49]

Anesthetic concerns for TAVR are the same as those for patients undergoing SAVR. The major differences are related to tailoring anesthetic toward early extubation at the end of the procedure, bearing in mind the patient's age, comorbidities, and hemodynamic goals. The literature does not strongly support which anesthetic type is better suited for patients undergoing transfemoral TAVR. Most procedures are performed under balanced general anesthesia (BGA), but reports exist on the use of monitoring anesthesia care (MAC) with the application of the local anesthetic to a puncture site on the groin.[51,70] Both anesthetic methods have their own advantages and disadvantages, and meticulous patient selection, experience, and expertise of the cardiac anesthesiologist is required to assure success (**Table 1**).

BGA offers secured airway, especially during critical procedural moments, if hemodynamic instability occurs or when the need for emergent surgical intervention arises.[28,63,64] Furthermore, BGA provides the ability to use TEE monitoring throughout the case.[51] Early postprocedural extubation is facilitated by careful titration of short-acting medications with no difference in procedural duration.[71,72] Disadvantages of BGA are related to the potential hemodynamic instability caused by anesthetic medications, producing a decrease in inotropy, chronotropy, and systemic vascular resistance with the need for inotropic and vasotropic support.[73] In addition, with BGA there is always chance of trauma during airway manipulation. Alternatively, MAC with noninvasive ventilation assistance[70] and local anesthetic infiltration provides for a responsive patient, enabling neurologic assessment during the procedure.[28,63,70,74–76] Furthermore, avoidance of anesthetics provides for more stable hemodynamics and

Table 1
Advantages and disadvantages of general anesthesia versus intravenous sedation with local anesthesia for transfemoral TAVR

	Advantages	Disadvantages
Balanced general anesthesia	TEE monitoring throughout procedure Secured airway at all times Ability to suspend mechanical ventilation Better pain control	Airway manipulation and potential damage Potential for prolonged intubation Hemodynamic instability throughout the procedure
Local anesthetic infiltration and IV sedation	Avoidance of airway manipulation Quicker emergence and recovery, shorter hospital stay Neurologic monitoring	Inability to use TEE Procedural need for lying in one position for prolonged period of time Intolerance to decrease in CBF with RVP Unprotected airway (with increase chance for sudden instability) Inability to suspend ventilation Local anesthetic toxicity Escalation in sedation reaching general anesthesia levels

Abbreviations: CBF, cerebral blood flow; RVP, rapid ventricular pacing; TEE, transesophageal echocardiography.

potentially shortens hospital stay.[74,77] If TEE guidance is required for the procedure, BGA is a better choice, but echocardiographic imaging can be obtained via TTE or a brief TEE-probe insertion in a sedated patient.[63,70,76] Conversion to BGA has been reported at the rate of 17%, with the potential for increased procedural morbidity.[71,77,78]

Transapical TAVR is commonly performed under general anesthesia because of the necessity for mechanical ventilation during anterolateral thoracotomy.[28,76] Nevertheless, epidural anesthetic in the spontaneously breathing, awake patient for the transapical approach has been reported.[79] The subclavian approach is performed via surgical cut-down, requiring deeper levels of sedation or BGA.[66,70]

If BGA is used for TAVR, before induction a large-bore peripheral intravenous line and a radial arterial line (either arm is suitable) for continuous blood-pressure monitoring is placed in addition to standard monitors. In the situation of the subclavian or axillary approach, a contralateral radial artery is accessed. With the transapical approach, the arterial line is preferentially placed in the right radial artery, leaving the left brachial artery free for potential insertion of a pigtail catheter used to obtain aortic root aortography.[35,80] Patients presenting with significant preexisting LV and/or right ventricular (RV) dysfunction and pulmonary hypertension may be optimized by placement of the central venous introducer and pulmonary artery catheter (PAC) before the induction of anesthesia. Furthermore, approximately 1 L of crystalloid is given to optimize preload and compensate for the nil-by-mouth (NPO) status (slower preload optimization in patients with RV failure guided by PAC values). Intravascular fluid management is tailored according to the patient's NPO status, insensible losses, and surgical bleeding. In most cases crystalloids and colloids are sufficient for adequate optimization of the intravascular volume status, but blood and blood-product transfusion may be required with profound bleeding. The incidence of blood transfusion varies from 11.6% of patients reported by Webb and colleagues[21] to 23% and 50% reported by Guinot and colleagues[64] and Covello and colleagues,[63] respectively. Significant blood loss may be encountered during the introduction and removal of the deployment device sheath from the femoral vascular access sites. Moreover, bleeding may be expected from the LV apex puncture site during the transapical approach and intrathoracic bleeding from the subclavian approach.[28,66] A contrast dye injection–guided fluoroscopy is used to assess for arterial dissection or leakage sites requiring vascular stent implantation or open vascular repair.[64] Intraprocedural normothermia is maintained by fluid warming as well as warm forced-air garments.

The hemodynamic goals during induction include maintenance of intravascular preload, contractility, and afterload. In the majority of TAVR cases, following induction and placement of the single-lumen endotracheal tube, an additional large-bore peripheral intravenous line is placed as well as a central venous introducer sheath and PAC to obtain baseline hemodynamic parameters (pulmonary artery systolic, diastolic, and mean pressures; cardiac output and index; wedge pressure). A transapical TAVR approach does not routinely require one-lung ventilation because the lung can easily be retracted.[28] The routine antibiotic prophylaxis is given before the surgical incision or vascular access. The anesthesia is maintained using volatile anesthetics such as isoflurane or sevoflurane, intermediate-acting muscle relaxants such as rocuronium or cis-atracurium, and smaller intermittent doses of fentanyl or infusions of remifentanil, alfentanil, and sufentanil.[62,64,81] During BGA, profound muscle paralysis is not needed for the entire duration of the procedure, but it is important to avoid any patient movement during valvuloplasty and stent-valve deployment. External defibrillation pads are placed in proper locations on the patient's chest. RVP has a negative hemodynamic effect because it decreases myocardial oxygen supply by decreasing cardiac output and, therefore, coronary perfusion pressure, and increases oxygen demand owing to tachycardia. Thus it is important to limit the duration of RVP to a minimum (10–15 seconds) and to provide adequate time for reperfusion of the heart between subsequent RVP episodes. Maintenance of mean systemic pressure of greater than 75 mm Hg is recommended.[28] In most cases the patient's heart rate, normal sinus rhythm, and blood pressure return to baseline levels spontaneously after an RVP episode (see **Fig. 9**). It is not clear whether a large and stiff deployment device introduced through the LV apex during the transapical approach introduces an additional change in LV geometry, potentially leading to exacerbation of LV dysfunction and/or mitral regurgitation caused by the tethering effect. The report by Webb and colleagues[21] has shown a higher need for CPB in the transapical than in the transfemoral approach. A recent report, however, showed that patients with preoperative mitral regurgitation grades 3+ and 4+ tolerated a transapical approach well, with the postprocedural mitral regurgitation grades staying the same or diminishing.[82] In the situation of inadequate return of hemodynamic parameters to baseline, aggressive support of the circulation may be required, using boluses and/or infusions of epinephrine and norepinephrine.[64] In addition to ischemia from RVP, unanticipated significant intravalvular or paravalvular aortic insufficiency (**Figs. 8 and 9**) may result in an acute increase in LV end-diastolic pressure, further diminishing myocardial oxygen supply. While the circulation is aggressively medically supported, a decision should be made for stent-valve reexpansion or deployment of a "valve-in-valve." Theoretical immediate postvalvuloplasty or postdeployment complications include obstruction of the coronary ostia, dislodgment of the valve-stent, pericardial tamponade, and hemodynamically significant ventricular arrhythmias.[21,36,37,63–65,83] The need for mechanical circulatory support via CPB is rare (<5%).[28] Anesthesiologists should have clear preprocedural communication with the cardiologist, surgeon, and perfusionist, with a focus on emergent cannulation strategy. Following successful deployment of the stent-valve and retraction of the deployment device sheaths, patients are prepared for emergence.

POSTPROCEDURE CARE

In approximately 81% of cases emergence from BGA is achieved at the end of the procedure in the catheterization suite,[64] unless contraindicated, in which case the

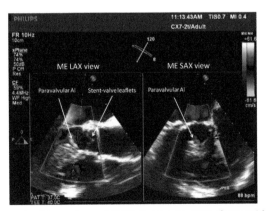

Fig. 8. Two orthogonal mid-esophageal (LAX, long-axis; SAX, short-axis) views with color-flow Doppler depicting the paravalvular insufficiency after stent-valve deployment.

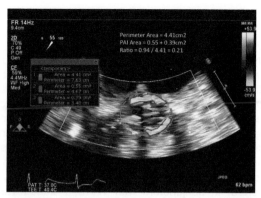

Fig. 9. Mid-esophageal short-axis view of the aortic valve with a color-flow Doppler demonstrating area percentage measurements of the paravalvular insufficiency jets compared with the stent-valve circumferential area. Note the multiple paravalvular jets with crescent-shaped irregular origin. The calculated ratio of measures areas is greater than 20%, suggesting moderate paravalvular insufficiency. Treatment options will include reexpansion and/or deployment of the second stent-valve (valve-in-valve). (*Modified from* Bloomfield GS, Gillam LD, Hahn RT, et al. A practical guide to multimodality imaging of transcatheter aortic valve replacement. JACC Cardiovasc Imaging 2012;5:441–55, with permission.)

patient is transported to the intensive care unit while intubated. The extubation criteria for TAVR procedures are no different from any other procedure whereby general anesthesia has been administered.[28] Before extubation, postoperative nausea and vomiting prophylaxis is administered as well as full reversal of muscle relaxants. Patients recovering from transfemoral TAVR are maintained in the supine position until the removal of the sheaths. Monitoring for groin hematoma, lower extremity ischemia, and retroperitoneal bleeding should be continued throughout the postprocedural period. Particular attention should be applied to prevent significant hypertension during extubation and immediately after the procedure to minimize chances for LV apex rupture in patients after transapical TAVR.[28] Postoperative analgesia for all approaches is managed initially with intermittent boluses of intravenous narcotics (fentanyl or morphine) and oral tramadol or acetaminophen, depending on the patient's needs and institutional preferences.[64] Unless femoral vascular access has been surgically obtained, incisional pain is fairly minimal particularly if infiltrated with local anesthetic (lidocaine, bupivacaine, or ropivacaine). Compared with the transfemoral approach, patients undergoing TAVR via the transapical approach were reported to receive larger doses of longer-acting narcotics[64]; they also experienced lower rates of extubations in the catheterization suite (81% vs 25%, $P<.001$) and longer duration of mechanical ventilation (505 vs 220 minutes, $P<.001$), despite having shorter procedure times (97 vs 120 minutes, $P<.001$).[64] Because of the observational character of the study, this result may represent a selection bias related to transapical patients being "sicker" and procedures being performed though a thoracotomy approach. Patients are given an antiplatelet medication regimen (clopidogrel and aspirin), which is continued throughout the perioperative time, obviating central neuraxial analgesia techniques. Therefore adequate analgesia following anterolateral thoracotomy is minimized by intercostal nerve blockade, under direct surgical vision, using bupivacaine or ropivacaine.[84]

AVOIDING COMPLICATIONS

Transfemoral Approach

Peripheral vascular injury

The reports of early TAVR experience from different registries and randomized trials used unstandardized definitions for outcomes and complications related to the procedure, preventing direct comparison. A recent report from Valve Academic Research Consortium (VARC) established definitions that can be used in research protocols as well as when comparing outcomes variables.[85] The most common complication associated with the transfemoral approach is a peripheral vascular insufficiency (PVI) (femoral and/or iliac), which may result in endothelial avulsion, dissection, rupture, and hemorrhage. In the PARTNER trial, the risk of PVI occurred in 11% of patients undergoing TAVR compared with 3.2% ($P<.001$) for SAVR patients.[24] Major vascular complications reported, in conjuncture with VARC, included vascular dissection (62.8%), vascular perforation (31.3%), access-site hematoma (22.9%), retroperitoneal bleeding (9.5%), false aneurysm (3.4%), and gastrointestinal ischemia (1.6%).[86] Severe atherosclerotic disease and tortuous or aneurysmatic appearance of the peripheral arterial vessels obviates the transfemoral approach altogether in favor of the transapical, transaortic, or subclavian/axillary artery approaches. Evaluation of the size, tortuosity, and calcification of the iliofemoral arteries is determined by CT or invasive angiography. Inadequate preoperative screening of the blood vessels' size and the relatively large size of the introducer is undesirable.[87] Furthermore, the gain in procedural experience over time in combination with smaller sheath sizes is directly related to the decreasing incidence of PVI.[86,88] Toggweiler and colleagues[88] reported a decrease in the incidence of PVI from 8% to 1% from the initial first-generation valve experience versus currently available technology. Analysis of the patients enrolled in the PARTNER trial demonstrated major vascular complications to be fairly frequent (15.3%) after transfemoral TAVR, associated with an almost 5-fold increase in 30-day mortality.[86] In addition, occurrence of major PVI was related to significantly increased risk of major bleeding, transfusions, and renal failure requiring dialysis, embolization or migration of the device, use of hemodynamic support devices, conversion to open heart surgery, greater use of contrast, and longer fluoroscopy times.[86] The attributable risk factors for major PVI include female sex[86,89] (independent of women having small-diameter vessels), femoral artery calcifications,[88,90] smaller diameter of vessels, and a higher sheath to femoral/external iliac artery ratio.[88,90]

Stroke

The rate of neurologic events associated with TAVR is concerning because the incidence of major stroke is higher in high-risk surgical candidates and inoperable patients,[9,24,26,27] with more than two-thirds of patients exhibiting silent cerebral ischemic lesions.[34] The early (30-day) stroke rate has been reported to be in the region of 2.4% in the high-risk PARTNER cohort[24] to 3% to 4% in the recent meta-analysis.[6,91] Furthermore, the rate of neurologic events and major stroke at 1 year in the high-risk surgical TAVR cohort was reported to be 8.3% and 5.1%, compared with 4.3% and 2.4% ($P = .04$ and $P = .07$) in the surgical arm, respectively.[24] In PARTNER A, the transfemoral patients had a 3-times higher incidence of stroke or transient ischemic event than the open control patients (4.6% vs 1.4%, $P = .04$).[24] In the substudy of the PARTNER trial, the risk of neurologic events in the early phase was higher after TAVR than after SAVR.[92] Contrary to the increased risk of stroke reported in the meta-analysis and PARTNER trial comparison of TAVR versus SAVR patients, recent STS database analysis of high-risk patients undergoing isolated SAVR revealed a 4% risk of stroke within 30 days after the procedure.[93] The patient-selection bias and superior outcomes from PARTNER trial have been postulated as factors related to the increased risk of stroke in SAVR patients. Whatever the incidence of the stroke may be, the mechanism and temporal relationship between the procedure and clinical neurologic deficit differ between TAVR and SAVR.

The early peaking high-hazard phase associated with TAVR occurs within the first week, suggesting embolization of the native calcified valve particles. Although the mechanism of the early stroke is mostly related to the volume of cerebral emboli occurring during the procedure,[94] almost half of the early major strokes occurred after 24 hours, suggesting an embolic mechanism different from the one related to catheter use and native valve stretching.[9] A smaller indexed AV area has been reported as a risk factor for early stroke, suggesting an abundance of calcium deposits.[92] Transcranial Doppler (TCD) has been used in TAVR patients to describe the association between cerebral embolism and intraprocedural stroke, reporting high-density transient signals in almost every patient undergoing a TAVR procedure.[95] However, it has been difficult to prove a direct correlation between high-intensity transient signals and stroke or biomarkers of neurologic injury.[96,97]

Following the early phase, the rate of stroke declined to constant late-hazard phase. In the late phase, the chance of a neurologic event is more likely linked to patient-related factors such as generalized atherosclerotic burden rather than procedural or treatment variability.[92] The data from TCD in TAVR patients reports the contribution of the different intraprocedural steps toward the risk of particulate cerebral microembolization.[95] Thus, balloon valvuloplasty has been associated with a progressive increase in risk from initial balloon dilation to postdeployment dilation. Furthermore, the greatest risk during stent-valve delivery occurs during crossing of the native calcified AV. However, the greatest overall source of microemboli is related to prosthesis deployment. Compared with the transfemoral approach, retrograde manipulation of the aorta and aortic arch with the wire and deployment device is avoided with the transapical approach, potentially decreasing the risk of neurologic events.

Two recent meta-analyses reported a decrease in the neurologic event rate (2.7% vs 4.2%) and stroke rate (2.2% vs 3.4%) with the transapical approach on comparison with the transfemoral approach.[6,91] However, in both meta-analyses the difference did not reach statistical significance. Furthermore, the recent analysis of neurologic events from the PARTNER trial revealed an increased risk in transapical compared with transfemoral patients.[92] However, after performing "bagging analysis" in "nontransfemoral" candidates, the investigators found neurologic events to be patient-related or disease-related rather than approach-related.[92] Compared with the transfemoral approach, the rate of major stroke is not lower with the transapical approach but is the same regardless of the approach.[34,66] TCD analysis of the rates of cerebral microemboli also found no difference between the 2 approaches,[95] as did brain magnetic resonance imaging analysis.[34] The lack of statistical difference between the approaches emphasizes the mechanism of solid-particle embolism during valve stretching as well as a higher chance of gaseous air embolism associated with larger catheters used in the transapical approach.[34,66] Certain devices offering protection against the embolic episodes are available, but their efficacy needs to be established.[66,98]

TCD analysis found similar rates but different timing of microemboli between Edwards SAPIEN and CoreValve stent-valves.[95] The higher-profile, unsheathed SAPIEN valve was related to embolic events during the crossing of the native valve and positioning of the stent-valve. By contrast, embolic events were more common during the deployment and repositioning of the sheathed CoreValve.

Annular rupture

Annular rupture, though rare, is a devastating complication. The possible predisposing factors include significant calcification, smaller annular and sinotubular dimensions, excessive balloon dilation, and a porcelain aorta. Smaller leaks may be managed with pericardiocentesis and blood transfusion. However, emergent surgical intervention necessitating initiation of CPB may be required.[28,99]

Coronary ostial obstruction, ischemia, and myocardial infarction

Coronary ostial obstruction can occur as a result of displacement of the native aortic leaflets during valve implantation. This risk is higher in patients with a heavily calcified AV, especially in patients with the effacement of the AV sinus, low implantation of the coronary ostia, and long AV leaflets.[66] Thorough preoperative evaluation using MDCT and 3D echocardiography is focused on determining patients with a shorter distance from the coronary ostia (particularly left coronary) to the AV annulus.[60,100] On identification of patients at increased risk, prophylactic angiography wires can be placed in the ostia, enabling prompt diagnosis of obstruction and percutaneous intervention. The rate of myocardial infarction associated with the procedure varies dramatically depending on the definition of periprocedural myocardial infarction.[66]

Low cardiac output syndrome

Hypertrophied noncompliant ventricles associated with severe AS are highly susceptible to myocardial ischemia. Short periods of RVP associated with a decrease in cardiac output and increase in LV end-diastolic volume pressure secondary to acute aortic insufficiency after valvuloplasty and stent-valve deployment may lead to LV decompensation, resulting in failure requiring inotropic as well as mechanical circulatory support.[28]

Post-TAVR aortic insufficiency

The hemodynamically significant paravalvular aortic insufficiency (PAI) occurs with an incidence of 2% and 8% after SAVR using a bioprosthesis or mechanical prosthesis, respectively.[101] Approximately 66% to 89% of TAVR patients exhibit some degree of aortic insufficiency, primarily paravalvular in location (see **Fig. 8**).[9,24,85,102–104] More than moderate grades of PAI are present in 10% to 12% of TAVR patients.[9,24,85,102–104] However, even moderate PAI after TAVR has been associated with a higher mortality, especially in patients with moderate to severe LV systolic dysfunction.[22,105] Contrary to the paravalvular location, aortic insufficiency originating from the middle of the stent-valve results from improper valve deployment, sizing, presence of a guide wire through the valve holding a leaflet open, or an overhanging leaflet material resulting in improper leaflet closure. Therefore, evaluation must be undertaken after the guide wires have been withdrawn. The valve can be significantly damaged during crimping, leading to significant valvular aortic insufficiency on deployment. This problem may be remedied by an immediate valve-in-valve deployment. The mechanisms of PAI after TAVR are different.

SAVR permits the excision of the diseased native tissue and conformation of the annulus to the appropriate sewing ring with suture material. By contrast, balloon valvuloplasty and deployment of the stent-valve results in nonuniform compression of the native tissue with extensive calcification preventing adequate stent expansion, leading to PAI.[106] Predisposing factors include heavy, irregular, asymmetric calcification in the annular plane, undersizing or underexpansion of the prosthesis, increased angulation of the LV outflow tract in relation to the aorta, and a less deeply seated valve.[28,99,107,108] The extent of the leak may be reduced by restretching the implanted valve to obtain a better apposition between the valve and aortic annular plane, but patients with an AV annulus larger than the largest available stent-valve should not be considered optimal candidates. Therefore, accurate sizing of the stent-valve is crucial for procedural success.

Sizing of the virtual annular plane with TAVR may be difficult for the following reasons. Compared with surgery (using valve sizers) the measurement during TAVR is indirect, using imaging modalities such as TTE, TEE, MDCT, and invasive angiography.[60,61,100,103,104,107,109–111] Anatomically the annular plane is oval and not a perfect circle.[112] While evaluating the annulus with 2D imaging the plane can be cut at various angles, resulting in variable measurements. Three-dimensional images obtained by either MDCT or 3D echocardiography may be of significant relevance in better defining the annular plane dimensions.[60,61,100,104,109] Some studies have demonstrated a probable underestimation of the annular size by echocardiography compared with MDCT, which may lead to implantation of an undersized valve and an increase in the risk for PAI.[60,61,100,113] Despite this, the measurement of the AV annulus obtained by 2D TTE or TEE modalities have proved to be adequately accurate, resulting in excellent overall procedural success.[59,110] Because the gold-standard is not yet established, a multimodality approach is recommended for the assessment of the AV annulus size and severity of PAI.[59,85]

Precise quantification of PAI severity is difficult, as there may be multiple jets with an origin that is crescent-shaped and eccentric in direction, which may all lead to underestimation of severity. The standard classification used for the assessment of aortic insufficiency after SAVR has also been adopted for TAVR. However, the VARC made an effort to standardize definitions for PAI after TAVR.[50,85] According to these definitions the PAI can be graded on the basis of the percentage of the total circumference of the deployed stent-valve (see **Fig. 9**; **Table 2**).

The successful implantation of the SAPIEN stent-valve strongly relies on an accurate positioning of the valve at the AV annulus before deployment and proper RVP during the deployment. By contrast, the self-expandable CoreValve enables slower, more controlled release of the valve. Nevertheless, PAI after CoreValve deployment has been reported, with the angle between and aortic root axis and LV outflow tract axis and the depth of implantation being the major predictors of PAI.[101] Although manipulations of the deployed stent-valve are possible, they are technically difficult. The successful treatment of PAI may be remedied by a second valve-in-valve deployment.[114]

Acute kidney injury

Acute kidney injury (AKI) has been associated with the 4-fold increase in mortality following TAVR.[115,116] Periprocedural AKI and the need for renal replacement therapy has been attributed to the preexisting renal dysfunction,[117] amount of intraoperative contrast agent used,[118] and periprocedural blood transfusions.[116,119] Maintaining

Table 2		
Grading criteria for paravalvular insufficiency based on the percentage of circumferential extent		
Paravalvular Insufficiency Based on Circumferential Extent		
Mild	Moderate	Severe
<10%	10%–29%	≥30%

Data from Kappetein AP, Head SJ, Genereux P, et al. Updated standardized endpoint definitions for transcatheter aortic valve implantation: the Valve Academic Research Consortium-2 consensus document. J Am Coll Cardiol 2012;60:1438–54.

euvolemia is beneficial for prevention of AKI countering for the preoperative deficits, blood loss and evaporation during the procedure. In addition, it is beneficial to use the smallest volume of contrast agents possible and avoid potential nephrotoxins such as nonsteroidal anti-inflammatory drugs or vancomycin.

Conduction abnormalities

Newly developed left bundle branch block has been reported in up to 45% of TAVR patients, with the need for a permanent pacemaker in 3% to 8% of patients.[85] The incidence of intraventricular conduction abnormalities with the resultant implantation of a permanent pacemaker is higher (up to 4-fold) with the use of the self-expandable CoreValve compared with the Edwards valve: 20% versus 5%.[66] It is possible that the nitinol frame of the CoreValve creates higher pressure on the interventricular septum than does the stainless steel or cobalt chromium used in the framework of the SAPIEN valve. This pressure may lead to an increased incidence of left bundle branch block that may become very significant in patients with preexisting right bundle branch block, necessitating a permanent pacemaker. The possible mechanism includes direct mechanical injury of the left bundle branch, stent-induced inflammation, and a deeper (ventricular) implantation of the prosthesis.[66] A permanent pacemaker was placed in about 4% of inoperable and high-risk patients in the PARTNER trial, although this rate was not significantly different from that with medical treatment or SAVR.[9,24]

Malposition and migration of device

Rarely the implanted device will assume a malposition or will migrate. Immediate deployment of another overlapping valve may salvage the procedure in the case of malposition. However, a valve that has migrated distally into the aorta may be of hemodynamic insignificance as long as leaflets stay in line with the forward blood flow. Ventricular embolization requires surgical extraction.[28]

Transapical Approach

Specific complications of the transapical approach are related to the left thoracotomy incision, with a potential for lung and chest-wall injury and pneumothorax.[99] Accessing the left ventricle during the transapical approach may result in potentially life-threatening bleeding. A short burst of RVP to decrease chamber pressure is used to safely take out the sheath at the end of the procedure. Pledgeted sutures are used to secure the LV access site. The formation of an LV pseudoaneurysm is another possible late complication.[99]

SUMMARY

The TAVR procedure has emerged as a successful and comparable treatment option for many patients with AS. However, advances in technology and accumulating experience are necessary for further improvements and broadening of the current indications. The key for successful procedural outcome involves thorough preparedness and knowledge of the pertinent procedural details. Thus, the skill set possessed by cardiac anesthesiologists makes them crucially important members of the multidisciplinary team of physicians managing these patients.

REFERENCES

1. Cribier A, Eltchaninoff H, Bash A, et al. Percutaneous transcatheter implantation of an aortic valve prosthesis for calcific aortic stenosis: first human case description. Circulation 2002;106:3006–8.

2. Webb JG, Chandavimol M, Thompson CR, et al. Percutaneous aortic valve implantation retrograde from the femoral artery. Circulation 2006;113:842–50.
3. Fassl J, Augoustides JG. Transcatheter aortic valve implantation—part 1: development and status of the procedure. J Cardiothorac Vasc Anesth 2010;24:498–505.
4. Webb JG, Wood DA. Current status of transcatheter aortic valve replacement. J Am Coll Cardiol 2012;60:483–92.
5. Webb J, Cribier A. Percutaneous transarterial aortic valve implantation: what do we know? Eur Heart J 2011;32:140–7.
6. Jilaihawi H, Chakravarty T, Weiss RE, et al. Meta-analysis of complications in aortic valve replacement: comparison of Medtronic-Corevalve, Edwards-Sapien and surgical aortic valve replacement in 8,536 patients. Catheter Cardiovasc Interv 2012;80:128–38.
7. Carabello BA, Paulus WJ. Aortic stenosis. Lancet 2009;373:956–66.
8. Bonow RO, Carabello BA, Kanu C, et al. ACC/AHA 2006 guidelines for the management of patients with valvular heart disease: a report of the American College of Cardiology/American Heart Association Task Force on Practice Guidelines (writing committee to revise the 1998 Guidelines for the Management of Patients with Valvular Heart Disease): developed in collaboration with the Society of Cardiovascular Anesthesiologists: endorsed by the Society for Cardiovascular Angiography and Interventions and the Society of Thoracic Surgeons. Circulation 2006;114:e84–231.
9. Leon MB, Smith CR, Mack M, et al. Transcatheter aortic-valve implantation for aortic stenosis in patients who cannot undergo surgery. N Engl J Med 2010;363:1597–607.
10. Schwarz F, Baumann P, Manthey J, et al. The effect of aortic valve replacement on survival. Circulation 1982;66:1105–10.
11. Bach DS, Siao D, Girard SE, et al. Evaluation of patients with severe symptomatic aortic stenosis who do not undergo aortic valve replacement: the potential role of subjectively overestimated operative risk. Circ Cardiovasc Qual Outcomes 2009;2:533–9.
12. Iung B, Baron G, Butchart EG, et al. A prospective survey of patients with valvular heart disease in Europe: the euro heart survey on valvular heart disease. Eur Heart J 2003;24:1231–43.
13. Astor BC, Kaczmarek RG, Hefflin B, et al. Mortality after aortic valve replacement: results from a nationally representative database. Ann Thorac Surg 2000;70:1939–45.
14. Edwards MB, Taylor KM. Outcomes in nonagenarians after heart valve replacement operation. Ann Thorac Surg 2003;75:830–4.
15. Vaquette B, Corbineau H, Laurent M, et al. Valve replacement in patients with critical aortic stenosis and depressed left ventricular function: predictors of operative risk, left ventricular function recovery, and long term outcome. Heart 2005;91:1324–9.
16. Brown JM, O'Brien SM, Wu C, et al. Isolated aortic valve replacement in North America comprising 108,687 patients in 10 years: changes in risks, valve types, and outcomes in the Society of Thoracic Surgeons National Database. J Thorac Cardiovasc Surg 2009;137:82–90.
17. Bucerius J, Gummert JF, Borger MA, et al. Stroke after cardiac surgery: a risk factor analysis of 16,184 consecutive adult patients. Ann Thorac Surg 2003;75:472–8.
18. ElBardissi AW, Shekar P, Couper GS, et al. Minimally invasive aortic valve replacement in octogenarian, high-risk, transcatheter aortic valve implantation candidates. J Thorac Cardiovasc Surg 2011;141:328–35.

19. Gilard M, Eltchaninoff H, Iung B, et al. Registry of transcatheter aortic-valve implantation in high-risk patients. N Engl J Med 2012;366:1705–15.

20. Rodes-Cabau J, Webb JG, Cheung A, et al. Transcatheter aortic valve implantation for the treatment of severe symptomatic aortic stenosis in patients at very high or prohibitive surgical risk: acute and late outcomes of the multicenter Canadian experience. J Am Coll Cardiol 2010;55:1080–90.

21. Webb JG, Altwegg L, Boone RH, et al. Transcatheter aortic valve implantation: impact on clinical and valve-related outcomes. Circulation 2009;119:3009–16.

22. Tamburino C, Capodanno D, Ramondo A, et al. Incidence and predictors of early and late mortality after transcatheter aortic valve implantation in 663 patients with severe aortic stenosis. Circulation 2011;123:299–308.

23. Svensson LG, Tuzcu M, Kapadia S, et al. A comprehensive review of the PARTNER trial. J Thorac Cardiovasc Surg, in press.

24. Smith CR, Leon MB, Mack MJ, et al. Transcatheter versus surgical aortic-valve replacement in high-risk patients. N Engl J Med 2011;364:2187–98.

25. Reynolds MR, Magnuson EA, Lei Y, et al. Health-related quality of life after transcatheter aortic valve replacement in inoperable patients with severe aortic stenosis. Circulation 2011;124:1964–72.

26. Kodali SK, Williams MR, Smith CR, et al. Two-year outcomes after transcatheter or surgical aortic-valve replacement. N Engl J Med 2012;366:1686–95.

27. Makkar RR, Fontana GP, Jilaihawi H, et al. Transcatheter aortic-valve replacement for inoperable severe aortic stenosis. N Engl J Med 2012;366:1696–704.

28. Holmes DR Jr, Mack MJ, Kaul S, et al. 2012 ACCF/AATS/SCAI/STS expert consensus document on transcatheter aortic valve replacement. J Am Coll Cardiol 2012;59:1200–54.

29. Lange R, Bleiziffer S, Mazzitelli D, et al. Improvements in transcatheter aortic valve implantation outcomes in lower surgical risk patients: a glimpse into the future. J Am Coll Cardiol 2012;59:280–7.

30. Piazza N, van Gameren M, Juni P, et al. A comparison of patient characteristics and 30-day mortality outcomes after transcatheter aortic valve implantation and surgical aortic valve replacement for the treatment of aortic stenosis: a two-centre study. EuroIntervention 2009;5:580–8.

31. Grube E, Buellesfeld L, Mueller R, et al. Progress and current status of percutaneous aortic valve replacement: results of three device generations of the CoreValve Revalving system. Circ Cardiovasc Interv 2008;1:167–75.

32. Himbert D, Descoutures F, Al-Attar N, et al. Results of transfemoral or transapical aortic valve implantation following a uniform assessment in high-risk patients with aortic stenosis. J Am Coll Cardiol 2009;54:303–11.

33. Johansson M, Nozohoor S, Kimblad PO, et al. Transapical versus transfemoral aortic valve implantation: a comparison of survival and safety. Ann Thorac Surg 2011;91:57–63.

34. Rodes-Cabau J, Dumont E, Boone RH, et al. Cerebral embolism following transcatheter aortic valve implantation: comparison of transfemoral and transapical approaches. J Am Coll Cardiol 2011;57:18–28.

35. Svensson LG, Dewey T, Kapadia S, et al. United States feasibility study of transcatheter insertion of a stented aortic valve by the left ventricular apex. Ann Thorac Surg 2008;86:46–54 [discussion: 54–5].

36. Grube E, Schuler G, Buellesfeld L, et al. Percutaneous aortic valve replacement for severe aortic stenosis in high-risk patients using the second- and current third-generation self-expanding CoreValve prosthesis: device success and 30-day clinical outcome. J Am Coll Cardiol 2007;50:69–76.

37. Webb JG, Pasupati S, Humphries K, et al. Percutaneous transarterial aortic valve replacement in selected high-risk patients with aortic stenosis. Circulation 2007;116:755–63.
38. Bleiziffer S, Ruge H, Mazzitelli D, et al. Results of percutaneous and transapical transcatheter aortic valve implantation performed by a surgical team. Eur J Cardiothorac Surg 2009;35:615–20 [discussion: 20–1].
39. Walther T, Simon P, Dewey T, et al. Transapical minimally invasive aortic valve implantation: multicenter experience. Circulation 2007;116:I240–5.
40. Ewe SH, Delgado V, Ng AC, et al. Outcomes after transcatheter aortic valve implantation: transfemoral versus transapical approach. Ann Thorac Surg 2011;92:1244–51.
41. Al-Attar N, Nataf P. Development of aortic valve implantation. Herz 2009;34: 367–73.
42. Rodes-Cabau J, Dumont E, De LaRochelliere R, et al. Feasibility and initial results of percutaneous aortic valve implantation including selection of the trans-femoral or transapical approach in patients with severe aortic stenosis. Am J Cardiol 2008;102:1240–6.
43. Cribier A, Eltchaninoff H, Tron C, et al. Treatment of calcific aortic stenosis with the percutaneous heart valve: mid-term follow-up from the initial feasibility studies: the French experience. J Am Coll Cardiol 2006;47:1214–23.
44. Payne DM, Rodes-Cabau J, Doyle D, et al. Prominent septal hypertrophy: a contra-indication for transapical aortic valve implantation? J Cardiovasc Surg 2012;27:309–11.
45. Piazza N, Grube E, Gerckens U, et al. Procedural and 30-day outcomes following transcatheter aortic valve implantation using the third generation (18 Fr) Corevalve revalving system: results from the multicentre, expanded evaluation registry 1-year following CE mark approval. EuroIntervention 2008;4: 242–9.
46. Carabello BA. Aortic valve replacement should be operated on before symptom onset. Circulation 2012;126:112–7.
47. Shah PK. Severe aortic stenosis should not be operated on before symptom onset. Circulation 2012;126:118–25.
48. Osswald BR, Gegouskov V, Badowski-Zyla D, et al. Overestimation of aortic valve replacement risk by EuroSCORE: implications for percutaneous valve replacement. Eur Heart J 2009;30:74–80.
49. Tommaso CL, Bolman RM 3rd, Feldman T, et al. Multisociety (AATS, ACCF, SCAI, and STS) expert consensus statement: operator and institutional requirements for transcatheter valve repair and replacement, part 1: transcatheter aortic valve replacement. J Am Coll Cardiol 2012;59:2028–42.
50. Kappetein AP, Head SJ, Genereux P, et al. Updated standardized endpoint definitions for transcatheter aortic valve implantation: the Valve Academic Research Consortium-2 consensus document. J Am Coll Cardiol 2012;60:1438–54.
51. Patel PA, Fassl J, Thompson A, et al. Transcatheter aortic valve replacement-part 3: the central role of perioperative transesophageal echocardiography. J Cardiothorac Vasc Anesth 2012;26:698–710.
52. Bleiziffer S, Ruge H, Horer J, et al. Predictors for new-onset complete heart block after transcatheter aortic valve implantation. JACC Cardiovasc Interv 2010;3:524–30.
53. Detaint D, Lepage L, Himbert D, et al. Determinants of significant paravalvular regurgitation after transcatheter aortic valve: implantation impact of device and annulus discongruence. JACC Cardiovasc Interv 2009;2:821–7.

54. Ewe SH, Ng AC, Schuijf JD, et al. Location and severity of aortic valve calcium and implications for aortic regurgitation after transcatheter aortic valve implantation. Am J Cardiol 2011;108:1470–7.

55. Koos R, Mahnken AH, Dohmen G, et al. Association of aortic valve calcification severity with the degree of aortic regurgitation after transcatheter aortic valve implantation. Int J Cardiol 2011;150:142–5.

56. Altiok E, Koos R, Schroder J, et al. Comparison of two-dimensional and three-dimensional imaging techniques for measurement of aortic annulus diameters before transcatheter aortic valve implantation. Heart 2011;97:1578–84.

57. Jayasuriya C, Moss RR, Munt B. Transcatheter aortic valve implantation in aortic stenosis: the role of echocardiography. J Am Soc Echocardiogr 2011; 24:15–27.

58. Jilaihawi H, Kashif M, Fontana G, et al. Cross-sectional computed tomographic assessment improves accuracy of aortic annular sizing for transcatheter aortic valve replacement and reduces the incidence of paravalvular aortic regurgitation. J Am Coll Cardiol 2012;59:1275–86.

59. Messika-Zeitoun D, Serfaty JM, Brochet E, et al. Multimodal assessment of the aortic annulus diameter: implications for transcatheter aortic valve implantation. J Am Coll Cardiol 2010;55:186–94.

60. Otani K, Takeuchi M, Kaku K, et al. Assessment of the aortic root using real-time 3D transesophageal echocardiography. Circ J 2010;74:2649–57.

61. Willson AB, Webb JG, Labounty TM, et al. 3-dimensional aortic annular assessment by multidetector computed tomography predicts moderate or severe paravalvular regurgitation after transcatheter aortic valve replacement: a multicenter retrospective analysis. J Am Coll Cardiol 2012;59:1287–94.

62. Billings FT, Kodali SK, Shanewise JS. Transcatheter aortic valve implantation: anesthetic considerations. Anesth Analg 2009;108:1453–62.

63. Covello RD, Maj G, Landoni G, et al. Anesthetic management of percutaneous aortic valve implantation: focus on challenges encountered and proposed solutions. J Cardiothorac Vasc Anesth 2009;23:280–5.

64. Guinot PG, Depoix JP, Etchegoyen L, et al. Anesthesia and perioperative management of patients undergoing transcatheter aortic valve implantation: analysis of 90 consecutive patients with focus on perioperative complications. J Cardiothorac Vasc Anesth 2010;24(5):752–61.

65. Ree RM, Bowering JB, Schwarz SK. Case series: anesthesia for retrograde percutaneous aortic valve replacement–experience with the first 40 patients. Can J Anaesth 2008;55:761–8.

66. Rodes-Cabau J. Transcatheter aortic valve implantation: current and future approaches. Nat Rev Cardiol 2012;9:15–29.

67. Giannini C, Petronio AS, De Carlo M, et al. The incremental value of valvuloarterial impedance in evaluating the results of transcatheter aortic valve implantation in symptomatic aortic stenosis. J Am Soc Echocardiogr 2012;25:444–53.

68. Sinning JM, Hammerstingl C, Vasa-Nicotera M, et al. Aortic regurgitation index defines severity of peri-prosthetic regurgitation and predicts outcome in patients after transcatheter aortic valve implantation. J Am Coll Cardiol 2012;59: 1134–41.

69. Walther T, Dewey T, Borger MA, et al. Transapical aortic valve implantation: step by step. Ann Thorac Surg 2009;87:276–83.

70. Guarracino F, Landoni G. Con: transcatheter aortic valve implantation should not be performed under general anesthesia. J Cardiothorac Vasc Anesth 2012;26: 736–9.

71. Bergmann L, Kahlert P, Eggebrecht H, et al. Transfemoral aortic valve implantation under sedation and monitored anaesthetic care—a feasibility study. Anaesthesia 2011;66:977–82.
72. Hantschel D, Fassl J, Scholz M, et al. Leipzig fast-track protocol for cardioanesthesia. Effective, safe and economical. Anaesthesist 2009;58:379–86 [in German].
73. Filipovic M, Michaux I, Wang J, et al. Effects of sevoflurane and propofol on left ventricular diastolic function in patients with pre-existing diastolic dysfunction. Br J Anaesth 2007;98:12–8.
74. Dehedin B, Guinot PG, Ibrahim H, et al. Anesthesia and perioperative management of patients who undergo transfemoral transcatheter aortic valve implantation: an observational study of general versus local/regional anesthesia in 125 consecutive patients. J Cardiothorac Vasc Anesth 2011;25:1036–43.
75. Fassl J, Kodavatiganti R, Ingerski MS. Anesthesia management for retrograde aortic valve replacement. Can J Anaesth 2009;56:336 [author reply: 7].
76. Fassl J, Seeberger MD, Augoustides JG. Transcatheter aortic valve implantation: is general anesthesia superior to conscious sedation? J Cardiothorac Vasc Anesth 2011;25:576–7.
77. Motloch LJ, Rottlaender D, Reda S, et al. Local versus general anesthesia for transfemoral aortic valve implantation. Clin Res Cardiol 2012;101:45–53.
78. Fassl J. Pro: transcatheter aortic valve implantation should be performed with general anesthesia. J Cardiothorac Vasc Anesth 2012;26:733–5.
79. Mukherjee C, Walther T, Borger MA, et al. Awake transapical aortic valve implantation using thoracic epidural anesthesia. Ann Thorac Surg 2009;88:992–4.
80. Lichtenstein SV, Cheung A, Ye J, et al. Transapical transcatheter aortic valve implantation in humans: initial clinical experience. Circulation 2006;114:591–6.
81. Behan M, Haworth P, Hutchinson N, et al. Percutaneous aortic valve implants under sedation: our initial experience. Catheter Cardiovasc Interv 2008;72:1012–5.
82. Ye J, Cheung A, Lichtenstein SV, et al. Transapical transcatheter aortic valve implantation: follow-up to 3 years. J Thorac Cardiovasc Surg 2010;139:1107–13, 1113.e1.
83. Kapadia SR, Goel SS, Svensson L, et al. Characterization and outcome of patients with severe symptomatic aortic stenosis referred for percutaneous aortic valve replacement. J Thorac Cardiovasc Surg 2009;137:1430–5.
84. Fassl J, Walther T, Groesdonk HV, et al. Anesthesia management for transapical transcatheter aortic valve implantation: a case series. J Cardiothorac Vasc Anesth 2009;23:286–91.
85. Leon MB, Piazza N, Nikolsky E, et al. Standardized endpoint definitions for Transcatheter Aortic Valve Implantation clinical trials: a consensus report from the Valve Academic Research Consortium. J Am Coll Cardiol 2011;57:253–69.
86. Genereux P, Webb JG, Svensson LG, et al. Vascular complications after transcatheter aortic valve replacement: insights from the partner (Placement of AoRTic TraNscathetER Valve) trial. J Am Coll Cardiol 2012;60:1043–52.
87. Krishnaswamy A, Tuzcu EM, Kapadia SR. Update on transcatheter aortic valve implantation. Curr Cardiol Rep 2010;12:393–403.
88. Toggweiler S, Gurvitch R, Leipsic J, et al. Percutaneous aortic valve replacement: vascular outcomes with a fully percutaneous procedure. J Am Coll Cardiol 2012;59:113–8.
89. Hayashida K, Lefevre T, Chevalier B, et al. True percutaneous approach for transfemoral aortic valve implantation using the Prostar XL device: impact of

learning curve on vascular complications. JACC Cardiovasc Interv 2012;5: 207–14.

90. Hayashida K, Lefevre T, Chevalier B, et al. Transfemoral aortic valve implantation new criteria to predict vascular complications. JACC Cardiovasc Interv 2011;4:851–8.

91. Eggebrecht H, Schmermund A, Voigtlander T, et al. Risk of stroke after transcatheter aortic valve implantation (TAVI): a meta-analysis of 10,037 published patients. EuroIntervention 2012;8:129–38.

92. Miller DC, Blackstone EH, Mack MJ, et al. Transcatheter (TAVR) versus surgical (AVR) aortic valve replacement: occurrence, hazard, risk factors, and consequences of neurologic events in the PARTNER trial. J Thorac Cardiovasc Surg 2012;143:832–843.e13.

93. Brennan JM, Edwards FH, Zhao Y, et al. Long-term survival after aortic valve replacement among high-risk elderly patients in the United States: insights from the society of thoracic surgeons adult cardiac surgery database, 1991 to 2007. Circulation 2012;126:1621–9.

94. Szeto WY, Augoustides JG, Desai ND, et al. Cerebral embolic exposure during transfemoral and transapical transcatheter aortic valve replacement. J Cardiovasc Surg 2011;26:348–54.

95. Kahlert P, Al-Rashid F, Dottger P, et al. Cerebral embolization during transcatheter aortic valve implantation: a transcranial Doppler study. Circulation 2012; 126:1245–55.

96. Ghanem A, Muller A, Nahle CP, et al. Risk and fate of cerebral embolism after transfemoral aortic valve implantation: a prospective pilot study with diffusion-weighted magnetic resonance imaging. J Am Coll Cardiol 2010;55:1427–32.

97. Reinsfelt B, Westerlind A, Ioanes D, et al. Transcranial Doppler microembolic signals and serum marker evidence of brain injury during transcatheter aortic valve implantation. Acta Anaesthesiol Scand 2012;56:240–7.

98. Webb JG, Barbanti M. Cerebral embolization during transcatheter aortic valve implantation. Circulation 2012;126:1567–9.

99. Masson JB, Kovac J, Schuler G, et al. Transcatheter aortic valve implantation: review of the nature, management, and avoidance of procedural complications. JACC Cardiovasc Interv 2009;2:811–20.

100. Tamborini G, Fusini L, Gripari P, et al. Feasibility and accuracy of 3DTEE versus CT for the evaluation of aortic valve annulus to left main ostium distance before transcatheter aortic valve implantation. J Am Coll Cardiol 2012;5:579–88.

101. Clavel MA, Webb JG, Pibarot P, et al. Comparison of the hemodynamic performance of percutaneous and surgical bioprostheses for the treatment of severe aortic stenosis. J Am Coll Cardiol 2009;53:1883–91.

102. Mor-Avi V, Lang RM, Badano LP, et al. Current and evolving echocardiographic techniques for the quantitative evaluation of cardiac mechanics: ASE/EAE consensus statement on methodology and indications endorsed by the Japanese Society of Echocardiography. J Am Soc Echocardiogr 2011;24:277–313.

103. Yared K, Garcia-Camarero T, Fernandez-Friera L, et al. Impact of aortic regurgitation after transcatheter aortic valve implantation: results from the REVIVAL trial. J Am Coll Cardiol 2012;5:469–77.

104. Zamorano JL, Badano LP, Bruce C, et al. EAE/ASE recommendations for the use of echocardiography in new transcatheter interventions for valvular heart disease. J Am Soc Echocardiogr 2011;24:937–65.

105. Abdel-Wahab M, Zahn R, Horack M, et al. Aortic regurgitation after transcatheter aortic valve implantation: incidence and early outcome. Results from the German transcatheter aortic valve interventions registry. Heart 2011;97:899–906.

106. Rajani R, Kakad M, Khawaja MZ, et al. Paravalvular regurgitation one year after transcatheter aortic valve implantation. Catheter Cardiovasc Interv 2010;75: 868–72.
107. Santos N, de Agustin JA, Almeria C, et al. Prosthesis/annulus discongruence assessed by three-dimensional transoesophageal echocardiography: a predictor of significant paravalvular aortic regurgitation after transcatheter aortic valve implantation. Eur Heart J Cardiovasc Imaging 2012;13(11):931–7.
108. Sherif MA, Abdel-Wahab M, Beurich HW, et al. Haemodynamic evaluation of aortic regurgitation after transcatheter aortic valve implantation using cardiovascular magnetic resonance. EuroIntervention 2011;7:57–63.
109. Bloomfield GS, Gillam LD, Hahn RT, et al. A practical guide to multimodality imaging of transcatheter aortic valve replacement. J Am Coll Cardiol 2012;5: 441–55.
110. Moss RR, Ivens E, Pasupati S, et al. Role of echocardiography in percutaneous aortic valve implantation. J Am Coll Cardiol 2008;1:15–24.
111. Naqvi TZ. Echocardiography in percutaneous valve therapy. J Am Coll Cardiol 2009;2:1226–37.
112. Piazza N, de Jaegere P, Schultz C, et al. Anatomy of the aortic valvar complex and its implications for transcatheter implantation of the aortic valve. Circ Cardiovasc Interv 2008;1:74–81.
113. Yano M, Nakamura K, Nagahama H, et al. Aortic annulus diameter measurement: what is the best modality? Ann Thorac Cardiovasc Surg 2012;18:115–20.
114. Ussia GP, Barbanti M, Ramondo A, et al. The valve-in-valve technique for treatment of aortic bioprosthesis malposition an analysis of incidence and 1-year clinical outcomes from the Italian CoreValve registry. J Am Coll Cardiol 2011; 57:1062–8.
115. Aregger F, Wenaweser P, Hellige GJ, et al. Risk of acute kidney injury in patients with severe aortic valve stenosis undergoing transcatheter valve replacement. Nephrol Dial Transplant 2009;24:2175–9.
116. Bagur R, Webb JG, Nietlispach F, et al. Acute kidney injury following transcatheter aortic valve implantation: predictive factors, prognostic value, and comparison with surgical aortic valve replacement. Eur Heart J 2010;31:865–74.
117. Elhmidi Y, Bleiziffer S, Piazza N, et al. Incidence and predictors of acute kidney injury in patients undergoing transcatheter aortic valve implantation. Am Heart J 2011;161:735–9.
118. Van Linden A, Kempfert J, Rastan AJ, et al. Risk of acute kidney injury after minimally invasive transapical aortic valve implantation in 270 patients. Eur J Cardiothorac Surg 2011;39:835–42 [discussion: 42–3].
119. Nuis RJ, Van Mieghem NM, Tzikas A, et al. Frequency, determinants, and prognostic effects of acute kidney injury and red blood cell transfusion in patients undergoing transcatheter aortic valve implantation. Catheter Cardiovasc Interv 2011;77:881–9.

A Review of Cardiac Transplantation

Sofia Fischer, MD, Kathryn E. Glas, MD, FASE, MBA*

KEYWORDS

- Cardiac transplantation • Circulatory support • Donor criteria • Recipient selection

KEY POINTS

- Medical therapy for congestive heart failure (CHF) has improved dramatically in the past decade.
- Recent advances in CHF management have included biventricular pacing or cardiac resynchronization therapy (CRT) frequently combined with implantable cardioverter-defibrillator (CRT-D).
- If, during optimal medical therapy, left ventricular ejection fraction (LVEF) is less than or equal to 35% and cardiac dyssynchrony as evidenced by a prolonged QRS duration is greater than 120 ms, CRT is indicated for patients with New York Heart Association (NYHA) functional class III or ambulatory class IV.
- Survival after cardiac transplantation has improved. An increasing number of patients are receiving LVAD as bridge to transplant. Donor and recipient matching is important to improving outcomes.

INTRODUCTION AND HISTORY

In the United States, 5.8 million people have CHF and approximately 300,000 people die of heart failure each year.[1] Advanced heart failure is an epidemic with an estimated 100,000 to 250,000 patients having refractory NYHA class IIIB or class IV symptoms.[2] In 2011, the registry of the International Society for Heart and Lung Transplantation (ISHLT) reported the 100,000th HT recipient registered in its database.[3] Today, cardiac transplantation is accepted for treatment of end-stage heart failure.

Cardiac transplantation began with successful autotransplantation of the canine heart by Willman and colleagues[4] at Stanford University. The investigators found that immune rejection was the major barrier to successful cardiac transplantation. Long-term survival of orthotopic cardiac allograft would be possible via chemical immunosuppression.[5] On December 3, 1967, Christian Barnard performed the first successful human HT at the Groote Schuur Hospital in Cape Town, South Africa.[6]

Department of Anesthesiology, Emory University School of Medicine, 550 Peachtree Street, Atlanta, GA 30308, USA
* Corresponding author.
E-mail address: kglas@emory.edu

Anesthesiology Clin 31 (2013) 383–403
http://dx.doi.org/10.1016/j.anclin.2013.01.003
1932-2275/13/$ – see front matter © 2013 Elsevier Inc. All rights reserved.

Barnard used local irradiation, azathioprine, prednisone, and actinomycin C for immunosuppression. Three days later, Kantrowitz and colleagues[7] used an anencephalic donor heart to replace the heart of a 3-week-old baby diagnosed with tricuspid atresia.

During the following few years, cardiac transplantation was attempted globally with poor results, mostly due to surgical inexperience and difficulties with rejection. At Stanford, experimental and clinical work began to produce better results. Introduced by Stanford in 1973, transvenous endomyocardial biopsy for diagnosis of graft rejection is today the primary means of diagnosis of rejection.[8]

The discovery of cyclosporin A by professor Jean-Francois Borel in 1976 and its Food and Drug Administration approval in 1983 contributed to graft survival and rapid decrease of rejection and, until 1990, an increase in the number of heart transplantion (HTs) in the United States.[1] Despite a more liberal use of donors, the number of HTs performed in the United States has plateaued at approximately 2200 per year since 1990.[9]

The Organ Procurement and Transplantation Network (optn.transplant.hrsa.gov) report provides the following statistics. There were 3402 patients on the waiting list for cardiac transplantation as of November 2012. There is a lack of sufficient donor hearts to meet demand. Approximately 52% of patients awaiting HT are aged 50 to 64 years.[10] Average waiting time in status I is now more than 6 months.[11] Prevalence of patients awaiting HT as status IB has grown substantially. This is most likely a reflection of growing left ventricular assist device (LVAD) use.[10] Despite downward trends in donations and increased waiting time, the mortality rate on the waiting list declined over 12 years (1998–2010), from 20.7% to 13.7%.

The leading causes of heart disease for adult transplant recipients, from 2005 to 2010, have been[3]

Nonischemic cardiomyopathy (53.3%)
Ischemic cardiomyopathy (37.7%)
Adult congenital heart disease (2.9%)
Valvular heart disease (2.7%)
Repeat transplantation (2.6%)

The distribution of leading diagnoses has shifted significantly over time with nonischemic cardiomyopathy becoming the leading indication versus ischemic etiology in the late 1980s. This shift likely reflects decreasing prevalence of nicotine use, new therapies for ischemic heart disease, and, in particular, additional treatment options provided by the evolving field of mechanical circulatory support (MCS).[3]

Medical therapy for CHF has improved dramatically in the past decade. Mortality benefit for patients with stable NYHA class III to class IV HF (**Box 1**) has been shown in controlled trials using angiotensin-converting enzyme inhibitor therapy, β-blocker therapy, aldosterone antagonist therapy, and, for African Americans, combination hydralazine/nitrate therapy.[12]

Recent advances in CHF management have included biventricular pacing or CRT-D. If, during optimal medical therapy, LVEF is less than or equal to 35% and cardiac dyssynchrony as evidenced by a prolonged QRS duration is greater than 120 ms, CRT is indicated for patients with NYHA functional class III or ambulatory class IV.[13,14]

Cardiac transplantation today

1. Patient survival after HT

2. Gains in survival and yearly mortality rates

3. Major causes of death

4. Quality of life and employment after HT
5. Federal reimbursement
6. Retransplantation
    a. Current incidence
    b. Survival
    c. Ethical issues
    d. Indications

CARDIAC TRANSPLANTATION TODAY

Data from 2009 show that patient survival rate has improved 93% at 3 months, 89% at 1 year, 73% at 5 years, and 55% at 10 years.[15] The first year after transplant continues

---

Box 1
Contraindications to cardiac transplantation

Absolute contraindications

Systemic illness with a life expectancy less than 2 years despite HT, including

Active or recent solid organ or blood malignancy within 5 y

AIDS with frequent opportunistic infections

Systemic lupus erythematosus, sarcoidosis, or amyloidosis that has multisystem involvement and is still active

Irreversible renal or hepatic dysfunction in patients considered for only HT

Significant obstructive pulmonary disease (forced expiratory volume in the first second of expiration [FEV_1] <1 L/min)

Fixed pulmonary hypertension

Pulmonary artery systolic pressure >60 mm Hg

Mean transpulmonary gradient >15 mm Hg

Pulmonary vascular resistance >6 Wood units

Relative contraindications

Age >72 y

Any active infection (except patients with infected ventricular assist device [VAD])

Active peptic ulcer disease

Diabetes mellitus with end-organ damage

Severe peripheral vascular or cerebrovascular disease

Morbid obesity (body mass index >35 kg/m^2) or cachexia (body mass index <18 kg/m^2)

Creatinine >2.5 mg/dL or creatinine clearance <25 mL/min

Bilirubin >2.5 mg/dL, serum transaminases >3×, international normalized ratio >1.5 off warfarin

Severe pulmonary dysfunction with FEV_1 <40% normal

Active mental illness or psychosocial instability

Drug, tobacco, or alcohol abuse within 6 months

to represent the period with the highest mortality. After the first year there is a constant mortality rate of approximately 3% to 4% per year. Median survival is currently 11 years. Almost 100 patients have now lived past 25 years since their transplant procedure. Major gains in survival have been largely limited to the first 6 to 12 months, whereas the mortality rate after the first year has not shown statistically significant improvement over the past 2 decades. The improvement in first-year survival reflects improved immunosuppression and prevention and treatment of infection.

During the first-year graft failure, multiple organ failure, noncytomegalovirus (non-CMV) infection, and acute rejection are leading causes of death. After 5 years, malignancy, allograft vasculopathy, and non-CMV infection represent major causes of death. Long-term survival seems limited because of transplant vasculopathy and side effects of chronic immunosuppressive therapy. Cardiac allograft vasculopathy (CAV) develops in 20% of patients after 3 years, 30% at 5 years, and up to 50% after 10 years. CAV is a diffuse process affecting large epicardial vessels, coronary veins, and microcirculation. Histologically, CAV is characterized by concentric fibrous intimal hyperplasia and smooth muscle proliferation. The diffuse nature of CAV suggests an immune etiology.

Data from ISHLT indicate that 75% of recipients report no limitations of activity at 1 year and 5 years after HT. Many patients return to work after HT. Among recipients aged 25 to 55 years old, approximately 50% were employed 5 years after transplantation. In the United States, barriers to employment may be mostly related to the structure of disability benefits and health insurance considerations.

RETRANSPLANTATION

Cardiac retransplantation is a controversial procedure and has provoked ethical debate due to disparity between donor heart demand and supply. Many patients do not survive on the waiting list to receive their primary HT[16] whereas others are receiving a second organ. Given the factors limiting long-term survival in cardiac transplant recipients and the increasing number of patients transplanted for congenital heart disease at early ages, however, some patients are considered candidates for retransplantation. As of 2009, retransplantation accounted for 2.6% of adult HT operations and 6% of pediatric HT operations.[17] One-year survival rates for retransplantation have improved from 52.7% from 1982 to 1991 to most recently 83% from 2007 to 2011.[18]

An analysis of long-term survival rates in 20,787 primary HTs and 594 repeat HTs from the United Network for Organ Sharing (UNOS) database (1987–2004) found 71% overall increased risk of death for retransplant versus primary transplant recipients.[16] Excluding patients with primary graft failure (PGF) and intractable acute rejection occurring less than 6 months after transplantation, however, 1-year, 2-year, and 4-year survival rates for retransplanted patients were comparable to those after primary transplantation.[19]

Retransplantation shortly after PGF is not advisable due to unacceptable operative mortality and shortage of donor organs.[20,21] From available data, retransplantation should only be considered in patients with chronic graft dysfunction.[22]

Left ventricular assist devices outline

1. Life support as a bridge to HT

2. LVAD introduction as means for end-stage heart disease treatment (Randomized Evaluation of Mechanical Assistance for the Treatment of Congestive Heart Failure [REMATCH] trial)

3. LVAD in treatment of CHF today (major indications)

4. LVAD as bridge to transplant and bridge to candidacy

5. Survival after HT bridged with LVAD

6. Mechanical circulatory support national registry development

7. Transition from pulsatile to continuous flow pumps

8. Development of third-generation pumps

9. Transcutaneous energy transfer systems

LEFT VENTRICULAR ASSIST DEVICES

Because of the shortage of available organs for HT, more than 64% of HT recipients require life support as a bridge to transplant. This includes intravenous inotropes, mechanical ventilation, intra-aortic balloon pumps (IABPs), total artificial hearts, and VADs, primarily in the form of LVADs. In addition, better survival rates have consistently been observed, with devices designed to assist, instead of replace, the left ventricles (LVs) and occasionally right ventricle (RVs).[23] LVADs are currently used for rescue therapy, bridge to transplant, or destination therapy. LVADs have also been used as a bridge to candidacy in patients with high but potentially reversible pulmonary vascular resistance. Such patients might be eligible for HT after several months when pulmonary pressures fall after LV unloading.[9,11]

Published in 2001, the REMATCH trial demonstrated a 48% relative reduction in the risk of death over a 2-year study period in the LVAD group, compared with medical therapy, and a mortality rate reduction of 27% at 1 year. The trial established the efficacy of device therapy for end-stage HF and dramatically increased the use of this technology.[24] In 2009, the proportion of all patients who were bridged to transplant with MCS exceeded 30%.[3] LVAD as a bridge to candidacy enabled 10% of patients to undergo cardiac transplantation by 12 months after LVAD implant[25]; 15% of the pediatric population used VAD as a bridge to transplantation.[17] Once a patient receives an HT, there is no longer a statistically significant difference in survival of patients bridged with pulsatile flow VADs or continuous flow VADs compared with patients not requiring LVAD bridging.[3,11,26]

Data regarding VAD use as a bridge to transplant are limited in the Organ Procurement and Transplantation Network database.[23] In 2006, a national registry, the Interagency Registry for Mechanically Assisted Circulatory Support (INTERMACS), was developed.[27] One-year survival results of data collected in this registry from 2006 to 2010 were 74% for continuous flow pumps versus 61% for pulsatile flow pumps. The first continuous flow axial pump (HeartMate II, Thoratec, Pleasanton, California) was approved as a bridge to transplant therapy in the United States in April 2008. In January 2010, 20 months later, the same device was approved for destination therapy. The HeartWare (HeartWare International, Framingham, Massachusetts) was approved as a bridge to transplant in November 2012. It is a full-support device that is implanted in the pericardial space. Third-generation pumps currently under development operate without bearings by use of either hydrodynamically or magnetically levitated rotors, which may allow even greater pump longevity.[11] Researchers are also working to develop a fully implantable device to decrease or eliminate the infectious complications that currently complicate some LVAD management.

Currently, more than 4000 patients have been entered into the database with primary device implant. Current actuarial survival rates with continuous flow pumps exceed 80% at 1 year and 70% at 2 years. After the approval of durable continuous axial flow pumps, the use of pulsatile technology drastically decreased. By the first half of 2011, more than 99% of LVAD implants were continuous flow devices. No pulsatile VADs have been implanted for destination therapy since January 2010.[26]

Device-related infection remains common with MCS. The majority of infections involve the percutaneous driveline. Device-related infections allow upgrade to UNOS status IA. Transcutaneous energy transfer systems that allow LVAD to be totally implantable may one day eliminate the need for a percutaneous driveline and associated infections.[11]

Recipient selection outline

1. Indications and contraindications for HT

2. Prognosis scores

3. Adult candidate status

4. Heart allocation policy changes in 2006

5. Alternate cardiac transplant recipient list

6. Congenital heart disease in HT population

RECIPIENT SELECTION

HT recipient selection requires an extensive multidisciplinary approach to estimate prognosis in patients with severe CHF, their ability to survive surgery, postoperative compliance with medical management, and identification of potentially reversible factors and adequacy of current medical therapy. According to the current American College of Cardiology/American Heart Association guidelines, updated in 2009, indications for cardiac transplantation focus on the identification of patients with severe functional impairment or dependence on intravenous inotropic support (**Box 2**).[14,18] Most candidates have severe LV systolic dysfunction. Refractory angina, life-threatening ventricular arrhythmias, and diastolic heart failure are less common.

Progress in modeling heart failure to establish a risk score for prognosis may allow better design of therapies to improve survival. The Seattle Heart Failure Model is a 21-variable model that incorporates the impact of new heart failure therapies, including implantable cardioverter-defibrillators (ICDs) and CRT, and accurately estimates 1-year, 2-year, and 3-year survival rates.[28]

Patients awaiting HT are assigned a status code according to the level of urgency and medical support they require. Currently, status IA patients meet 1 or more of the following criteria:

1. MCS (defined as either an RVAD and/or LVAD, with 30 days of status IA time allocated; IABP; total artificial heart or extracorporeal membrane oxygenation [ECMO])
2. MCS for more than 30 days with device-related complication
3. Mechanical ventilation
4. High-dose or multiple inotropes with continuous monitoring of LV filling pressures

Status IB patients have either and/or right VAD (RVAD) for more than 30 days without evidence of device-related complication or (2) continuous infusion of inotropes without hemodynamic monitoring.

Status II patients are all others who do not meet status IA or IB criteria.[23]

Distance of transplant center from donor hospital is delineated into 5 zones (in nautical miles): zone A to 500, zone B 500 to 1000, zone C 1000 to 1500, zone D 1500 to 2500, and zone E beyond 2500. On July 12, 2006, UNOS implemented an

---

Box 2
Indications for cardiac transplantation

Absolute indications

Hemodynamic compromise due to HF

Refractory cardiogenic shock

Dependence on intravenous inotropic support to maintain adequate organ perfusion

Peak oxygen consumption (Vo_2) <10 mL/kg/min

Severe symptoms of ischemia limiting routine activity and not amenable to revascularization

Recurrent symptomatic ventricular arrhythmias refractory to therapy

Relative indications

Peak Vo_2 11–14 mL/kg/min (or 55% of predicted) and major limitation of patient daily activities

Recurrent unstable ischemia not amenable to other intervention

Recurrent instability of fluid balance/renal function not due to noncompliance with therapy

Insufficient indications

Low LVEF

History of functional class III or class IV symptoms of HF

Peak Vo_2 >15 mL/kg/min (and >55% predicted) without other indications

From Hunt SA, Abraham WT, Chin MH, et al. Focused update incorporated into the ACC/AHA 2005 guidelines for the diagnosis and management of heart failure in adults: a report for the diagnosis and management of heart failure in adults: a report of the ACC Foundation/AHA Task Force on Practice Guidelines. J Am Coll Cardiol 2009;53:e1–90.

---

allocation policy change prioritizing zone A status IA and status IB patients ahead of local status II patients.[23] The intent of this change was to direct donor hearts to the most critically ill patients and decrease waiting list mortality rates. In the 2 years after policy change, the waitlist mortality rates for status IA patients decreased by 34% and for status IB patients by 27%. Despite that donor hearts were allocated to sicker recipients, the predicted increase in post-transplant mortality has not occurred.[29]

For marginal HT candidates, several large-volume programs in the United States offer an alternate cardiac transplant recipient list where suboptimal donor hearts that otherwise would go unused (donor age >55 y, moderate *Left ventricular hypertrophy (LVH), regional wall motion abnormalities*, single-vessel coronary artery disease, history of cocaine use, or prolonged ischemic time >4 h) are offered to alternate recipients with clinical outcomes still significantly better than the natural history of end-stage HF.[30–32]

Donor evaluation and selection

- Donor demographics
- Donor heart evaluation: coronary angiography and impact of transmitted coronary artery disease
- Donor and recipient matching
- Donor characteristics associated with negative outcome (older age, LVH, gender mismatch, cause of donor death, donor inotropic support)
- Ischemic time (described later)

DONOR EVALUATION AND SELECTION

Due to organ shortage, the criteria for donor hearts have been eased. The median donor age in 2009 was 35 versus 27 years in 1990; 14% of donors in 2009 were aged 50 to 60 years. In Europe, 22% of donors are 50 years or older, a higher proportion than in other locations.[3] The most common causes of death are head trauma (50.2%) and stroke (28.8%).

Donors must meet national/regional criteria for brain death. Donor age, height and weight, gender, ABO blood type, chest radiograph, ECG, echocardiogram, and cause of death are required. Laboratory data include CMV, HIV status, and hepatitis B, and hepatitis C, and arterial blood gas results. Donor contraindications include intractable ventricular arrhythmias, excessive inotropic support, discreet regional wall motion abnormalities or LVEF less than 40% despite optimization of hemodynamics, congenital heart disease, transmissible diseases, systemic malignancies. Coronary angiography is recommended for male donors over 45 years old and female donors over 50 years old.[33] With an aging donor pool, significant coronary artery disease may be as high as 20%, the risk of transmitted coronary atherosclerosis without angiography 5% to 10%, and the risk for early graft failure with more than 1 coronary artery involved is 3 times higher.[34]

Matching suitable donors to recipients uses several important factors: ABO blood group compatibility, HLA typing, and compatibility of body size. As a general rule, the use of hearts from donors whose body weight is no more than 30% below the recipient weight is safe. A male donor of average weight, 70 kg, can be safely used for any size recipient irrespective of weight.[35] In recipients with significant pulmonary hypertension, use of a larger donor heart is advised.[19] The final decision to accept the heart is made by the procurement team during harvesting and direct examination.

Donor characteristics that have been associated with negative outcome include older age, presence of LVH, gender mismatches, donor cause of death, and donor inotropic support. Use of donor hearts greater than 40 years of age is associated with reduction in survival and a higher incidence of CAV.[19] Donor hearts with LVH greater than 14 mm have been associated with lower survival in recipients.[36] Transplanting a female donor heart into a male recipient is associated with significantly higher risk of PGF and worse 5-year and 10-year survival rates.[37] Donor cause of death due to spontaneous intracranial hemorrhage is associated with significantly increased coronary vasculopathy.[38] Preharvest high donor inotropic support is associated with PGF.[39]

Donor heart harvest and preservation outline

- Brain death–induced damage
- Surgical technique of donor heart harvest, including congenital details
- Impact of ischemic time
- Current preservative solutions
- Continuous warm perfusion for cardiac preservation

DONOR HEART HARVEST AND PRESERVATION

Brain death leads to profound metabolic and hemodynamic derangements. Acute brain death is associated with intense vagal discharge with bradycardia and hypertension followed by a catecholamine storm. Adrenaline and norepinephrine levels rise more than 100-fold and arterial blood pressure rises up to 400 mm Hg, leading to sub-endocardial ischemia, necrosis, and myocardial depression with regional wall motion abnormalities. This is followed by pronounced vasodilation as vasculature becomes refractory to vasoconstrictor support and loss of temperature control.[34] Overall, brain death leads to myocardial dysfunction, loss of central thermoregulation with resultant arrhythmias, central diabetes insipidus with hypovolemia, and frequent development of neurogenic pulmonary edema. Invasive monitoring and inotropic support might be required to maintain filling pressures as well as high inspired oxygen concentration and positive end-expiratory pressure ventilation.[33]

Donor heart is harvested through a median sternotomy. After pericardiotomy, the heart is examined for any evidence of regional wall motion abnormalities, previous infarctions, myocardial contusion, and coronary calcifications. Donor is systemically heparinized. Great veins are ligated and heart exsanguinated by opening the inferior vena cava. The ascending aorta is clamped just proximal to the innominate artery and the heart is arrested with cardioplegia infused into the aortic root. During cardiectomy, the ascending aorta is divided proximal to the innominate artery together with pulmonary artery, pulmonary veins, and vena cava. Some complex forms of congenital heart disease may require extensive reconstruction of pulmonary arteries, aortic arch, or inferior vena cava in a recipient and necessitate harvesting of extended portions of great vessels and great veins.[40] On explantation, the graft is examined for presence of patent foramen ovale and valvular abnormalities. Cold static preservation with crystalloid solutions is the current gold standard for donor heart myocardial protection. It allows safe overall ischemic time of up to 4 hours with a PGF rate less than 2%.[41]

Ischemic time for the donor heart starts with aortic cross-clamp during the harvest and ends with removal of the cross-clamp from the recipient aorta. In the situations when ischemic times longer than 4 hours are expected, donor hearts should only be accepted from young donors with normal cardiac function and no inotropic support.[42] The data from the 2010 ISHLT registry showed a statistically significant increase in acute graft failure and in 1-year and 5-year mortality rates with ischemic times longer than 210 minutes.[41]

The length of ischemic time can be influenced by the experience of the harvesting and operating surgeons, distance between donor hospital and transplant center, and experience of transplant team and coordinator.[34] In the United States, median ischemic graft times of 197 minutes have been reported.

In an effort to circumvent the length of ischemic time as a limiting factor, the Trans-Medics portable warm blood perfusion system, the Organ Care System (TransMedics, Andover, Massachusetts), a transportable commercial system that allows a new type of organ transplant, called a living organ transplant, has recently been developed. The organ care system consists of a miniature pulsatile pump with an inline heater and oxygenator. Proprietary solution for organ maintenance consists of a crystalloid part combined with oxygenated warm donor blood with hematocrit of 20% to 25%. This allows maintenance of the donor heart in a warm functioning beating state outside the body.[43] The Organ Care System allows monitoring of cardiac output, aortic pressure, blood temperature, saturation, and hematocrit. It also allows direct visual and echocardiographic surveillance and ex vivo coronary angiography of a donor heart.[41,44] Two phase I trials, 1 in Europe and 1 in the United States, evaluated the Organ Care System in HT. Thirty-day patient survival rate was 93%. In both trials, the cold ischemic time was reduced to approximately 60 to 80 minutes. In 1 case with perfusion time of 7 hours and 32 minutes, the Organ Care System allowed a transplant with excellent primary graft function.[43]

Preanesthetic considerations outline

- HT is an urgent or emergent procedure
- HT depends on donor availability and requires minimal ischemic time
- Preoperative evaluation of recipient
- Ideal time for induction and incision
- Preoperative device interrogation
- Approach to preoperative anticoagulation
- Lines
- Preparations for redo sternotomy
- Antibiotics and immunosuppression

PREANESTHETIC CONSIDERATIONS

HT occurs on an urgent or emergent basis, frequently during night hours. Timing of transplantation depends on when donor surgery can be done, and any delay of the recipient implantation due to preparation or difficulties with recipient cardiectomy should be avoided to minimize the ischemic time. Close communication between the harvesting team and the team preparing the recipient is essential.

Preoperative evaluation and preparation of the recipient must be expeditious. Preanesthetic evaluation should focus on nothing by mouth status, airway examination, level of cardiovascular support (inotropic infusions, chronic medications for heart failure, and presence of LVAD), presence of hemodynamic monitoring lines, and antiarrhythmic devices (pacemaker, ICD, CRT, or CRT-D). Recent chest radiographs and laboratory studies must be reviewed to assess pulmonary, hepatic, and renal compromise associated with CHF.

Antiarrhythmic devices need to be interrogated and reprogrammed to a mode that is not affected by electrocautery interference. The ICD function should be turned off and external defibrillator pads placed on the patient. These devices are typically surgically removed at the end of surgical procedure before the chest closure. Patients with end-stage heart disease are frequently taking angiotensin-converting enzyme inhibitors that can increase the risk of intraoperative hypotension or chronically anticoagulated with warfarin that can increase risk of bleeding. Vasopressin infusion can be beneficial for treatment of angiotensin-converting enzyme inhibitor-induced hypotension, and fresh frozen plasma should be ordered if the international normalized ratio is elevated. History of prior sternotomy, presence of LVAD, or history of difficult airway can increase recipient preparation time.

Ideally, induction of anesthesia and recipient surgical incision begin when the harvesting team has examined the donor heart and made the final determination that the organ is acceptable. Optimally, the recipient is placed on cardiopulmonary bypass (CPB) and the heart is excised as soon as the donor heart arrives at the recipient hospital.

Large-bore intravenous access and arterial lines are placed before induction of general anesthesia. It is often helpful to have both a radial arterial catheter and a femoral arterial catheter for the procedure because of abnormal pressure gradients that frequently develop between the radial artery and aorta, resulting in misdiagnosis of hemodynamic instability during or after CPB.[45,46] Many anesthesiologists prefer continuous cardiac output–mixed venous oxygen saturation (MvO_2) pulmonary artery catheters' placement before the induction for complete hemodynamic assessment. The pulmonary artery catheter needs to be withdrawn during the removal and implantation process. For this reason, it is important to ensure the sterile sheath encompasses at least 80 cm of the catheter when it is inserted. The catheter is typically removed to the 20-cm mark to ensure the scissors does not catch the tip during heart removal. The catheter can be readvanced in to the pulmonary artery once the superior vena cava cannula has been removed.

If a recipient has a preexisting central venous access, the site should be examined for evidence of infection and chart reviewed for the time of placement. Consideration should be given to changing the site of the catheter. Central venous catheters that were placed urgently should also be replaced.[45] Patients presenting for HT often have a history of multiple ICU admissions with previous arterial punctures and central lines insertions, making arterial and central venous access challenging. Placement of an arterial line can also be difficult in patients with an axial flow LVAD because no arterial pulse can be palpated.[47] Ultrasound evaluation of the central veins and peripheral arteries before attempted insertion of catheters may be helpful to determine vessel patency and to guide lines insertion.[48] Adherence to sterile techniques is particularly important because of postoperative immunosuppression.

In patients with prior sternotomy, the usual precautions and preparations include immediate availability of blood before sternotomy, multiple large-bore peripheral intravenous access or additional central catheter, application of external defibrillator pads, and preparation for peripheral cannulation by surgical team.

The surgical team requests antibiotics specific to donor and recipient infection patterns and immunosuppressive medications. Some of the immunosuppressive agents are given before incision. CMV status of the donor and of the recipient is needed to determine whether CMV-negative packed red blood cells should be ordered. Products are typically irradiated. Availability of FFP, platelets, and cryoprecipitate should be confirmed at the start of the procedure.

Induction and maintenance of general anesthesia outline

- Timing of arrival to the operating rrom
- Prior inotropic mechanical support continuation
- Choice of drugs for induction
- Postinduction transesophageal echocardiography (TEE) examination
- Intraoperative approach to anticoagulation

INDUCTION AND MAINTENANCE OF GENERAL ANESTHESIA

HT recipients usually arrive at the operating room with hemodynamic monitors in place at the time or just before the final acceptance of the donor heart. Any prior inotropic support, IABP counterpulsation, and mechanical circulatory assistance have to be maintained during induction until the institution of CPB. Because of the emergency nature of these cases, it is common that patients have recently eaten, and rapid sequence induction may be necessary.[49]

High-dose narcotic techniques have been used for induction and maintenance of cardiac transplant patients for many years with good results.[50] The choice of drugs is less important than the way they are used, with the main goal to provide stable hemodynamic state. Anesthetic induction in patients with poor ventricular function can be complicated by hemodynamic instability with cardiovascular collapse. Balanced anesthetic techniques, using small titrated doses of an induction agent, such as etomidate, fentanyl, or midazolam, and inhalational anesthetic, facilitated with fast-acting muscle relaxant (succinylcholine or rocuronium), are recommended.[51]

The presence of LVAD is highly instrumental in counteracting myocardial depression associated with general anesthesia. Instituting or increasing inotrope infusions can be beneficial in patients without LVAD support. Hypotension may not respond to ephedrine or phenylephrine, and rapidly escalating doses of inotropic support (epinephrine, norepinephrine, or dobutamine) should be promptly instituted because most patients with end-stage heart disease have significant down-regulation of the β-receptors.[52]

A comprehensive TEE examination should be performed after anesthetic induction. The biventricular contractility of the native heart and regurgitant valvular lesions can be monitored before institution of CPB for changes. TEE guidance allows early detection of deterioration and facilitates rapid therapeutic intervention to maintain hemodynamic stability. The left atrium and LV should be carefully examined for the presence of intracardiac thrombus. Manipulation of the heart is minimized before aortic cross-clamping if thrombus is noted. Absence of patent foramen ovale should be confirmed. The ascending aorta, aortic arch, and descending aorta are examined for presence of atheromatous plaque before aortic cannulation.

Heparin (300–400 units per kg) is administered before aortic cannulation unless there is documentation of heparin-induced thrombocytopenia (HIT). Patients with end-stage heart disease can develop HIT from previous repeated heparin exposures related to the use of IABPs, LVAD insertion, heparin-coated pulmonary artery catheters, and interventional cardiology procedures. The incidence of HIT is approximately 0.5% to 5%, with HIT antibodies usually decreasing to negative titers within 3 months.[53]

If the operation cannot be delayed until HIT antibodies become negative, alternative anticoagulation is recommended, such as with direct thrombin inhibitors (bivalirudin, argatroban, lepirudin, or danaparoid). Use of direct thrombin inhibitors has been associated with severe perioperative bleeding due to lack of pharmacologic reversibility.[54,55]

If heparin antibodies are negative, current guidelines recommend the use of heparin over direct thrombin inhibitors or platelet inhibitors that may cause profound hypotension. Heparin use should be confined to intraoperative period only, with alternative anticoagulation used postoperatively as needed.[56,57] If HIT antibodies are present and risk of intraoperative and postoperative bleeding deemed too high for use of nonantagonizable direct thrombin inhibitors, some investigators recommend preoperative plasmapheresis to reduce HIT antibodies and allow intraoperative heparin use.[58–60]

Heart transplantation techniques

1. Orthotopic HT
   a. Prebypass period
   b. Three types of orthotopic HT and advantages
2. Heterotopic HT

HEART TRANSPLANTATION TECHNIQUES
Orthotopic Heart Transplantation

Incision is via median sternotomy for orthotopic HT. Cannulation of the aorta is performed high along the ascending aorta, near the aortic arch. The superior and inferior vena cavae are cannulated individually and encircled with tourniquets, leaving the surgical field bloodless. The aorta is cross-clamped close to the aortic arch. Prior to resection of the native heart, the pulmonary artery catheter is withdrawn from the surgical field.

There are 3 surgical techniques for orthotopic HT: the classic or biatrial approach, the bicaval approach, and the total transplantation technique.

Shumway and colleges at Stanford University describe the classic or biatrial method.[61] After initiation of CPB, the recipient heart is excised, aorta and pulmonary artery are transected above the semilunar commissures, and atria are incised along the atrioventricular grooves, leaving cuffs for donor heart implantation. Atrial appendages are removed to decrease the risk of postoperative thrombus formation. The 4 anastomoses in biatrial technique include left and right atrial cuffs and end-to-end pulmonary artery and aortic anastomoses.

The bicaval method was described in 1991 by Sievers and colleagues.[62] In this technique, recipient right atrium is totally excised and the donor right atrium attached directly to the inferior and superior vena cava requiring 5 anastomoses: left atrial cuff, individual end-to-end inferior vena cava and superior vena cava, and pulmonary artery and aorta. The bicaval approach was reported associated with better short-term results, such as perioperative mortality, preservation of sinus rhythm, less tricuspid and mitral regurgitation, and lower atrial pressures.[63] An analysis of the UNOS database found the use of the bicaval anastomosis the most commonly used technique today (62% in 2007) and associated with fewer pacemaker insertions and a small but significant survival advantage.[64]

To decrease ischemic time for distant procurements, the additional surgical strategies include performing the left atrial anastomosis and the aortic anastomosis in a recipient first, followed by the releasing the cross-clamp to reperfuse the transplanted heart. The subsequent pulmonary artery and right atrial or bicaval anastomoses can be performed on a perfused and beating heart.[29]

The total transplantation technique, described by Yacoub and colleagues[65] involves total preservation of donor heart and 8 anastomoses: 4 pulmonary veins, separate inferior vena cava and superior vena cava, and pulmonary artery and aorta. This approach is associated with increased ischemic time and used in 2.6% of HTs.

Heterotopic Heart Transplantation

Heterotopic HT is a virtually abandoned procedure today. It was first described by Carrel and Guthrie[66] and performed by Christian Barnard in 1974. It involves preservation of recipient heart in orthotopic position and placement of donor heart in the right thorax attached in parallel with the native heart. Before the introduction of cyclosporine and MCS, heterotopic HT allowed a recipient to maintain some cardiac output if the allograft began to fail. It was also an option for HT recipients with pulmonary hypertension and high probability of postoperative donor RV failure. With introduction of LVAD as a bridge to candidacy, the indications for heterotopic HT are probably limited to immunosuppressed patients with significant pulmonary hypertension requiring retransplantation in whom LVAD represents high risk for infection. Heterotopic transplantation is also indicated for pediatric transplant recipients with significant donor-to-recipient size mismatch.[9,19]

Weaning from CPB
• Rewarming
• TEE assessment
• Deairing
• Inotropes
• Role of pacing
• CPB discontinuation
• PGF

Weaning from Cardiopulmonary Bypass

Weaning from CPB proceeds similarly to any other cardiac cases. Patients are rewarmed and deeply anesthetized to prevent an excessive increase of pulmonary vascular resistance and RV afterload associated with pain response. The lungs are suctioned and ventilated with 100% oxygen, tidal volumes 6 mL/kg to 8 mL/kg and positive end-expiratory pressure 5 mm Hg to 6 mm Hg to prevent mechanical compression of the pulmonary capillary bed and increase in PVR.[47] Routine deairing maneuvers are performed. Placing patients in steep Trendelenburg position before removal of the cross-clamp is considered beneficial by many investigators as is temporary occlusion of the carotid vessels to prevent air or debris from embolizing to the head.

The heart is re-evaluated with TEE with attention to retention of air in ostia of pulmonary veins, LV apex, intraventricular septum and left atrium, and left atrial appendage. A brief evaluation of ventricular and valvular function and confirmation of no intracardiac shunts should be performed as soon as a rhythm is present and there is some flow through the heart. Depending on the surgical technique, atrial suture lines and excess atrial tissue may be seen.

Half of patients require electrical defibrillation. It usually takes several minutes for spontaneous rhythm to return. Bradycardia and junctional rhythms may occur due to ischemic injury to sinus and atrioventricular nodes.[67] A recipient's residual atrial tissue may continue to have electrical activity, seen clinically as 2 P-waves on ECG. The native P-wave has no physiologic effect on the donor heart.

Denervated donor heart lacks normal physiologic feedback loops controlling inotropy and chronotropy. Isoproterenol or dobutamine is used frequently for its direct effect on cardiac β-receptors to increase heart rate. Use of temporary epicardial pacing should be initiated in the setting of relative bradycardia until the intravenous chronotropic agent has achieved the desired heart rate. Heart rate should be maintained within high normal range 90 to 110 beats per minute to augment cardiac output, increase RV contractility, and overpace possible arrhythmias.

Temporary pacing wires are placed on donor right atrium and ventricle even if the initial rhythm is sinus.[35,68] Some patients need temporary pacing in the immediate intraoperative and short-term postoperative period. However, 4% to 12% of patients require permanent pacemaker implantation due to the loss of sinus node function.[1] It has recently been found that when the heart is procured with lungs, the heart recipient is twice as likely to need a permanent pacemaker, probably due to injury to the conduction system during harvesting.[69]

The heart is carefully loaded not to exceed central venous pressure more than 10 mm Hg to 12 mm Hg and CPB flow is slowly decreased to approximately half of initial value while monitoring arterial and central venous pressure and biventricular function with TEE and direct observation of RV contractility in the surgical field. After several minutes of sustainable hemodynamic state, consideration should be given to gradual discontinuation of CPB. The pulmonary artery catheter can be readvanced after removal of superior vena cava cannula.

Postbypass contractility of the donor heart may range from excellent (requiring minimal support) to very poor. In extreme cases PGF can occur. This highly lethal complication, although uncommon (2.5% incidence in large case series),[69] is responsible for more than 30% of early deaths after cardiac transplantation.[17] PGF manifests as severe biventricular dysfunction with hypotension, low cardiac output, and high filling pressures. Risk factors associated with PGF include prolonged ischemic time, donor-recipient gender mismatch, donor-recipient weight ratio less than 0.8, presence of ECMO or extracorporeal LVAD at the time of transplantation, congenital etiology of heart failure, and retransplantation. Concurrent lung harvest in a donor may also cause PGF, likely due to ventricular distention and injury after administration of additional cardioplegia for lung procurement.[69]

Right heart failure

- RV failure as a cause of mortality after HT
- Incidence
- What causes it
- Manifestation
- Patients at risk
- Therapy goals
- Inotropic agents
- Pacing role
- Pulmonary vasodilators
- Role of sildenafil
- MCS choice

RIGHT HEART FAILURE

Right heart failure is a common occurrence and a cause of morbidity and mortality after cardiac transplantation. Contemporary registry data from ISHLT indicate that approximately 20% of early deaths after cardiac transplantation are attributable to RV failure.

Causes of RV Failure

RV failure is of multifactorial origin; preexisting increased pulmonary vascular resistance, ischemia-reperfusion injury of the myocardium associated with graft preservation, and prolonged ischemic times are 3 of the main causes.[70] Pulmonary hypertension may be additionally aggravated due to adverse inflammatory effects of the CPB, hypoxemia, and administration of blood products and protamine.[68]

The donor right heart, especially when it is young and comparably small, is not accustomed to high pulmonary vascular resistance. The nonadapted thin-walled RV is able to maximally produce pressures of 45 mm Hg to 50 mm Hg after which it may fail acutely.[47,68]

Manifestations

Clinically RV failure is evidenced by failure to wean a recipient from CPB and low cardiac output in the face of rising central venous pressure. The right heart can be seen in the surgical field to dilate and contract poorly. TEE shows a dilated, poorly contracting RV as evidenced by measurement of RV fractional area change in the midesophageal 4-chamber view[71] and an underfilled vigorously contracting LV.[52] Severe tricuspid regurgitation secondary to dilatation of the tricuspid valve annulus might be seen.

RV failure can in turn cause a decrease in LV end-diastolic volume with septal shift to the left that further limits early diastolic LV filling. This vicious cycle results in a low cardiac output syndrome with hypotension and shock.[68,72]

Patients at Risk

Patients with an increased systolic pulmonary artery pressure of greater than 60 mm Hg and/or a *pulmonary artery vascular resistance* greater than 200 dyne/s/cm^{-5} and/or a transpulmonary gradient of greater than 15 mm Hg before transplantation are considered at high risk for developing early perioperative RV failure.[47]

Pulmonary artery hypertension and elevated PVR should be considered relative contraindications to HT when the PVR is greater than 5 Wood units or the PVR index is greater than 6 or the transpulmonary gradient exceeds 16 mm Hg to 20 mm Hg. If the pulmonary artery systolic pressure exceeds 60 mm Hg in conjunction with any of these 3 variables, the risk of right heart failure and early death is increased. If the PVR can be reduced to less than 2.5 Wood units with a vasodilator but the systolic blood pressure falls to less than 85 mm Hg, the patient remains at high risk of right heart failure and mortality after HT.[12]

Therapy

Therapy is directed at preventing a low cardiac output syndrome. The goal is to optimize RV preload, increase RV contractility, decrease RV afterload, and improve coronary perfusion. MCS should be applied early before secondary organ damage or profound metabolic acidosis occurs. MCS includes implantation of intraaortic balloon pump, RVAD or ECMO in RV failure resistant to inotropic agents, and pulmonary vasodilators.[47,68]

Systemic vasodilators with pulmonary vasodilating properties, including nitroglycerine and sodium nitroprusside, can be used in the absence of systemic hypotension.[35] Novel selective inhaled pulmonary vasodilators, such as inhaled nitric oxide, prostaglandins (prostaglandin E1, alprostadil, and prostaglandin I2, epoprostenol/prostacyclin) can be used in the management of perioperative RV dysfunction with systemic hypotension, such that combined pulmonary and systemic vasodilators are not indicated.[15,35,73–75] In patients who have undergone heart and lung transplantation, it has been suggested that inhaled prostacyclin is as effective as inhaled nitric oxide for treatment of RV failure.[76] Once inhaled therapy is initiated, it should not be weaned rapidly but slowly, typically over hours or days in an ICU setting. Rapid weaning of selective pulmonary vasodilators can precipitate life-threatening rebound pulmonary hypertension with acute RV failure.[15] In a recent clinical trial, use of oral sildenafil was proved an effective bridging strategy in the weaning of intravenous and inhaled pulmonary vasodilators after HT.[77]

Inotropic Agents

Inotropic agents that can be used to augment RV function include isoproterenol, milrinone, dobutamine, and epinephrine.[35] Levosimendan has also been reported to reverse low cardiac output after HT. Levosimendan is currently approved for use in acute heart failure in Europe but not in the United States.[78,79]

Levothyroxine increases cyclic adenosine monophosphate levels and should be considered with a loading dose of 0.8 µg/kg after removal of the aortic cross-clamp, followed by infusion of 0.12 µg/kg/h for 6 hours during prolonged CPB courses associated with decreased triiodothyronine levels.[47,80]

Pacing

Preservation of sinus rhythm is important. To increase RV contractility, the heart rate can be elevated by pacing to maintain a heart rate of approximately 100 to 120 beats per minute to increase RV output and overpace possible arrhythmias.[47,68]

Mechanical Circulatory Support for Right Ventricular Failure and Primary Graft Failure

MCS is indicated for continuing or worsening hemodynamic deterioration, such as decreasing cardiac index or MvO_2 less than 50% refractory to medical management. If IABP does not maintain coronary perfusion pressure, an RVAD, biventricular assist device, or ECMO should be considered.[35] The choice of MCS modality depends on whether isolated RV failure versus biventricular failure is present and on adequacy of lung function.[76]

In isolated RV failure, small VADs, such as Levitronix CentriMag (Pharos, Waltham, Massachusetts), can be used for temporary RV support.[35] Patients requiring implantation of an RVAD for RV failure after HT face an in-hospital mortality rate of 73% to 100%.[70] Some investigators advocate the use of peripheral venoarterial ECMO in HT recipients with RV failure, reporting better in-hospital survival and graft survival rates versus with isolated RVAD use.[70,81,82] In cases of PGF, the choice depends on the adequacy of lung function.[76] Devices, such as TandemHeart (CardiacAssist, Inc Pittsburgh, PA) and Levitronix Centrimag, can provide biventricular support.[35] If lung function is also inadequate, venoarterial ECMO support is preferred.[76]

ECMO can be instituted from the peripheral vascular access, allowing sternal wound closure and obviating reopening the chest to remove support devices.[20,76] Postoperative bleeding is a major issue with ECMO because of need for systemic anti-coagulation with ECMO. The alternative is to convert the CPB cannulas to ECMO cannulas and leave the chest open. Recent studies report in-hospital survival rates with the use of ECMO in the adults from 20% to 50% and mortality rates from 50% to 70%.[20,70] Contrary to the experience and practice in adults, the first choice for support in the setting of PGF in the pediatric setting should be ECMO.[35]

REFERENCES

1. Boilson BA, Raichlin E, Park SJ, et al. Device therapy and cardiac transplantation for end-stage heart failure. Curr Probl Cardiol 2010;35:8–64.
2. Miller LW. Left ventricular assist devices are underutilized. Circulation 2011;123: 1552–8.
3. Stehlik J, Edwards LB, Kucheryavaya AY, et al. The registry of the International Society for Heart and lung transplantation: twenty-eighth adult heart transplant report—2011. J Heart Lung Transplant 2011;30:1078–94.
4. Willman VL, Cooper T, Cian LG, et al. Auto-transplantation of the canine heart. Surg Gynecol Obstet 1962;115:299–302.
5. Lower RR, Dong E, Shumway NE. Suppression of rejection crisis in the cardiac homograph. Ann Thorac Surg 1965;1:645–9.

6. Barnard CN. The operation. A human cardiac transplant: an interim report of a successful operation performed at Groote Schuur Hospital, Cape Town. S Afr Med J 1967;41:1271–4.

7. Kantrowitz A, Haller JD, Joos H, et al. Transplantation of the heart in an infant and an adult. Am J Cardiol 1968;22(6):782–90.

8. Cauls PK, Stinson EB, Billingham ME, et al. Diagnosis of human cardiac allograft rejection by serial cardiac biopsy. J Thorac Cardiovasc Surg 1973;66:461–6.

9. Milla F, Pinney SP, Anyanwu AC. Indications for heart transplantation in the current of left ventricular assist devices. Mt Sinai J Med 2012;79:305–16.

10. 2010 Annual Report of the U.S. Organ Procurement and Transplantation Network and the scientific registry of transplant recipients: 1998-200. Department of Health and Human Services, Health Resources and Services Administration, Healthcare Systems Bureau, Division of Transplantation, Rockville, MD; United Network for Organ Sharing, Richmond, VA.

11. Stewart GC, Givertz MM. Mechanical circulatory support for advanced heart failure: patients and technology in evolution. Circulation 2012;125:1304–15.

12. Mehra MR, Kobashigawa J, Starling R, et al. Listing criteria for heart transplantation: International Sciety fo Heart and Lung Transplantation guidelines for the care of cardiac transplant candidates – 2006. J Heart Lung Transplant 2006;25: 1024–42.

13. Nicolini F, Gherli T. Alternatives to transplantation in the surgical therapy for heart failure. Eur J Cardiothorac Surg 2009;35:214–28.

14. Hunt SA, Abraham WT, Chin MH, et al. 2009 Focus update incorporated into the ACC/AHA 2005 guidelines for the diagnosis and management of heart failure in adults. Circulation 2009;53:e1–90.

15. Augoustides JG, Rhia H. Recent progress in heart failure treatment and heart transplantation. J Cardiothorac Vasc Anesth 2009;23:738–48.

16. Shuhaiber JH, Kim JB, Hur K, et al. Comparison of survival in primary and repeat heart transplation from 1987 through 2004 in the United States. Ann Thorac Surg 2007;83:2135–41.

17. Kirk R, Edwards LB, Kucheryavaya AY, et al. The registry of the International Society for Heart and lung Transplantation: fourteenth pediatric heart transplantation report—2011. J Heart Lung Transplant 2011;30:1095–103.

18. Mancini D, Lietz K. Selection of cardiac transplant candidates in 2010. Circulation 2010;122:173–83.

19. Hunt SA, Haddad F. The changing face of heart transplantation. J Am Coll Cardiol 2008;52:587–98.

20. Bittner HB. Extra-corporeal membrane oxygenation support in cardiac transplantation. Appl Cardiopulm Pathophysiol 2011;15:272–7.

21. Ibrahim M, Hendry P, Masters R, et al. Management of acute severe perioperative failure of cardiac allografts: a single-centre experience with a review of the literature. Can J Cardiol 2007;23:363–7.

22. Johnson MR, Aaronson KD, Canter CE, et al. Heart retransplantation. Am J Transplant 2007;7:2075–81.

23. Vega JD, Moore J, Murray S, et al. Heart transplantation in the United States, 1998-2007. Am J Transplant 2009;9:932–41.

24. Rose EA, Gelijns AC, Moskowitz AJ, et al. Long-term use of a left ventricular assist device for end-stage heart failure. N Engl J Med 2001;345:1435–43.

25. Kirlin JK, Naftel DC, Kormos RL, et al. Third INTERMACS annual report: the evolution of destination therapy in the United States. J Heart Lung Transplant 2011;30: 115–23.

26. John R, Pagani FD, Naka Y, et al. Post-cardiac transplant survival after support with a continuous-flow left ventricular assist device: impact of duration of left ventricular assist device support and other variables. J Thorac Cardiovasc Surg 2010;140:174–81.
27. Kirlin JK, Naftel DC, Kormos RL, et al. The fourth INTERMACS annual report: 4,000 implants and counting. J Heart Lung Transplant 2012;31:117–26.
28. Levy WC, Mozaffarian D, Linker DT, et al. The Seattle heart failure model: prediction of survival in heart failure. Circulation 2006;113:1424.
29. Vega JD. The change in heart allocation policy in the United States: is it working as designed? J Heart Lung Transplant 2010;29:255–6.
30. Felker GM, Milano CA, Yager EE, et al. Outcomes with an alternate list strategy for heart transplantation. J Heart Lung Transplant 2005;24:1781–6.
31. Chen JM, Russo MJ, Hammond KM, et al. Alternate waiting list strategies for heart transplantation maximize donor organ utilization. Ann Thorac Surg 2005;80:224–8.
32. Laks H, Marelli D, Fonarow GC, et al. Use of two recipient lists for adults requiring heart transplantation. J Thorac Cardiovasc Surg 2003;125:49–59.
33. Ramakrishna H, Jaroszewski DE, Arabia FA. Adult cardiac transplantation: a review of perioperative management part-I. Ann Card Anaesth 2009;12:71–8.
34. Grauhan O. Screening and assessment of the donor heart. Appl Cardiopulm Pathophysiol 2011;15:191–7.
35. Costanzo MR, Taylor D, Hunt S, et al. The International Society of Heart and Lung Transplantation guideline for the care of heart transplant recipients. J Heart Lung Transplant 2010;29:914–56.
36. Kuppahally SS, Valantine HA, Weisshaar D, et al. Outcome in cardiac recipients of donor hearts with increased left ventricular wall thickness. Am J Transplant 2007;7:2388–95.
37. Weiss ES, Allen JG, Patel ND, et al. The impact of donor-recipient sex matching on survival after orthotopic heart transplantation – analysis of 18,000 transplants in the modern era. Circ Heart Fail 2009;2:401–8.
38. Yamani MH, Erinc K, Starling RC, et al. Donor intracranial bleeding is associated with advanced transplant coronary vasculopathy: evidence from intravascular ultrasound. Transplant Proc 2004;36:2564–6.
39. D'ancona G, Santise G, Falleta C, et al. Primary graft failure after heart transplantation: the importance of donor pharmacological management. Transplant Proc 2010;42:710–2.
40. Conway J, Dipchand AI. Heart transplantation in children. Pediatr Clin North Am 2010;57:353–73.
41. Wagner FM. Donor heart preservation and perfusion. Appl Cardiopulm Pathophysiol 2011;15:198–206.
42. Russo MJ, Chen JM, Sorabella RA, et al. The effect of ischemic time on survival after heart transplantation varies by donor age: an analysis of the United Network for Organ Sharing database. J Thorac Cardiovasc Surg 2007;133:554–9.
43. Yeter R, Hubler M, Pasic M, et al. Organ preservation with the organ care system. Appl Cardiopulm Pathophysiol 2011;15:207–12.
44. Ghodsizad A, Bordel V, Ungerer M, et al. Ex vivo coronary angiography of a donor heart in the Organ Care System. Heart Surg Forum 2012;15(3):E161–3.
45. Gaitan BD, Thunberg CA, Stansbury LG, et al. Development, current status, and anesthetic management of the implanted heart. J Cardiothorac Vasc Anesth 2011;25:1179–92.
46. Denault A, Deschamps A. Abnormal aortic-to-radial arterial pressure gradients resulting in misdiagnosis of hemodynamic instability. Can J Anaesth 2009;56:534–6.

47. Koster A, Diehl C, Dongas A, et al. Anesthesia for cardiac transplantation: a practical overview of current management strategies. Appl Cardiopulm Pathophysiol 2011;15:213–9.
48. Troianos CA, Hartman GS, Glas KE, et al. Guidelines for performing ultrasound guided vascular cannulation: recommendation of the American Society of Echocardiography and the Society of Cardiovascular Anesthesiologists. J Am Soc Echocardiogr 2012;114:46–69.
49. Waterman PM, Bjerke R. Rapid-sequence induction technique in patients with severe ventricular dysfunction. J Cardiothorac Anesth 1988;2:602–6.
50. Hensley F, Martin DE, Larach DR, et al. Anesthetic management for cardiac transplantation in North America – 1986 survey. J Cardiothorac Anesth 1987;1:429.
51. Demad K, Wyner J, Mihm FG, et al. Anaesthesia for heart transplantation. A retrospective study and review. Br J Anaesth 1986;58:1357.
52. Shanewise J. Cardiac transplantation. Anesthesiol Clin North America 2004;22: 753–65.
53. Levy JH, Winkler AM. Heparin-induced thrombocytopenia and cardiac surgery. Curr Opin Anaesthesiol 2010;23:74–9.
54. Wadia Y, Cooper JR, Bracey AW, et al. Intraoperative anticoagulation management during cardiac transplantation. Tex Heart Inst J 2008;35:62–5.
55. Christiansen S, Hammel D, Schmidt C, et al. Heparin in patients with heparin-induced thrombocytopenia type II requiring LVAD implantation and cardiac transplantation. J Heart Lung Transplant 2000;19:510–2.
56. Warkentin TE, Greinacher A, Koster A, et al. Treatment and prevention of heparin-induced thrombocytopenia: American College of Chest Physicians Evidence-Based Clinical Practice Guidelines (8th edition). Chest 2008;133:340S–80S.
57. Levy JH, Tanaka KA, Hursting MJ, et al. Reducing thrombotic complications in perioperative setting: an update on heparin-induced thrombocytopenia. Anesth Analg 2007;105:570–82.
58. Welsby IJ, Um J, Milano CA, et al. Plasmapheresis and heparin reexposure as a management strategy for cardiac surgical patients with heparin-induced thrombocytopenia. Anesth Analg 2010;110:30–5.
59. Robinson JA, Lewis BE. Plasmapharesis in the management of heparin induced thrombocytopenia. Semin Hematol 1999;36:29–32.
60. Abdel-Razeq HN, Bajouda AA, Khalil MM, et al. Treating heparin-induced thrombocytopenia the unconventional way! Saudi Med J 2004;25:1258–60.
61. Shumway NE, Lower R, Stofer RC. Transplantation of the heart. Adv Surg 1966;2: 265–84.
62. Sievers HH, Weyand M, Kraatz EG, et al. An alternative technique for orthotopic cardiac transplantation, with preservation of the normal anatomy of the right atrium. J Thorac Cardiovasc Surg 1991;39:70–2.
63. Schnoor M, Schafer T, Luhmann D, et al. Bicaval versus standard technique in orthotopic heart transplantation: a systematic review and meta-analysis. J Thorac Cardiovasc Surg 2007;134:1322–31.
64. Davies RR, Russo MJ, Morgan JA, et al. Standard versus bicaval techniques for orthotopic transplantation: an analysis of the United Network for Organ Sharing database. J Thorac Cardiovasc Surg 2010;140:700–8.
65. Yacoub M, Mankad P, Ledingham S, et al. Donor procurement and surgical technique for cardiac transplantation. Semin Thorac Cardiovasc Surg 1990;2:153–61.
66. Carrel A, Guthrie CC. the transplantation of veins and organs. Am Med 1905;10: 1101–2.

67. Jacquet L, Ziady G, Stein K, et al. Cardiac rhythm disturbances early after ortho-topic heart transplantation: prevalence and clinical importance of the observed abnormalities. J Am Coll Cardiol 1990;16:832–7.

68. Wagner F. Monitoring and management of right ventricular function following cardiac transplantation. Appl Cardiopulm Pathophysiol 2011;15:220–9.

69. Russo MJ, Iribarne A, Hong KM, et al. Factors associated with primary graft failure after heart transplantation. Transplantation 2010;90:444–50.

70. Taghavi S, Zuckermann A, Ankersmit J, et al. Extracorporeal membrane oxygen-ation is superior to right ventricular assist device for acute right ventricular failure after heart transplantation. Ann Thorac Surg 2004;78:1644–9.

71. Anavekar NC, Gerson D, Skali H, et al. Two-dimensional assessment of right ventricular function: an echocardiographic MRI correlative study. Echocardiog-raphy 2007;24:452–6.

72. Augoustides JG, Ochroch EA. Inhaled selective pulmonary vasodilators. Int Anesthesiol Clin 2005;43(2):101–14.

73. Mubarak KK. A review of prostaglandin analogs in the management of patients with pulmonary arterial hypertension. Respir Med 2010;104:9–21.

74. Khan TA, Schnickel G, Ross D, et al. A prospective randomized, crossover pilot study of inhaled nitric oxide versus inhaled prostacyclin in heart transplant and lung transplant recipients. J Thorac Cardiovasc Surg 2009;138:1417–24.

75. Creagh-Brown BC, Griffiths MJ, Evans TW. Bench-to-bedside review:inhaled nitric oxide therapy in adults. Crit Care 2009;13:212.

76. Vlahakes GJ. Right ventricular failure after cardiac surgery. Cardiol Clin 2012;30: 283–9.

77. Boffini M, Sansone F, Ceresa F, et al. Role of oral sildenafil in the treatment of right ventricular dysfunction after heart transplantation. Transplant Proc 2009;41: 1353–6.

78. Weis F, Beiras-Fernandez A, Kaczmarek I, et al. Levosimendan: a new thera-peutic option in the treatment of primary graft dysfunction after heart transplanta-tion. J Heart Lung Transplant 2009;28:501–4.

79. Petersen JW, Felker GM. Inotropes in the management of acute heart failure. Crit Care Med 2008;36:S106–11.

80. Ranasinghe AM, Bonser RS. Thyroid hormone in cardiac surgery. Vascul Pharma-col 2010;52:131–7.

81. Takhavi S, Ankersmit A, Zuckerman GA, et al. A retrospective analysis of extra-corporeal membrane oxygenation versus right ventricular assist device in acute graft failure after heart transplantation. Transplant Proc 2003;35:2805–7.

82. Marasco SF, Esmore DS, Negri J, et al. Early institution of mechanical support improves outcomes in primary cardiac allograft failure. J Heart Lung Transplant 2005;24:2037–42.

Anesthetic Considerations for Adults Undergoing Fontan Conversion Surgery

Emad B. Mossad, MD[a,b,*], Pablo Motta, MD[a,b],
David F. Vener, MD[a,b]

KEYWORDS

- Adult congenital heart disease • Fontan operation • Venous capacitance
- Protein-losing enteropathy

KEY POINTS

- Adults with congenital heart disease are a growing population with residual defects that require repeat interventions. The care of these patients will increasingly require a care team with an understanding of the unique physiology and anatomy of these patients.
- The Fontan conversion operation is an evolution in surgical intervention for patients with single ventricles and failed prior operations.
- Patients with single ventricular repair have significant comorbidities and unique physiologic status that must be considered by the anesthesiologist.

INTRODUCTION

Patients more than 18 years of age now represent the largest group of patients with congenital heart defects (CHDs), with a population growing at a rate of 5% to 7% annually.[1,2] The most common operations in the Society of Thoracic Surgery (STS) Congenital Heart Surgery Database for patients more than 18 years old for the years 2008 to 2011 are outlined in **Table 1**. During this period, 6234 procedures were performed on 5892 patients.[3] Although these numbers remain small compared with the overall number of adult cardiac operations, they represent one of the only adult cardiac surgical populations that is continuing to grow.

The first groups of children with surgically repaired cyanotic defects, primarily those with tetralogy of Fallot, as well as those with more straightforward defects

Disclosures: The authors have all contributed equally to the article. None of the authors have any conflict of interest related to this work.
[a] Baylor College of Medicine, Houston, TX, USA; [b] Division of Pediatric cardiovascular Anesthesia, Texas Children's Hospital, 6621 Fannin Street, Suite W17417, Houston, TX 77030, USA
* Corresponding author. Texas Children's Hospital, 6621 Fannin Street, Suite W17417, Houston, TX 77030.
E-mail address: ebmossad@texaschildrens.org

Table 1
STS congenital heart surgery data 2008 to 2011 for adults (>18 years old)

Primary Procedure	Total Number	% of ACHS	30-d Mortality (%)
Pulmonary valve replacement: RV to PA conduit	1081	39	2.6
Pacemaker procedure	628	23	1.7
ASD repair	255	9	0
Arrhythmia surgery	248	9	2.8
Aortic aneurysm	158	6	3.2
Mitral valve repair/replacement	147	5	1.4
Fontan conversion	123	4	10.6
Others	152	5	1.3

Abbreviations: ACHS, adult congenital heart surgery cases; PA, pulmonary artery.
Data from Society of Thoracic Surgeons Congenital Heart Surgery Executive Summary, Duke Clinical Research Institute. Available at: http://www.sts.org/sites/default/files/documents/STSExecSummary_Adults.pdf. Accessed December 19, 2012.

such as atrial septal defects, are now more than 50 years of age. In addition, a growing cohort of patients with more complex lesions is now surviving into their 20s and 30s, and potentially beyond, although their lifespan remains significantly shorter than those without CHD.[3] With the progress of care and long-term follow-up, it is now evident that many of the patients who had complete repairs as infants and children require ongoing monitoring throughout their lifetime and may require subsequent surgeries to repair progressive disease processes such as conduit failure or dilatation, valve insufficiency, aneurysm development, or residual defects. In addition, many of these patients, particularly those with right ventricular outflow lesions and those with single-ventricle physiology, require repeat operations or planned surgical modifications, including conduit revisions, Fontan conversion surgery, or heart transplantation because of progressive heart failure. A large cohort of these patients require multiple interventions in both the operating room and cardiac catheterization laboratories for electrophysiology investigations and ablations for arrhythmia management, percutaneous valve insertion, placement and dilations of stents, and other procedures.[4] Because of the complexity of their diseases and the need for reoperations, the risk profile for these patients significantly exceeds that of patients without CHDs.[5]

Adult patients with CHDs are often still followed and treated by pediatric specialists, including cardiologists, surgeons, and anesthesiologists in children's hospitals. These patients comprise 5% to 10% of the annual surgical volume in many children's hospitals and a significant number of catheter interventions in these hospitals (**Fig. 1**). These patients are increasingly seen by adult providers, including adult cardiac anesthesiologists. There are now a few programs around the country that have begun to specialize in the treatment of this unique population.[5,6] Caring for this population requires familiarity with congenital cardiac defects, their surgical and medical treatment, and the underlying physiology in order to safely manage their perioperative course. Giamberti and colleagues[5] showed that the training and experience of the surgical and anesthesia care team may affect patient outcomes. Most of the procedures that require repeat sternotomy, such as conduit revisions or aortic aneurysm repairs, have perioperative mortalities no higher than 3.2%, but each subsequent reoperation carries increasing morbidity (**Fig. 2**).[5]

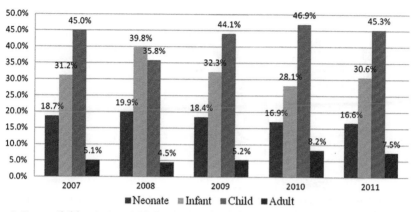

Fig. 1. Texas Children's Hospital Heart Center cardiovascular and thoracic surgery case volume by age (2007–2011). (*Data from* Texas Children's Hospital. Heart Center Outcomes Book 2011. Available at: http://www.texaschildrens.org/uploadedFiles/2011-Heart-Center-Outcomes.pdf. Accessed March 12, 2013.)

EVOLUTION AND OUTCOMES OF THE FONTAN CONVERSION SURGERY
History

The first successful single-ventricle surgeries were described independently in the early 1970s by Fontan and Baudet[7] in France and Kreutzer and colleagues[8] in Argentina for the treatment of tricuspid atresia. These single-ventricle repairs involved creating a direct anastomosis between the right atrium (RA) and pulmonary artery, bypassing the right ventricle (RV) and creating a passive pulmonary blood flow pattern, typically using the right atrial appendage as a conduit to the pulmonary artery (**Fig. 3**A). Variations on this surgery have become the treatment of choice for single-ventricle anatomy of all types, including hypoplastic left heart syndrome and its variants as well as complex atrioventricular canal defects and others. With advances in surgical

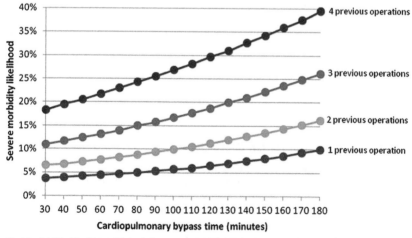

Fig. 2. Morbidity likelihood in adult congenital heart surgery as it relates to cardiopulmonary bypass duration and number of previous cardiac operations. (*Data from* Giamberti A, Chessa M, Abella R, et al. Morbidity and mortality risk factors in adults with Congenital Heart Disease Undergoing Cardiac Reoperations. Ann Thorac Surg 2009;88:1284–90; with permission.)

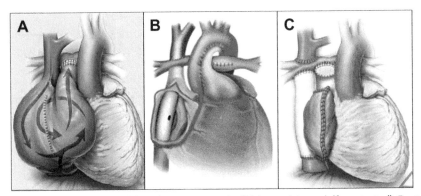

Fig. 3. (*A*) Atriopulmonary (classic) Fontan repair. (*B*) Lateral tunnel (fenestrated) Fontan repair. (*C*) Extracardiac Fontan repair. ([*A, C*] *From* Texas Children's Hospital. Heart Center Outcomes Book 2011. Available at: http://www.texaschildrens.org/uploadedFiles/2011-Heart-Center-Outcomes.pdf. Accessed March 12, 2013; and [*B*] *From* Gaca AM, Jaggers JJ, Dudley LT, et al. Repair of congenital heart disease: a primer – part 1. Radiology 2008;247: 617–31; with permission.)

techniques and experience, modifications in surgical strategy were developed to account for variations in anatomy as well as to minimize complications associated with the original surgery that became more obvious as patients survived into adulthood.

The most frequent complications following the atriopulmonary Fontan include massive right atrial dilatation, atrial arrhythmia development, protein-losing enteropathy (PLE) and progressive heart failure, particularly in patients with a functional RV acting as the systemic chamber. Late surgical complications such as progressive anastomotic stenosis may also contribute to the need for reoperations. Nonetheless, many of the surviving patients have a reasonable quality of life.[9]

Subsequent surgical improvements after the initial reports by Fontan and Baudet[7] and Kreutzer and colleagues[8] included staging the procedure by the creation of a Glenn shunt (bidirectional connection from the superior vena cava to the pulmonary artery) followed by completion of the Fontan with an intracardiac lateral tunnel (LT) or hemi-Fontan and now more commonly the extracardiac (EC) Fontan (see **Fig. 3**B, C).[10] In addition, some circumstances such as a high pulmonary artery resistance may indicate the need for a fenestration within the repair to allow a pop-off of the systemic venous pathway and preservation of cardiac output. During the period of 2008 to 2011 in the STS Database, Fontan completion, in its most common variants, accounted for 3.8% of all operations performed and 10.4% in children between the ages of 1 and 18 years.[3]

Indications and Benefits of Fontan Conversion

Following the initial success of the original Fontan repairs, long-term follow-up showed premature decline in survival and functional status of these patients.[11] Despite a perfect Fontan operation, patients followed for a median of 12.2 years had an actuarial freedom from death or transplantation of less than 80% at 20 years, with many patients suffering debilitating arrhythmias (10%), thromboembolic events (7.9%), and heart failure–related symptoms (7%).[12] These consequences identify the palliative rather than curative nature of the Fontan state, primarily because progressive atrial dilatation results in fluid energy loss, effective pressure decrease, and fluid resistance along the pathway.[13] This condition is manifested by worsening exercise capacity, lower anaerobic thresholds, and increased endothelin-1 and brain and atrial natriuretic peptides.[14]

Fontan conversion surgery refers to procedures in which the original systemic venous-to-pulmonary-artery anastomosis is taken down and a modified pathway is constructed to decompress the RA in an attempt to enhance forward flow through the passive Fontan pathway, decrease the risk of arrhythmias and thromboembolic events, and improve survival. These procedures are most commonly performed in the late teenage years and beyond, when the complications of the original surgery become intolerable. Fontan conversion surgery is particularly high risk because of multiple factors, including repeat sternotomy, advanced heart failure, and significant arrhythmias. It is commonly accompanied by arrhythmia surgery with intraoperative cryoablation of the atrial endocardium in a maze operation and may also involve valvuloplasty of insufficient atrioventricular valves. Of the most frequent procedures in the latest STS Congenital Heart Surgery Database report (2008–2011), Fontan revision or conversion is the 10th most common performed on adult patients, but it carries the highest mortality (123 procedures reported with a 10.6% 30-day mortality) (see **Table 1**).

LT Versus EC Repairs

Indications for Fontan conversion in an adult who has previously undergone a classic atriopulmonary Fontan include a combination of increasing symptoms of systemic ventricular failure, refractory arrhythmias, and other complications related to obstructed or sluggish flow in the Fontan pathway. Surgical options for the Fontan conversion include LT and EC repairs with/without arrhythmia surgery and pacemaker placement. Although there are theoretic advantages to each of the two approaches (**Table 2**), most reports show a similar short and intermediate follow-up conduct, including similar in-hospital mortality, hospital length of stay, improvement in New York Heart Association (NYHA) class, recurrence of arrhythmias, and late death.[15,16]

Texas Children's Hospital Fontan Conversion Data

The experience of several institutions with the Fontan conversion surgery for adults suffering from a variety of sequelae of the original repair is encouraging. Survivors

Table 2
Comparison of LT and EC Fontan

	LT Fontan	EC Fontan
Potential advantages	Positive growth potential, especially in young patients Ease of fenestration when indicated Avoidance of conduit-related issues (stenosis, thrombosis)	Flexibility in anatomically variable morphology (heterotaxy) Avoidance of sinus node manipulation Fewer atrial incisions and suture lines (low risk for arrhythmias) Potential for a shorter cardiopulmonary bypass and avoidance of aortic cross-clamp and cardioplegic arrest
Potential disadvantages	Higher incidence of sinus node dysfunction, IART, and SVT Need for cross-clamp and cardioplegic arrest to complete the repair	Rigid, fixed-size conduit with potential for obstruction and/or stenosis Higher risk of thromboembolism

Abbreviations: IART, intra-atrial reentrant tachycardia; SVT, supraventricular tachycardia.

of the conversion experience an improvement in functional status, decreased debilitating arrhythmias, and reduced need for medical therapy.[17,18] Our experience at
Texas Children's Hospital over the past 15 years with 61 Fontan conversions is
summarized in **Box 1**. Timing of referral of these patients is critical for a favorable
outcome, and should be considered with the early onset of arrhythmia and other
markers of a failing Fontan pathway. The success of this complicated procedure
requires the involvement of the cardiac anesthesiologist in the preoperative risk
assessment and understanding of the impact of the interventions on Fontan
physiology.

PERIOPERATIVE CONSIDERATIONS FOR THE ADULT UNDERGOING FONTAN CONVERSION
Risk Stratification

Adults presenting for Fontan conversion are at significant risk for early intraoperative
and postoperative complications. The preoperative anesthetic evaluation should
focus on the variables that contribute to increased morbidity. These variables include
the presence of preoperative arrhythmias, functional class and single-ventricular
morphology, desaturation caused by a fenestration, baffle leak or decompressing
collaterals, presence of PLE, and history of stroke or other thromboembolic events.
A proposed risk score identifies these variables as the FACET score (**Box 2**).[19]

Transesophageal Echocardiography Before and After Repair

Two-dimensional transesophageal echocardiography (TEE) helps to define the type of
single-ventricle morphology based on the atrioventricular (AV) connection, the ventriculoarterial connection, and the ventricular morphology. The type of AV connection

---

Box 1
Outcomes for Fontan conversion (Texas Children's Hospital 1997–2012)

Total Fontan conversion cases	61
Time from previous Fontan repair (y)	14 ± 6
Age at operation (y)	21 ± 10 (range 3.6–48.7)
Male gender (%)	61
Preoperative arrhythmias (%)	75% of all patients
	Atrial flutter/IART 74
	Atrial fibrillation 14
	Sinus node dysfunction 21
	Ventricular dysfunction 9
Immediate Operative Results	
Duration of inotropic support (d)	1.6 ± 1.4
Postoperative mechanical ventilation (d)	1.3 ± 0.5
Duration of chylous chest tube drainage (d)	5 ± 3.8
Hospital length of stay (d)	10 ± 7
Reoperation for bleeding, neurologic complications, sternal infection (%)	0
Hospital mortality (%)	0
Midterm Follow-up (Median 5.4 y)	
NYHA class I/II (% of patients)	93
Recurrence of atrial arrhythmias (%)	18
1-y, 5-y, and 8-y survival and freedom from transplantation (%)	94, 86, and 79 respectively

Box 2
FACET risk stratification for Fontan conversion

F	Functional class (NYHA)
	Systolic function: normal (1), mild (2), moderate (3), severe (4)
A	Arrhythmia
C	Desaturation (Spo$_2$<90%)
E	PLE:
	Recurrent chylous effusions
	Hypoalbuminemia (<3 g/dL for >3 months)
T	Thrombosis or stroke

can help to diagnose double-inlet ventricle (>50% of both AV valves [AVV] open into a single ventricle), unbalanced AV canal defect (>75% of a common AV valve opening into 1 ventricle), and the AV valve atresia if there is lack of connection between atrium and ventricle (tricuspid atresia or mitral atresia). The ventriculoarterial connection differentiates between double-outlet RV, transposition of the great arteries, and great vessel atresia when there is only 1 ventricular outlet (right-side lesion, pulmonary atresia; left-side lesion, aortic atresia). The ventricular morphology based on its relationship with AV valves (tricuspid is committed to RV, mitral to left ventricle [LV]), moderator band and trabeculations (RV hallmarks) help to differentiate the morphologic RV from LV in transposition cases.[20]

Doppler interrogation is important to assess the Fontan connections (inferior vena cava to RA/conduit, superior vena cava to RA/conduit), AV and semilunar valves for obstruction/regurgitation, confirm unrestrictive atrial level shunting (**Fig. 4**A, B) and unobstructed pulmonary venous flow, and estimation of gradient across any outflow tract obstruction. All these abnormal flow patterns should be addressed during the Fontan palliation and/or Fontan conversion and require aortic cross-clamping. Other complications of Fontan circulation that need to be ruled out are cavoatrial shunting, thrombus formation, and obstruction of the systemic venous pathways. Unobstructed cavopulmonary anastomosis or conduit flow shows a normal biphasic flow pattern of moderate velocity (0.2–0.5 m/s). Pulsed-wave Doppler interrogation showing a velocity of greater than 1.5 m/s indicates obstruction. Pulsed-wave Doppler in the pulmonary artery should show increase in flow with inspiration during spontaneous ventilation.[21]

Pulmonary reverse flow patterns may be associated with postoperative morbidity such as length of chest tube drainage but did not predict mortality.[22] Baffle leak evaluation is essential because it is a common cause of desaturation in these patients. Color Doppler flow mapping showing continuous right to left shunting with turbulent flow at the atrial level is characteristic (see **Fig. 4**C).

Obstructed pulmonary vein flow has been described as a complication of LT Fontan (especially right upper pulmonary vein) and all 4 pulmonary veins should be interrogated before and after the repair. Gradients more than 5 mm Hg may require surgical revision by enlarging the communication between the pulmonary veins and the atrium, or adjusting the position of the Fontan baffle.[23]

Patients with single ventricles are at risk of progressive systemic ventricular diastolic and systolic dysfunction.[24] Standard methods of examining wall motion, calculating ejection fraction, and evaluating function are difficult to apply with the single-ventricular morphology of the Fontan conversion candidate. However, ventricular function should always be examined intraoperatively and compared with prior studies. Patients with severely decreased ventricular function have a greater incidence of early death than those with normal function (35% vs 4%, respectively).[25]

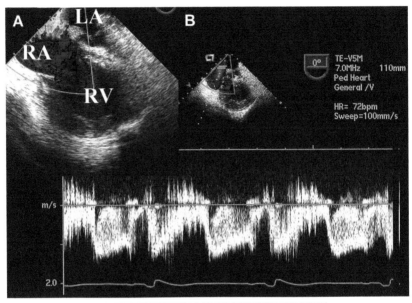

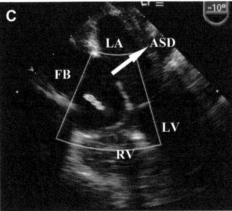

Fig. 4. (A) Doppler color image showing flow acceleration at the atrial septal communication in a patient with Fontan repair for hypoplastic left heart syndrome. Note the absent LV cavity. LA, left atrium. (B) Pulse wave Doppler interrogating the flow acceleration at the atrial septal communication with a velocity of 1.5 m/s. (C) Midesophageal 4-chamber view of a patient with tricuspid atresia palliated with a Fontan procedure. Note the color flow through the Fontan baffle (FB) to the common atrium and the atretic RV. ASD, atrial septal defect.

Anesthetic Considerations

Venous capacitance and tone

Single-ventricle physiology is a peculiar circulation, in which the pulmonary ventricle is absent as an effective pump and thus unable to provide pulsatile blood flow to the pulmonary arteries. Systemic venous return to the lungs is a passive phenomenon and depends on blood volume, peripheral venous capacitance, and the gradient between central venous pressure, pulmonary vascular resistance, and atrial pressure.

The energy generated by the single ventricle needs to overcome peripheral vascular resistance and contribute to propulsion of venous return from the lower extremities to the pulmonary vascular bed. Venous vascular capacitance and compliance are decreased in Fontan physiology to sustain the increased venous pressure needed to perfuse the pulmonary circulation and provide enough preload to the single ventricle (**Fig. 5**). This increased resting peripheral venous and vasomotor tone in Fontan patients is associated with a slightly increased plasma norepinephrine level.[26] This is an adaptive mechanism developed in response to chronic exposure to the Fontan circulation, preventing the onset of edema. Fontan patients have an attenuated cardiac output response to exercise caused by the increased resting venous tone, which limits their ability to mobilize blood from capacitance vessels and contributes to impaired cardiovascular response to exertion. In situations of Fontan circulation failure, venous hypertension develops, causing generalized edema and PLE.

The anesthetic goals are to maintain an adequate preload and to avoid sudden venous pooling with sedation and induction of anesthesia. Fontan patients are volume dependent, so prolonged nil-by-mouth status should be avoided and liberal fluid intake encouraged. Patients should optimally be scheduled as the first case of the day and/or have an intravenous (IV) catheter placed to provide fluid intake during the nil-by-mouth period. Volume load before induction is indicated in most Fontan patients. Selection of induction, hypnotic, and muscle-relaxant agents must consider the impact on venous vasodilatation resulting in sudden hypotension.[27] Etomidate is commonly used for induction because of its stable cardiovascular profile, whereas agents such as propofol that significantly affect arterial and venous tone should be administered cautiously, if at all.

Once positive-pressure ventilation is initiated after induction of anesthesia, passive venous return diminishes because of positive intrathoracic pressure, causing desaturation and decreased cardiac output. A ventilatory strategy should be used that preserves pulmonary blood flow and optimizes oxygen delivery, which is achieved

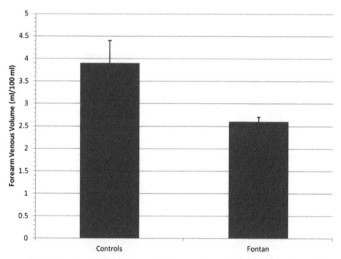

Fig. 5. Increased forearm venous volume during 40 mm Hg venous congestion of control and Fontan subjects ($P<.05$). (*Data from* Kelley JR, Mack GW, Fahey JT. Diminished vascular capacitance in patients with univentricular hearts after the Fontan operation. Am J Cardiol 1995;76:158–63; with permission.)

by limiting peak inspiratory pressure (<20 cm H_2O), using low respiratory rates (<20 breaths per minute) and short inspiratory times, avoiding excessive positive end-expiratory pressure, and incorporating higher tidal volumes (10–15 mL/kg).

Arrhythmia

Supraventricular arrhythmias are a common complication in Fontan physiology. Fifty percent of the patients experience atrial tachycardia at 20-year follow-up.[28] Atrial contribution to ventricular filling (atrial kick) is important in patients with single-ventricle physiology, especially those with impaired diastolic relaxation. The limited contractile and preload reserves increase the dependency on heart rate to increase cardiac output.

The mechanism of the arrhythmia is most commonly macro reentry within atrial muscle caused by extensive suture lines, stretched atrial tissue, and damaged sino-atrial node artery flow. Residual hemodynamic abnormalities such as AVV regurgitation causing chronic atrial hypertension may also contribute to arrhythmia generation. Fontan patients are at increased risk of sudden death caused by either intra-atrial reentrant tachycardia with 1:1 conduction, or ventricular arrhythmias.

Arrhythmias that are hemodynamically compromising should be quickly addressed by cardioversion because circulatory collapse is imminent. Most of these patients are anticoagulated, avoiding the need for TEE before cardioversion. An electrophysiologic evaluation should be considered preoperatively, and radiofrequency ablation of the reentrant pathway in the cardiac electrophysiology laboratory is possible but is a challenging procedure because of the anatomic variations. Medical treatment with antiarrhythmic drugs should be used with the goal of rate control and/or cardioversion. Despite being a common preoperative finding in patients presenting for Fontan conversion, there is no consensus on the optimal medical treatment of arrhythmias, or the timing to refer a patient with a failing Fontan to avoid further progression of arrhythmias.[29]

During Fontan conversion surgery, most patients require a right atrial maze for reentrant atrial tachycardia, and/or a Cox maze III for atrial fibrillation.[17] Pacemaker insertion is necessary in 50% of patients.

PLE

PLE is a condition related to gastrointestinal venous congestion resulting in impaired lymphatic drainage and malabsorption. The reported prevalence of PLE in patients with a failed atriopulmonary Fontan ranges from 2.5% to 24% with 50% mortality within 5 years after diagnosis.[30] Patients presenting with PLE for Fontan conversion have undergone multiple treatment strategies including diuretics, afterload reduction, supplemental high-protein/low-fat diet, and attempts at halting intestinal protein leak with heparin or steroids, creation of a fenestration, or atrial pacing. Silvilairat and colleagues[30] described the following as risk factors for mortality in Fontan patients with PLE: symptomatic depressed ventricular function (NYHA class III or IV), low serum albumin level (<2.5 g/dL), and/or short atrioventricular flow deceleration time (<120 milliseconds). The effect of protein loss on maturation has been documented in patients whose growth and development is impaired, or with delayed onset of puberty.

The diagnosis of PLE requires the following criteria: hypoproteinemia (≤6.0 g/dL), hypoalbuminemia (≤3.0 g/dL) for more than 3 months, and/or increased fecal alpha1-antitrypsin clearance (>27 mL/d) in the absence of liver or renal disease, and accompanying ascites, pleural effusions, edema, diarrhea, or abdominal pain for 3 months or longer. In addition, lymphocytopenia has been observed in PLE but it has not been related with recurrent infection or sepsis. The cause of PLE in the failing Fontan is postulated to be related to activation of the renin-angiotensin system, with high mesenteric resistance and low pulmonary vascular compliance.[31]

PLE has been associated with gastrointestinal bleeding. The mechanism is not clear, and several factors have been implicated such as increased venous pressure, infection, or immune-mediated inflammation along with antiplatelet and/or anticoagulant therapy.

PLE leads to severe hypoalbuminemia and consideration must be given to the alteration in action and duration of anesthetic drugs that are highly protein bound.[32] Albumin is a major carrier for acidic drugs such as etomidate. Hypoalbuminemia-reduced binding to etomidate (normally 76% bound) increases its unbound fraction, thus enhancing its effects.

Coagulation and bleeding risk

Baseline coagulation defects exist in patients with Fontan physiology. Most Fontan patients have an increased risk of thrombosis caused by increased factor VIII and decreased anticoagulant protein C and S concentrations.[33] Factor VIII levels greater than 150% of normal are observed in patients with a failing Fontan, and are associated with a 5-fold to 6-fold increased risk for venous thrombosis. Thrombotic events occur in up to 33% of Fontan patients, with increasing risk in those with a failing pathway. It has been suggested that the increase of plasma factor VIII concentrations may be caused by upregulation of factor VIII synthesis by inflamed liver sinusoidal endothelium. PLE may also contribute to the increased incidence of thromboembolism as a consequence of anticoagulant proteins C and S, and antithrombin III loss.[34]

In contrast, patients with a failed Fontan have bleeding propensity caused by increased systemic venous pressure, liver congestion, the presences of collateral vessels, and the frequent use of antithrombotic therapy. Anticoagulant therapy (aspirin or warfarin) is frequently used in the failing Fontan presenting for Fontan conversion, thus increasing the risk of postoperative coagulopathy and transfusion requirements. The decision for longer-term anticoagulation therapy is influenced by the anticipated risk for thrombosis, often based on the surgical technique, presence of arrhythmias, and a patient's functional status.

The use of antifibrinolytics is controversial in Fontan patients. As mentioned previously, Fontan patients are at risk for thrombosis but hyperfibrinolysis is possible in patients with failing Fontan physiology and liver congestion who undergo surgical revision on bypass. Fontan circulation is prone to endothelial dysfunction indicated by raised levels of von Willebrand factor, and fibrinolysis is preserved.[35] Antifibrinolytic usage was not associated with early baffle fenestration closure after the modified Fontan procedure and they should be administered judiciously.[36]

Lactic acidosis

Hyperlactatemia (HL) during cardiopulmonary bypass (CPB) is common in adults following repair of CHDs and is associated with an increased postoperative morbidity. HL seems to be related mainly to insufficient oxygen delivery (type A). HL correlates with bypass duration and low oxygen delivery (<260 mL/min/m^2) and is associated with hyperglycemia.[37]

Late onset HL (>3 mmol/L) in the intensive care unit is common (>44%) following Fontan repair. The incidence in Fontan patients is significantly higher than in a group of mixed congenital surgeries despite similar CPB times, and may be related to increased catecholamine use. Late-onset HL has not been associated with adverse

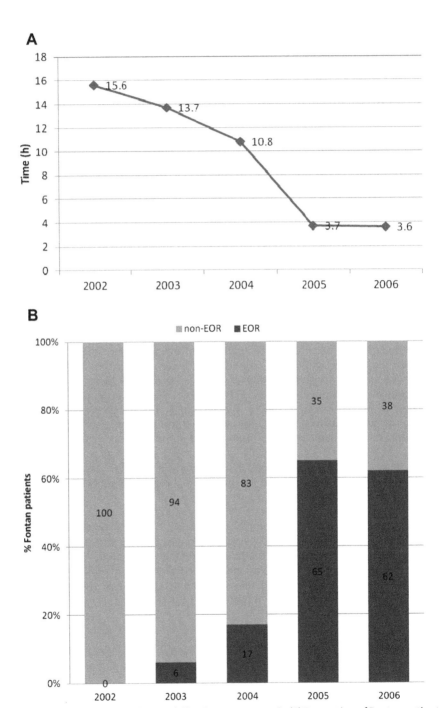

Fig. 6. (*A*) Mean time to extubation following Fontan repair. (*B*) Proportion of Fontan patients extubated in the operating room (EOR). (*Data from* Morales DL, Carberry KE, Heinle JS et al. Extubation in the operating room after Fontan's procedure: effect on practice and outcomes. Ann Thorac Surg 2008;86:576–82; with permission.)

outcomes, and thus should be interpreted carefully.[38] Hyperglycemia should be corrected and, if possible, catecholamine use limited.

Early extubation

There are several clinical benefits for early extubation following Fontan repair or conversion. First, it decreases the complications from mechanical ventilation and intubation such as laryngotracheal trauma, nosocomial pneumonia, and hypertensive crises caused by airway manipulation. In addition, Fontan physiology benefits from negative inspiratory pressure to improve pulmonary blood flow. Early extubation also decreases intensive care unit and hospital stay, decreasing the cost per admission.[39]

However, there are considerations for remaining intubated in the immediate postoperative period, such as avoiding hemodynamic instability or the risk of atelectasis and lung collapse causing hypoxia. Criteria for early extubation include an otherwise healthy patent with few comorbidities and an uneventful surgery with short CPB and aortic cross-clamp times (<90 minutes). Ongoing coagulopathy precludes early extubation because of the potential need for surgical reexploration. The anesthetic should be tailored to allow extubation in the operating room by limiting the total amount of narcotics, sedatives, and muscle relaxants.

At Texas Children's Hospital we embarked on a program to achieve safe early extubation in the operating room for patients undergoing Fontan repair and revision starting in 2002 (**Fig. 6**). The average time to extubation decreased (15.6 hours in 2002 to 3.6 hours in 2006), and the proportion of Fontan patients extubated in the operating room increased from 0% to 62%.[40] Our current practice relies on inhalation anesthetics, short-acting narcotics, judicious use of muscle relaxants, and the use of dexmedetomidine for postoperative sedation. However, although the Fontan conversion patient presents with more comorbidities, a higher risk of postoperative bleeding, and the need for a more cautious approach to early extubation, with adherence to a similar team approach for the postoperative care of these patients, the average mechanical ventilation duration has decreased to 3.6 hours in children undergoing a primary Fontan, and 1.5 ± 0.3 days in our series of adults undergoing redo Fontan conversion surgery."

SUMMARY

The growing population of adults with CHD requires surgical and catheter interventions and revisions of their initial repairs. These patients require the expertise of a team of surgeons, cardiologists, anesthesiologists, and intensive care physicians who are familiar with their lesions, the options and evolution of repairs, and the consequences of their disease. This requirement is clearly shown in the adult with single ventricular physiology with a failed primary Fontan repair presenting for a Fontan conversion surgery.

REFERENCES

1. Mascio C, Pasquali S, Jacobs J, et al. Outcomes in adult congenital heart surgery: analysis of the Society of Thoracic Surgeons database. J Thorac Cardiovasc Surg 2011;142:1090–7.
2. Marelli AJ, Mackie AS, Ionescu-Ittu R, et al. Congenital heart disease in the general population: changing prevalence and age distribution. Circulation 2007;115:163–72.

3. Society of Thoracic Surgeons, STS Congenital Heart Surgery Database Executive Summary - Adults, [Online]. Available at: http://www.sts.org/sites/default/files/documents/STSExecSummary_Adults.pdf. Accessed October 29, 2012.
4. Dearani J, Mavroudis C, Quintessenza J, et al. Surgical advances in the treatment of adults with congenital heart disease. Curr Opin Pediatr 2009;21:565–72.
5. Giamberti A, Chessa M, Abella R, et al. Morbidity and mortality risk factors in adults with congenital heart disease undergoing cardiac reoperations. Ann Thorac Surg 2009;88:1284–90.
6. Karamlou T, Diggs B, Ungerleider R, et al. Adults or big kids: what is the ideal clinical environment for management of grown-up patients with congenital heart disease? Ann Thorac Surg 2010;90:573–9.
7. Fontan F, Baudet E. Surgical repair of tricuspid atresia. Thorax 1971;4:240–8.
8. Kreutzer G, Galindez E, Bono H, et al. An operation for the correction of tricuspid atresia. J Thorac Cardiovasc Surg 1973;66:613–21.
9. Angeli E, Napoleone C, Balducci A, et al. Natural and modified history of single-ventricle physiology in adult patients. Eur J Cardiothorac Surg 2012;42(6): 996–1002.
10. Petko M, Myung R, Wernovsky G, et al. Surgical reinterventions following the Fontan procedure. Eur J Cardiothorac Surg 2003;24:255–9.
11. Fontan F, Kirklin JW, Fernandez G, et al. Outcome after a "perfect" Fontan operation. Circulation 1990;81:1520–36.
12. Khairy P, Fernandes SM, Mayer JE, et al. Long term survival, modes of death, and predictors of mortality in patients with Fontan surgery. Circulation 2008;117:85–92.
13. Lardo AC, del Nido PJ, Webber SA, et al. Hemodynamic effect of progressive right atrial dilatation in atriopulmonary connections. J Thorac Cardiovasc Surg 1997;114:2–8.
14. D'Udekem Y, Cheung MM, Setyapranata S, et al. How good is a good Fontan? Quality of life and exercise capacity of Fontans without arrhythmias. Ann Thorac Surg 2009;88:1961–89.
15. Morales DL, Dibardino DJ, Braud BE, et al. Salvaging the failing Fontan: lateral tunnel versus extracardiac conduit. Ann Thorac Surg 2005;80:1445–52.
16. Backer CL, Deal BJ, Kaushal S, et al. Extracardiac versus intra-atrial lateral tunnel Fontan: extracardiac is better. Semin Thorac Cardiovasc Surg Pediatr Card Surg Annu 2011;14:4–10.
17. Mavroudis C, Backer CL, Deal BJ. Late reoperations for Fontan patients: state of the art invited review. Eur J Cardiothorac Surg 2008;34:1034–40.
18. Takahashi K, Fynn-Thompson F, Cecchin F, et al. Clinical outcomes of Fontan conversion surgery with and without associated arrhythmia intervention. Int J Cardiol 2009;137:260–6.
19. Koh M, Yagihara T, Uemura H, et al. Optimal timing of the Fontan conversion: change in the P-wave characteristics precedes the onset of atrial tachyarrhythmias in patients with atriopulmonary connection. J Thorac Cardiovasc Surg 2007;133:1295–302.
20. Gologorsky E, Gologorsky A, Rosenkranz E. An adult patient with Fontan physiology: a TEE perspective. Anesthesiol Res Pract 2012;475015:1–5.
21. Russell IA, Rouine-Rapp K, Stratmann G, et al. Congenital heart disease in the adult: a review with internet-accessible transesophageal echocardiographic images. Anesth Analg 2006;102:694–723.
22. Leyvi G, Bennett HL, Wasnick JD. Pulmonary artery flow patterns after the Fontan procedure are predictive of postoperative complications. J Cardiothorac Vasc Anesth 2009;23:54–61.

23. Padalino MA, Saiki Y, Tworetzky W, et al. Pulmonary venous pathway obstruction from recurrent restriction at atrial septum late after Fontan procedure. J Thorac Cardiovasc Surg 2004;127:281–3.

24. Moniotte SLJ, Barrea C. Functionally univentricular heart. In: Lai WW, Mertens LL, Cohen MS, et al, editors. Echocardiography in pediatric congenital heart disease. 1st edition. West Sussex (United Kingdom): Wiley-Blackwell; 2009. p. 459–75.

25. Piran S, Veldtman G, Siu S, et al. Heart failure and ventricular dysfunction in patients with single or systemic right ventricles. Circulation 2002;105:1189–94.

26. Kelley JR, Mack GW, Fahey JT. Diminished vascular capacitance in patients with univentricular hearts after the Fontan operation. Am J Cardiol 1995;76:158–63.

27. Krishnan US, Taneja I, Gewitz M, et al. Peripheral vascular adaptation and orthostatic tolerance in Fontan physiology. Circulation 2009;120:1775–83.

28. Weipert J, Noebauer C, Schreiber C, et al. Occurrence and management of atrial arrhythmia after long-term Fontan circulation. J Thorac Cardiovasc Surg 2004; 127:457–64.

29. Anderson PA, Breitbart RE, McCrindle BW, et al. The Fontan patient: inconsistencies in medication therapy across seven Pediatric Heart Network centers. Pediatr Cardiol 2010;31:1219–28.

30. Silvilairat S, Cabalka AK, Cetta F, et al. Protein-losing enteropathy after the Fontan operation: associations and predictors of clinical outcome. Congenit Heart Dis 2008;3:262–8.

31. Yu JJ, Yun TJ, Yun SC, et al. Low pulmonary vascular compliance predisposes post-Fontan patients to protein-losing enteropathy. Int J Cardiol 2011. [Epub ahead of print].

32. Trojnarska O, Cieplucha A. Challenges of management and therapy in patients with a functionally single ventricle after Fontan operation. Cardiol J 2011;18: 119–27.

33. Odegard KC, McGowan FX Jr, Zurakowski D, et al. Procoagulant and anticoagulant factor abnormalities following the Fontan procedure: increased factor VIII may predispose to thrombosis. J Thorac Cardiovasc Surg 2003;125:1260–7.

34. Odegard KC, Zurakowski D, DiNardo JA, et al. Prospective longitudinal study of coagulation profiles in children with hypoplastic left heart syndrome from stage I through Fontan completion. J Thorac Cardiovasc Surg 2009;137:934–41.

35. Binotto MA, Maed NY, Lopes AA. Altered endothelial function following the Fontan procedure. Cardiol Young 2008;18:70–4.

36. Gruber EM, Shukla AC, Reid RW, et al. Synthetic antifibrinolytics are not associated with an increased incidence of baffle fenestration closure after the modified Fontan procedure. J Cardiothorac Vasc Anesth 2000;14:257–9.

37. Ranucci M, De Toffol B, Isgrò G, et al. Hyperlactatemia during cardiopulmonary bypass: determinants and impact on postoperative outcome. Crit Care 2006;10: 1–9.

38. Hamamoto M, Imanaka H, Kagisaki K, et al. Is an increase in lactate concentration associated with cardiac dysfunction after the Fontan procedure? Ann Thorac Cardiovasc Surg 2005;11:301–6.

39. Mutsuga M, Quiñonez LG, Mackie AS, et al. Fast-track extubation after modified Fontan procedure. J Thorac Cardiovasc Surg 2012;144:547–55.

40. Morales DL, Carberry KE, Heinle JS, et al. Extubation in the operating room after Fontan's procedure: effect on practice and outcomes. Ann Thorac Surg 2008;86: 576–82.

Critical Care of the Cardiac Patient

Avery Tung, MD, FCCM

KEYWORDS

- Critical care • Mechanical ventilation • Hemodynamic monitoring
- Ventricular assist devices

KEY POINTS

- New advances in core critical care therapies such as mechanical ventilation have allowed physicians to deliver supportive care in a less harmful and more sustainable way.
- Advances include low(er) tidal volume ventilation, prioritizing airway pressure over maximal Po_2, and selective use of sigh breaths in place of higher tidal volumes for sustaining oxygenation.
- Advances in techniques for hemodynamic monitoring and central line insertion have dramatically reduced complications referable to invasive monitoring.
- The increased diagnostic complexity of patients with ventricular assist devices has made the diagnosis of low cardiac output more challenging. In addition to right ventricular failure, tamponade, bleeding, sepsis, and aortic insufficiency must all be considered.

INTRODUCTION

As the spectrum of cardiac surgeries has grown, the diversity and complexity of postoperative cardiac surgical care has also increased. Cardiac surgery in 2012 now involves not only traditional revascularization and valve procedures but also ventricular assist device (VAD) implantation, transplant, percutaneous valve insertions, and extracorporeal approaches to cardiopulmonary support. In addition, advanced minimally invasive and robotic techniques have allowed cardiac surgery to be performed on patients formerly considered too ill to survive. The combination of these novel procedures, and an overall sicker patient population, have challenged intensivists caring for cardiac surgery patients to develop new care strategies to adapt to the changing patient population and surgical environment.

A comprehensive review of postoperative critical care for cardiac surgery is beyond the scope of this article, which instead examines 4 areas in critical care where clinical practice is evolving rapidly. Among these are management of mechanical ventilation, thresholds for blood transfusion, strategies for hemodynamic monitoring, and

Disclosures: None.

Conflicts of Interest: None.

Department of Anesthesia and Critical Care, University of Chicago, 5841 South Maryland Avenue, MC4028, Chicago, IL 60637, USA

E-mail address: atung@dacc.uchicago.edu

Anesthesiology Clin 31 (2013) 421–432

http://dx.doi.org/10.1016/j.anclin.2012.12.008

processes for central line insertion. In addition, current approaches to common dilemmas in postoperative cardiac care are reviewed: diagnosis of tamponade, and the diagnosis and management of low cardiac output states in patients with a VAD.

EVOLVING STRATEGIES IN CURRENT CRITICAL CARE
Mechanical Ventilation

The development of the multi-institution ARDSnet research network in 1994 has led to a much richer understanding of the epidemiology of lung injury and the value of specific therapeutic approaches. Although the most widely publicized finding from ARDSnet research is the correlation between tidal volume and mortality in patients with lung injury,[1] several other observations relating to mechanical ventilation have led to modifications in current clinical practice. Taken together, these results have noticeably altered ventilator management of patients with lung injury and have contributed to lower mortality in this patient population.

The most surprising epidemiologic observation from multiple studies of patients with acute respiratory distress syndrome (ARDS) is that partial pressure of oxygen (Po_2) is not a risk factor for adverse outcome.[2,3] In the original ARDSnet study comparing 6 mL/kg and 12 mL/kg tidal volumes, for example, mortality was decreased in the 6-mL/kg group whereas Po_2 was the same in both tidal volume groups.[1] This finding is counterintuitive, as known causes of hypoxemia are clearly present in ARDS, and derangements in lung function such as pulmonary edema appear to be markers for greater severity of disease.[4]

When viewed in light of other empiric observations about ARDS, however, the lack of relationship between Po_2 and outcome becomes clearer. One common strategy for improving Po_2 in patients with lung injury is by increasing positive end-expiratory pressure (PEEP). However, although PEEP improves oxygenation, several high-profile trials have found no outcome benefit of high (13–15 cm H_2O) over low (5–7 cm H_2O) PEEP levels.[5,6] This lack of outcome benefit with PEEP may result in part from the inhomogeneous effect of ARDS on lung tissue. Because damaged alveoli are also less compliant, adding PEEP may overdistend normal, functional alveoli, ultimately inducing lung damage and worsening outcomes. A similar "unintended consequences" argument can be made for prone ventilation and the use of nitric oxide. Both interventions improve oxygenation, but the increased complexity involved in their use may limit any benefit resulting from higher Po_2, resulting ultimately in no effect on mortality.[7,8] One possible explanation for the absence of a relationship between Po_2 and outcome may be that any benefit from greater oxygenation is almost completely offset by detrimental effects of the ventilator strategies needed to generate a higher Po_2.

Exotic ventilator modes such as pressure control or airway pressure release ventilation have thus become less common as intensive care unit (ICU) physicians move away from blood gas values to target ventilator parameters such as airway pressure and compliance. One current question is whether the combination of ventilator settings resulting in barely adequate oxygenation and intermittent "recruitment maneuvers" affects outcome. Such maneuvers involve periodic, scheduled, large tidal volume breaths occurring throughout the day to boost oxygenation by "recruiting" alveoli that collapse during low tidal volume ventilation. In principle, because the newly recruited tidal volumes are intermittent, a benefit from chronically low tidal volumes may be harnessed without unacceptably low oxygenation. Existing literature, however, is mixed. Although recruitment maneuvers clearly improve oxygenation, no strong outcome signal has yet been found.[9]

For patients in the cardiac surgery ICU, ARDS is an infrequent complication. The incidence of ARDS after cardiac surgery is 0.4% versus 24% in a mechanically ventilated mixed surgical/medical ICU population.[10,11] Nevertheless, patients status post cardiopulmonary bypass with aortic cross-clamp have by definition sustained some degree of lung injury merely by excluding the lung from the circulation. Cardiac surgery patients also frequently receive blood and undergo large positive fluid shifts. Both interventions increase the incidence of ARDS. One important question is thus whether cardiac surgery patients should routinely be ventilated with low tidal volume strategies. Such a strategy would not only involve reducing tidal volumes to 6 mL/kg (or even lower) but also the relatively high respiratory rates ($\sim$30 breaths/min) needed to maintain CO_2 homeostasis and increased PEEP levels to maintain oxygenation. Potential downsides to such a ventilator strategy include derangements in acid-base balance, a greater need for sedation owing to the rapid shallow breathing pattern and high levels of partial carbon dioxide pressure (Pco_2), and greater complexity for ICU caregivers. Because of such concerns, literature-reported compliance with low tidal volume ventilation hovers at approximately 30% to 50%.[12] In light of the relatively brief periods of postoperative mechanical ventilation required by most cardiac surgery patients, the benefits of a low tidal volume strategy are unclear.

Existing studies in patients without lung injury are equivocal. Whereas some find a shorter time to extubation after cardiac surgery,[13] others find no benefit.[14] Further work in this area to identify potential high-risk groups may clarify whether aggressive low tidal volume strategies can meaningfully affect cardiac surgery outcomes. Changes in clinical practice, however, do provide some information for the ICU physician caring for cardiac surgery patients. In part as a result of aggressive education regarding tidal volumes, most critical care physicians are setting tidal volumes lower than 10 mL/kg and finding no adverse effects.[15] Such an "intermediate" tidal volume setting (7–8 mL/kg) may provide most of the benefit of lower tidal volumes without the technical challenges of managing hypercarbia, high respiratory rates, and agitation.

Transfusion

Existing evidence suggests considerable heterogeneity with respect to transfusion practice in cardiac surgery.[16] The likelihood of receiving blood during cardiac surgery may vary as much as 3- to 4-fold from one institution to another.[17] Survey data also support a wide variation in transfusion practice among cardiac surgery caregivers, with different protocols and thresholds for product use.[18] These observations suggest that identifying an optimal strategy for the management of blood products is a frustratingly elusive goal.

Even the (apparently) simple question of what hemoglobin trigger to use for transfusion in patients with coronary artery disease is extremely difficult to answer. Early studies[19] found an adverse effect of low hematocrit on outcome in patients with known coronary artery disease, suggesting a different hematocrit threshold for such patients. A large 2002 multicenter trial in critically ill patients[20] found worse outcomes for patients transfused to hemoglobin (Hb) levels between 10 and 12 g/dL versus 7 to 9 g/dL, but no difference in the subgroup with coronary artery disease, also raising the possibility that patients with coronary artery disease may have unique hematocrit requirements. In 2007 a large retrospective trial evaluating the relationship between preoperative anemia and outcome after coronary bypass grafting found increased morbidity and mortality, with preoperative anemia starting at a surprisingly high Hb level (11 g/dL)[21] Although an emerging consensus exists today that critically ill patients without coronary artery disease do not need an Hb level of 10 mg/dL to optimize critical care outcomes, a target Hb for those with coronary artery disease is less clear.

Recent literature fails to completely resolve this lack of clarity. A recent comparison of high (10 g/dL) versus low (8 g/dL) Hb in patients undergoing hip replacement with known coronary disease and low hematocrit found no benefit to maintaining a higher hematocrit.[22] Other recent studies in patients with acute coronary syndrome or those undergoing urgent/emergent stenting for acute coronary syndrome are similarly mixed. While anemia before percutaneous coronary intervention appears to predict adverse outcome,[23] transfusion for low hematocrits during acute coronary syndromes also appears to worsen outcomes,[24] even showing worsened outcomes for patients receiving blood transfusion. One recent study in cardiac surgery patients, however, found an inverse relationship between nadir hematocrits during bypass and perioperative mortality, with higher hematocrits corresponding to lower mortality. This relationship was particularly strong in patients with EuroSCOREs higher than 4.[25]

Although the mechanisms leading to such diverse outcomes are unclear, a paradigm similar to that for oxygenation during mechanical ventilation may be partly responsible. Although augmenting oxygen-carrying capacity by transfusing blood may benefit some patients, adverse immunologic effects from blood transfusion may counteract this benefit in others. Another recent propensity-adjusted Korean study in critically ill surgical patients found a benefit to blood transfusion that increased with lower pretransfusion Hb.[26] This study, possibly done with a more genetically homogeneous population than is typical in the United States, may suggest that immunologic effects of blood transfusion account in part for their adverse effects on survival. Overall, these data suggest that centers using more blood than is normal during cardiac surgery may be able to modestly reduce their transfusion thresholds without significantly affecting outcome in either direction. Further work is needed to better identify the relevance of Hb level and blood transfusion to outcomes in critically ill patients.

Central Line Management

Because of the frequent need for vasopressors and invasive hemodynamic monitoring, cardiac surgery patients often require a central line during the postoperative period. Fortunately, techniques for insertion and management of central lines have evolved dramatically in the past 10 years. Widespread use of ultrasonography for central line placement and the increasing use of checklists have both contributed to a dramatically lower incidence of central line complications and central line–associated bloodstream infections.

Since the 2006 multicenter study validating the use of checklists to reduce central line infections,[27] checklists have been adopted in some form by many hospitals to reduce the incidence of line infections. Although the mechanism(s) linking checklist use to improved rates of central line infection are unclear, one clear accomplishment of the original 2006 validation study was to demonstrate to clinicians that it was possible to dramatically reduce the rates of central line infection. Whether because of or despite checklists, it is clear that since 2006 the rates of central line infection have fallen dramatically, so much so that the Centers for Disease Control and Prevention dedicated the March 4, 2011 issue of the *Morbidity and Mortality Weekly Report* to this success story about quality and safety.[28]

The use of ultrasonography for central line insertion has also allowed clinicians more freedom to steer clear of situations whereby central line infections are most likely. Because the pre-ultrasonography risk of inserting a new central line was higher relative to the risk of central line infection, clinicians would be more likely to leave an old central line in place rather than replace it with a new stick. In fact, studies of routine line changes in the pre-ultrasonography era frequently found no benefit.[29] However, with ultrasonography the risk and difficulty of new central line placement has gone down significantly, allowing clinicians to reduce the risk of a new insertion, particularly in difficult patients with thick necks, prior neck surgery, or other examples of difficult anatomy.

Other advances have also contributed to safer strategies for venous access, including the use of ultrasonography to identify peripheral veins, an increasing use of peripherally inserted central lines,[30] hemodynamic monitoring strategies that do not require central lines,[31] and better techniques for maintenance of central line dressing. Taken together, these approaches have significantly improved the use of central access in cardiac surgery patients.

Hemodynamic Monitoring

Considerable debate exists regarding how best to identify the optimal fluid balance or choice of vasoactive agent for critically ill patients.[32] Postoperative cardiac surgery patients increase the complexity of this task by adding uncertainty regarding cardiac function. Against this background, clinicians have most commonly relied on pulmonary artery (PA) catheterization and invasive arterial monitoring. In light of accumulating evidence that traditional interpretations of PA catheter data may mislead,[33] however, and to address monitoring needs of newer surgeries such as left ventricular assist device (LVAD) insertion, new strategies for hemodynamic monitoring after cardiac surgery are becoming available.

One ongoing challenge is the differential diagnosis of a postoperative state of low cardiac output. Both the diagnosis of the low-output state and its cause can be difficult to ascertain. Traditional indicators such as perioperative urine output and mentation may not accurately reflect cardiac output, particularly if the surgery itself has caused kidney injury and/or the patient remains intubated. Similarly, use of vasoconstrictors may produce a seemingly normal blood pressure while obscuring an inadequate cardiac output. Finally, many patients with advanced cardiac disease present for surgery already in a low-output state, and may remain so well into the postoperative period. For this reason, ICU clinicians caring for complex cardiac surgery patients have historically measured cardiac output directly using PA catheterization. Although thermodilution cardiac output remains the most common approach to cardiac output monitoring in cardiac surgery patients, physicians are increasingly supplementing direct measurements of cardiac output with dynamic, arterial waveform–derived cardiac output and volume responsiveness measurements, and lactate and venous oxygen saturation monitoring.

One area where new hemodynamic monitoring tools have contributed to the clinical diagnosis has been the diagnosis of low cardiac output immediately after cardiac surgery. In this time frame, potential causes of low cardiac output states include hypovolemia, systolic and diastolic heart failure, ischemia, valvular dysfunction, and cardiac tamponade. Of these, one of the most difficult challenges with traditional monitoring is distinguishing tamponade from acute postoperative right ventricular dysfunction. In tamponade, external compression of the heart limits diastolic filling, causing stroke volumes and cardiac output to decrease. In right ventricular failure, transient right ventricular systolic dysfunction due to intracoronary air or debris, hypotension, or inadequate preservation during cross-clamp leads to inadequate left ventricular filling. In both situations, cardiac output and blood pressure are low, and the patient is only intermittently responsive to fluid. In addition, PA and right atrial pressures are high, consistent with either right ventricular dysfunction or external compression of the heart. Not infrequently, acute right ventricular dysfunction can present with the same equalization of pressures that signals cardiac tamponade.

Clarifying whether tamponade or right ventricular dysfunction is the cause of hemodynamic compromise after cardiac surgery is important because of the consequences.

Although the only definitive treatment for tamponade is operative reexploration, current evidence suggests that a take-back is associated with a higher incidence of infection and worsened outcomes.[34] If the cause is right ventricular failure, however, a conservative approach using vasoconstrictors to support blood pressure may suffice without the need to explore.

One new solution for this diagnostic dilemma is the use of surface or transesophageal echocardiography. Simple 2-dimensional echocardiography machines are now frequently used for vascular access, and may be easily repurposed for rapid diagnostic evaluation of the heart. Although complex Doppler analysis is usually beyond the scope of these devices, a quick 4-chamber view of the heart can often distinguish between tamponade and right ventricular failure. Although pericardial effusions are common after cardiac surgery, and may not by themselves be diagnostic for cardiac tamponade,[35] other echocardiographic signs (diastolic collapse of the right atrium or ventricle) can add diagnostic clarity. In addition, visualizing both a large, poorly contracting right ventricle and a small, normally contracting left ventricle in the setting of equalization of pressures is strongly suggestive of right ventricular failure and may thus make tamponade less likely. Surface echo is currently more readily available than transesophageal echocardiography (TEE) for emergent hemodynamic diagnosis, although its images can often be insufficiently clear for diagnostic purposes. TEE, however, is also becoming increasingly more accessible to critical care physicians, with newer probes able to remain in the esophagus for days at a time.

For most patients after complex cardiac surgery, cardiac output measurement via a PA catheter remains a critical tool in hemodynamic monitoring. No other monitor affords the ability to simultaneously measure right and left ventricular filling pressures and cardiac output.

CHALLENGES AND STRATEGIES FOR NEW PROCEDURES

In addition to incremental improvements in postoperative critical care, ICU physicians have also adapted to a new spectrum of cardiac surgical procedures. The most prominent of these is the use of cardiac assist devices. Over the past decade, the role of VADs has transitioned from rescue therapy to mainstay in the surgical treatment of heart failure. Early versions of these devices were pneumatically driven pumps that withdrew blood from the left (or right) ventricle and pumped it into the aorta (or PA) in a pulsatile fashion. More recent "axial-flow" devices are continuous, nonpulsatile, magnetic rotor-driven devices that continuously pump blood from the ventricle to the aorta. Both devices add complexity to hemodynamic management and postoperative critical care. This section briefly reviews the diagnosis and management of patients with hemodynamic instability readmitted to the ICU after LVAD implantation.

Readmission to the hospital after LVAD placement is common. In early trials of pulsatile devices,[35] patients in the (pulsatile) LVAD group were significantly more likely to be readmitted to the hospital than those in the control arm. Although fewer rehospitalizations occur in patients with nonpulsatile devices, more than 50% of patients will require readmission to the hospital.[36] Although most readmissions do not require ICU care, patients readmitted for hemodynamic instability comprise a subset that often requires ICU-level diagnosis and monitoring.

Coagulation-induced complications are a common reason for hemodynamic instability with a VAD. Both bleeding (by decreasing preload) and LVAD thrombosis (by reducing cardiac output) may precipitate hemodynamic instability. Studies of early pulsatile assist devices such as the Thoratec HeartMate I found relatively low rates of thromboembolism[37] despite using warfarin for only 8.2% of the total study duration. These results suggested that these devices would not need systematic anticoagulation, and prolonged trials of pulsatile devices found few thrombotic or bleeding events despite not using routine anticoagulation for study patients.[35]

In patients with newer, nonpulsatile axial-flow assist devices, monitoring and managing coagulation is considerably more difficult. Bleeding complications after nonpulsatile LVAD insertion are higher, with reported incidences ranging from 5% to 30%.[36,38] The challenge of managing coagulation with nonpulsatile devices is exacerbated by the relative lack of abnormalities in standard clotting parameters. In a large retrospective study of HeartMate II LVAD patients,[39] 50% experienced a bleeding event within 2 months. At the time of bleed, the average international normalized ratio was 1.67 and the average platelet count was 237,000.

Several factors contribute to the higher incidence of bleeding in patients on axial-flow devices. First, because initial trials of HeartMate II insertion[40] found significantly higher (3%) incidences of thrombotic events when anticoagulation was not used, patients on axial-flow devices are routinely anticoagulated. In addition, 2 pathophysiologic mechanisms contribute to the difficulty in coagulation management. The first is a loss of large von Willebrand factor (vWF) multimers, owing to shearing by the LVAD pump mechanism. Direct measurements of vWF multimers demonstrate that nearly all patients with nonpulsatile LVADs have depleted levels of vWF multimers,[39] and that patients bridged to transplantation with an LVAD had similarly low vWF levels even if they had no concurrent evidence of gastrointestinal (GI) bleeding. Unfortunately, no clear threshold vWF level could be identified as a predictive factor, and the variability in vWF levels is high.[41]

The other unique coagulation abnormality in LVAD patients is a decrease in platelet aggregation. A study of 16 patients who had undergone HeartMate II insertion, 11 had impaired platelet aggregation and a history of bleeding episodes.[42] Because the suppression of platelet aggregation exceeded the decreased vWF activity, the investigators concluded that a platelet aggregation was due to more than just depleted vWF levels. Other studies of platelet dysfunction with LVAD insertion[43] have reached similar conclusions.

Although bleeding in LVAD patients is common and can cause hypotension, the diagnosis and management are fairly straightforward. Decreased LVAD flows, a decreased pulse index, a low hematocrit, and hyponatremia are all signs suggestive of a bleeding-induced low-output state. Although mediastinal and thoracic bleeding are most common overall, such bleeding usually occurs earlier and is easy to diagnose. In particular tamponade may occur, with literature-reported incidences as high as 28%.[38] By contrast, lower and upper GI bleeding[44] are a frequent cause of occult GI bleeding and hypovolemia. Because axial-flow devices have an active suction effect, left ventricular volumes in hypovolemic VAD patients may become sufficiently small that flow into the VAD is obstructed. These "suction events" may then result in increased power as the VAD struggles to generate flow against an occluded inflow cannula.

A more difficult diagnosis to make is that of device thrombosis. Intradevice clot may partially or completely inactivate the assist device, essentially returning the patient to his or her predevice status. Although this complication is infrequent[40] it is difficult to diagnose and treat, and may require replacing the device. Device thrombosis may be suspected clinically when power readings spike transiently more than 14 days after implantation, chronically increasing power requirements of at least 2 W, elevated or rising lactate dehydrogenase levels, and clinical signs of left heart failure including low output and pulmonary edema.[45] Unlike tamponade or aortic insufficiency, echocardiography may often fail to clearly identify device thrombosis because residual flow may remain, and clot that does not project into the left ventricle may not be seen. Similarly, angiography may also not be able to visualize flow inside the device.

Most current evidence recommends a "ramp" test to increase diagnostic certainty regarding the likelihood of device thrombosis. In this test, pump speed is gradually increased ("ramped up") while left ventricular end-diastolic dimensions (LVEDD) and pulsatility index are monitored.[45] A pattern of decreasing pulsatility index and LVEDD with increased pump speed suggests a functioning LVAD, whereas no change in pulsatility index or LVEDD indicates device thrombosis. In 17 patients suspected of VAD thrombosis and tested in this way, 10 tests were positive and device thrombosis was confirmed in 8 of 10 cases at the time of device exchange.[45]

Three other causes of low output with an axial-flow device deserve mention: sepsis, right ventricular failure, and aortic insufficiency. All can occur as late complications of VAD insertion and require ICU care. Of these, sepsis is the most common. Nearly half of all LVAD patients develop an infection by day 60, and almost all patients develop an infection by the end of the first year after implantation. Although one 2009 study found that drive-line and pocket infections did not affect mortality, overt bloodstream sepsis correlated with a 3-fold increased mortality.[46]

Clinically, sepsis in a patient with an axial-flow device presents similarly to hypovolemia, with the exception that the pulsatility index may not be decreased and that VAD flows may be unchanged. Fever may not be present, and the clinical presentation may consist only of worsening renal insufficiency, altered mental status, or other signs of end-organ dysfunction.

Right ventricular failure can occur with a 10% to 15% incidence in patients receiving an axial-flow LVAD.[38] Because VAD insertion results in an acute increase in cardiac output, and because patients undergoing LVAD implantation may have coexisting pulmonary hypertension, inadequate right ventricular systolic function and consequent dilation may acutely result in inadequate flow delivery to the LVAD and low cardiac output. As noted earlier, right ventricular failure may mimic tamponade hemodynamically, with high central venous pressure (CVP) and PA pressures in addition to low cardiac output. Detailed strategies to diagnose and manage right ventricular failure are beyond the scope of this article, but include echocardiography to make the diagnosis and adjustment of VAD flows to normalize the position of the interventricular septum. Inotropic support, vasoconstrictors to maintain a sufficiently high mean arterial pressure to preserve right ventricular perfusion, modulation of pulmonary vascular resistance, and limiting right ventricular dilation (usually measured by CVP as a proxy) are other components of acute right ventricular failure.

Finally, aortic insufficiency may occur as a late de novo complication of continuous-flow LVAD insertion. The overall incidence is reported as between 25% and 38%.[47,48] Although the mechanism of new-onset aortic insufficiency associated with continuous flow is unclear, several studies have found that an aortic valve that does not open during systole is a significant predictor of de novo aortic sufficiency at 1 year (odds ratio 6–10).[49] For this reason, many LVAD centers adjust axial flow and blood pressure to allow the aortic valve to open periodically. Such patients commonly present with pulmonary edema, low output, normal VAD flows, right ventricular failure, and end-organ dysfunction. No consensus yet exists regarding definitive treatment of this complication. Medically, diuresis and afterload reduction can minimize pulmonary edema and optimize forward flow. Both transcatheter aortic valve closure and aortic valve implantation have been reported in the literature,[49,50] but whether such therapies can be widely applied is unclear.

SUMMARY

Driven in part by ongoing evolution of basic critical care strategies, and by unique challenges posed by new cardiac surgical procedures, the critical care of cardiac surgery patients continues to evolve. New advances in core critical care therapies such as mechanical ventilation have allowed physicians to deliver supportive care in a less harmful and more sustainable way. Advances include low(er) tidal volume ventilation, prioritizing airway pressure over maximal Po_2, and selective use of sigh breaths in place of higher tidal volumes for sustaining oxygenation. In addition, advances in techniques for hemodynamic monitoring and central line insertion have dramatically reduced complications referable to invasive monitoring, with increased use of ultrasound imaging for line placement. Similarly, critical care physicians are now armed with significantly more data to inform their use of blood products, and the transfusion thresholds most likely to result in benefit.

In addition, the changing landscape of cardiac surgery procedures has led to new challenges and solutions for the cardiac intensivist. With the increased availability of transesophageal and transthoracic echocardiography, complex diagnostic challenges such as tamponade or right ventricular failure have become easier to navigate. On the other hand, the increased diagnostic complexity of patients with VADs has made the diagnosis of low cardiac output more challenging. In addition to right ventricular failure, tamponade, bleeding, sepsis, and aortic insufficiency must all be considered. With the rapid introduction of new cardiac surgery techniques, critical care will likely need to continue to adapt to changing patients and procedures.

REFERENCES

1. ARDSnet investigators. Ventilation with lower tidal volumes as compared with traditional tidal volumes for acute lung injury and the acute respiratory distress syndrome. The Acute Respiratory Distress Syndrome Network. N Engl J Med 2000;342:1301–8.
2. Nuckton TJ, Alonso JA, Kallet RH, et al. Pulmonary dead-space fraction as a risk factor for death in the acute respiratory distress syndrome. N Engl J Med 2002; 346:1281–6.
3. Brun-Buisson C, Minelli C, Bertolini G, et al, ALIVE Study Group. Epidemiology and outcome of acute lung injury in European intensive care units. Results from the ALIVE study. Intensive Care Med 2004;30:51–61.
4. ARDS Definition Task Force, Ranieri VM, Rubenfeld GD, Thompson BT, et al. Acute respiratory distress syndrome: the Berlin Definition. JAMA 2012;307:2526–33.
5. Brower RG, Lanken PN, MacIntyre N, et al, National Heart, Lung, and Blood Institute ARDS Clinical Trials Network. Higher versus lower positive end-expiratory pressures in patients with the acute respiratory distress syndrome. N Engl J Med 2004;351:327–36.
6. Briel M, Meade M, Mercat A, et al. Higher vs lower positive end-expiratory pressure in patients with acute lung injury and acute respiratory distress syndrome: systematic review and meta-analysis. JAMA 2010;303:865–73.
7. Pelosi P, Brazzi L, Gattinoni L. Prone position in acute respiratory distress syndrome. Eur Respir J 2002;20:1017–28.
8. Adhikari NK, Burns KE, Friedrich JO, et al. Effect of nitric oxide on oxygenation and mortality in acute lung injury: systematic review and meta-analysis. BMJ 2007;334:779.
9. Fan E, Wilcox ME, Brower RG, et al. Recruitment maneuvers for acute lung injury: a systematic review. Am J Respir Crit Care Med 2008;178:1156–63.

10. Milot J, Perron J, Lacasse Y, et al. Incidence and predictors of ARDS after cardiac surgery. Chest 2001;119:884–8.

11. Gajic O, Dara SI, Mendez JL, et al. Ventilator-associated lung injury in patients without acute lung injury at the onset of mechanical ventilation. Crit Care Med 2004;32:1817–24.

12. Walkey AJ, Wiener RS. Risk factors for underuse of lung-protective ventilation in acute lung injury. J Crit Care 2012;27:323.e1–9.

13. Sundar S, Novack V, Jervis K, et al. Influence of low tidal volume ventilation on time to extubation in cardiac surgical patients. Anesthesiology 2011;114(5):1102–10.

14. Determann RM, Royakkers A, Wolthuis EK, et al. Ventilation with lower tidal volumes as compared with conventional tidal volumes for patients without acute lung injury: a preventive randomized controlled trial. Crit Care 2010;14(1):R1.

15. Checkley W, Brower R, Korpak A, et al, Acute Respiratory Distress Syndrome Network Investigators. Effects of a clinical trial on mechanical ventilation practices in patients with acute lung injury. Am J Respir Crit Care Med 2008;177(11):1215–22.

16. Bennett-Guerrero E, Zhao Y, O'Brien SM, et al. Variation in use of blood transfusion in coronary artery bypass graft surgery. JAMA 2010;304(14):1568–75.

17. Karkouti K, Wijeysundera DN, Beattie WS, et al, Reducing Bleeding in Cardiac Surgery (RBC) Research Group. Variability and predictability of large-volume red blood cell transfusion in cardiac surgery: a multicenter study. Transfusion 2007;47:2081–8.

18. Likosky DS, FitzGerald DC, Groom RC, et al. Effect of the perioperative blood transfusion and blood conservation in cardiac surgery clinical practice guidelines of the Society of Thoracic Surgeons and the Society of Cardiovascular Anesthesiologists upon clinical practices. Anesth Analg 2010;111(2):316–23.

19. Carson JL, Duff A, Poses RM, et al. Effect of anaemia and cardiovascular disease on surgical mortality and morbidity. Lancet 1996;348(9034):1055–60.

20. Hébert PC, Wells G, Blajchman MA, et al. A multicenter, randomized, controlled clinical trial of transfusion requirements in critical care. Transfusion Requirements in Critical Care Investigators, Canadian Critical Care Trials Group. N Engl J Med 1999;340(6):409–17.

21. Kulier A, Levin J, Moser R, et al, Investigators of the Multicenter Study of Perioperative Ischemia Research Group, Ischemia Research and Education Foundation. Impact of preoperative anemia on outcome in patients undergoing coronary artery bypass graft surgery. Circulation 2007;116(5):471–9.

22. Carson JL, Terrin ML, Noveck H, et al, FOCUS Investigators. Liberal or restrictive transfusion in high-risk patients after hip surgery. N Engl J Med 2011;365(26): 2453–62.

23. McKechnie RS, Smith D, Montoye C, et al, Blue Cross Blue Shield of Michigan Cardiovascular Consortium (BMC2). Prognostic implication of anemia on in-hospital outcomes after percutaneous coronary intervention. Circulation 2004; 110(3):271–7.

24. Garfinkle M, Lawler PR, Filion KB, et al. Red blood cell transfusion and mortality among patients hospitalized for acute coronary syndromes: a systematic review. Int J Cardiol 2012. [Epub ahead of print].

25. Loor G, Li L, Sabik JF 3rd, et al. Nadir hematocrit during cardiopulmonary bypass: end-organ dysfunction and mortality. J Thorac Cardiovasc Surg 2012; 144(3):654–62.

26. Park DW, Chun BC, Kwon SS, et al. Red blood cell transfusions are associated with lower mortality in patients with severe sepsis and septic shock: a propensity-matched analysis. Crit Care Med 2012;40:3140–5.

27. Pronovost P, Needham D, Berenholtz S, et al. An intervention to decrease catheter-related bloodstream infections in the ICU. N Engl J Med 2006;355(26): 2725–32.

28. Centers for Disease Control and Prevention Morbidity and Mortality Weekly Report. 2011. Available at: http://www.cdc.gov/mmwr/preview/mmwrhtml/mm6008a4.htm?s_cid=mm6008a4_w. Accessed December 1, 2012.

29. Cook D, Randolph A, Kernerman P, et al. Central venous catheter replacement strategies: a systematic review of the literature. Crit Care Med 1997;25(8): 1417–24.

30. Gunst M, Matsushima K, Vanek S, et al. Peripherally inserted central catheters may lower the incidence of catheter-related blood stream infections in patients in surgical intensive care units. Surg Infect (Larchmt) 2011;12(4):279–82.

31. Marik PE, Cavallazzi R, Vasu T, et al. Dynamic changes in arterial waveform derived variables and fluid responsiveness in mechanically ventilated patients: a systematic review of the literature. Crit Care Med 2009;37(9):2642–7.

32. Chong PC, Greco EF, Stothart D, et al. Substantial variation of both opinions and practice regarding perioperative fluid resuscitation. Can J Surg 2009;52(3): 207–14.

33. Kumar A, Anel R, Bunnell E, et al. Pulmonary artery occlusion pressure and central venous pressure fail to predict ventricular filling volume, cardiac performance, or the response to volume infusion in normal subjects. Crit Care Med 2004;32(3):691–9.

34. Biancari F, Mikkola R, Heikkinen J, et al. Estimating the risk of complications related to re-exploration for bleeding after adult cardiac surgery: a systematic review and meta-analysis. Eur J Cardiothorac Surg 2012;41(1):50–5.

35. Rose EA, Gelijns AC, Moskowitz AJ, et al, Randomized Evaluation of Mechanical Assistance for the Treatment of Congestive Heart Failure (REMATCH) Study Group. Long-term use of a left ventricular assist device for end-stage heart failure. N Engl J Med 2001;345(20):1435–43.

36. Slaughter MS, Rogers JG, Milano CA, et al. Advanced heart failure treated with continuous-flow left ventricular assist device. N Engl J Med 2009;361(23): 2241–51.

37. Slater JP, Rose EA, Levin HR, et al. Low thromboembolic risk without anticoagulation using advanced-design left ventricular assist devices. Ann Thorac Surg 1996;62(5):1321–7.

38. Genovese EA, Dew MA, Teuteberg JJ, et al. Incidence and patterns of adverse event onset during the first 60 days after ventricular assist device implantation. Ann Thorac Surg 2009;88(4):1162–70.

39. Uriel N, Pak SW, Jorde UP, et al. Acquired von Willebrand syndrome after continuous-flow mechanical device support contributes to a high prevalence of bleeding during long-term support and at the time of transplantation. J Am Coll Cardiol 2010;56(15):1207–13.

40. Boyle AJ, Russell SD, Teuteberg JJ, et al. Low thromboembolism and pump thrombosis with the HeartMate II left ventricular assist device: analysis of outpatient anti-coagulation. J Heart Lung Transplant 2009;28(9):881–7.

41. Miller LW. The development of the von Willebrand syndrome with the use of continuous flow left ventricular assist devices: a cause-and-effect relationship. J Am Coll Cardiol 2010;56(15):1214–5.

42. Klovaite J, Gustafsson F, Mortensen SA, et al. Severely impaired von Willebrand factor-dependent platelet aggregation in patients with a continuous-flow left ventricular assist device (HeartMate II). J Am Coll Cardiol 2009;53:2162–7.

43. Steinlechner B, Dworschak M, Birkenberg B, et al. Platelet dysfunction in out-patients with left ventricular assist devices. Ann Thorac Surg 2009;87(1):131–7.
44. Suarez J, Patel CB, Felker GM, et al. Mechanisms of bleeding and approach to patients with axial-flow left ventricular assist devices. Circ Heart Fail 2011;4: 779–84.
45. Uriel N, Morrison KA, Garan AR, et al. Development of a novel echocardiography ramp test for speed optimization and diagnosis of device thrombosis in continuous-flow left ventricular assist devices: the Columbia ramp study. J Am Coll Cardiol 2012;60(18):1764–75.
46. Topkara VK, Kondareddy S, Malik F, et al. Infectious complications in patients with left ventricular assist device: etiology and outcomes in the continuous-flow era. Ann Thorac Surg 2010;90(4):1270–7.
47. Pak SW, Uriel N, Takayama H, et al. Prevalence of de novo aortic insufficiency during long-term support with left ventricular assist devices. J Heart Lung Transplant 2010;29(10):1172–6.
48. Toda K, Fujita T, Domae K, et al. Late aortic insufficiency related to poor prognosis during left ventricular assist device support. Ann Thorac Surg 2011;92(3):929–34.
49. Russo MJ, Freed BH, Jeevanandam V, et al. Percutaneous transcatheter closure of the aortic valve to treat cardiogenic shock in a left ventricular assist device patient with severe aortic insufficiency. Ann Thorac Surg 2012;94(3):985–8.
50. D'Ancona G, Pasic M, Buz S, et al. TAVI for pure aortic valve insufficiency in a patient with a left ventricular assist device. Ann Thorac Surg 2012;93(4): e89–91.

Blood Management

Ajay Kumar, MD, SFHM[a],*, Moises Auron, MD, SFHM[b],
Mark Ereth, MD, MA[c]

KEYWORDS

- Blood management program • Evidence-based medicine • Blood transfusion
- Multidisciplinary approach

KEY POINTS

- Blood management is a system-based, comprehensive approach using evidence-based medicine to facilitate an environment to encourage an appropriate use of blood products in the hospital setting.
- The ultimate goal of a blood-management program is to improve patient outcomes by integrating all available techniques to ensure safety, availability, and appropriate allocation of blood products.
- It is a patient-centered, multidisciplinary, multimodal, planned approach to the management of patients and blood products.

INTRODUCTION

Blood management is a system-based, comprehensive approach that uses evidence-based medicine to facilitate an environment to encourage an appropriate use of blood products. With increasing evidence supporting a restrictive strategy of blood transfusion, there has been a renewed effort to implement blood management programs, particularly in the perioperative setting.

COMPONENTS OF A BLOOD-MANAGEMENT PROGRAM

Establishment of a blood management program requires use of evidence-based criteria for blood administration and an implementation process that can create an accountable culture to affect changes. In an era of electronic health records and extensive data management, the ability to track blood utilization has markedly improved. Key factors to consider when establishing a blood management program are:

- Standardized treatment protocol
- Preoperative optimization of patients
- Identifying and mitigating risk of blood exposure before surgery

[a] Division of Hospital Medicine, Hartford Hospital, Hartford, CT, USA; [b] Department of Hospital Medicine and Department of Pediatric Hospital Medicine, Cleveland Clinic, Cleveland, OH, USA; [c] Department of Anesthesiology, Mayo Clinic, Rochester, MN 55902, USA
* Corresponding author.
E-mail address: drajaykumar@gmail.com

Anesthesiology Clin 31 (2013) 433–450
http://dx.doi.org/10.1016/j.anclin.2013.02.001
1932-2275/13/$ – see front matter © 2013 Elsevier Inc. All rights reserved.

- Data collection regarding transfusion practice
- Transparency of data
- Intraoperative measures to reduce blood transfusion
- Education regarding blood safety

PREOPERATIVE EVALUATION

Preoperative anemia should be identified and treated to minimize the risk of perioperative transfusion. Identification of symptoms of anemia, transfusion history, underlying diseases, dietary deficiencies and factors that increase the likelihood of bleeding in the perioperative period should be thoroughly investigated.[1,2]

Clinical findings suggestive of anemia include palpitations, tachycardia, fatigue, angina, and dyspnea, all of which may suggest tissue hypoxia and cardiovascular decompensation. Bone pain and deformities may suggest underlying myeloproliferative disorder or metastatic cancer. Enlarged lymph nodes and hepatosplenomegaly may suggest lymphoproliferative disorders and malignancy. Skin findings include most commonly pallor; however, petechiae can reflect hemolysis or use of antiplatelet agents, and jaundice suggests underlying hemolysis.

Evaluation of current medications should target those which predispose to perioperative bleeding and anemia, such as nonsteroidal anti-inflammatory agents, aspirin, clopidogrel, and anticoagulants.

The goal of laboratory workup of anemia is to identify those conditions for which short-term interventions can be implemented for preoperative optimization such as iron, folate, and vitamin B_{12} deficiencies. Findings suggestive of other conditions require further evaluation with a hematologist. Surgery should be delayed unless the anemia is related to the condition for which surgery is to be performed.[3]

The initial evaluation includes a complete blood count, peripheral smear, and corrected reticulocyte count, to determine whether anemia is a result of loss or destruction of red blood cells (RBCs) or a decrease in bone marrow production. Additional tests include iron (Fe), total iron-binding capacity (TIBC), transferrin saturation, ferritin, serum RBC folate, and serum vitamin B_{12} levels.[2]

- Fe and TIBC are low in anemia arising from chronic disease.
- Fe is low and TIBC is high in iron-deficiency anemia.
- Ferritin levels less than 30 ng/mL in men and less than 20 ng/mL in women suggest iron-deficiency anemia.
- Upper endoscopy and colonoscopy should be pursued in elderly patients with iron-deficiency anemia.
- A celiac panel should be obtained in patients younger than 50 years with iron-deficiency anemia.

In patients with vitamin B_{12} deficiency, the evaluation and investigation for causation should include measurement of intrinsic factors and parietal cell antibodies, in pursuit of diagnosis of pernicious anemia or autoimmune gastritis.

A blood type and screen provides information about the patient's blood type and the presence of RBC antibodies. If the antibody screen is positive, further identification of the antibodies to RBC antigens is pursued.

PREOPERATIVE PHARMACOLOGIC OPTIMIZATION OF ANEMIA
Intravenous Iron Supplementation

The most common cause of asymptomatic anemia in surgical patients is iron deficiency. Patients undergoing orthopedic surgery have received more attention, given the frequency of the procedures and attempts to minimize intraoperative blood transfusions; however, preoperative anemia with iron deficiency is not uncommon in other surgical settings.[4]

Indications of intravenous iron

Oral iron supplementation provides inadequate bioactive iron levels to support erythropoiesis in ongoing iron-loss environments such as surgery. In addition, enteral absorption and bioavailability of iron is affected in cases of: bacterial overgrowth, chronic gastrointestinal bleeding, platelet dysfunction, use of antacids, celiac disease, short bowel syndrome in postbariatric surgery patients, and so forth.[5,6]

A prospective cohort study of patients undergoing orthopedic surgery found no hemoglobin improvement in 87 patients who received preoperative oral ferrous sulfate, 300 mg 3 times daily administered for 3 weeks before surgery; the investigators noted a poor compliance rate (67%) and an increased incidence of gastrointestinal adverse effects.[7]

The safety and efficacy of parenteral iron has been demonstrated in patients with end-stage renal disease (ESRD) on dialysis,[8] patients with inflammatory bowel disease,[9] as well as in multiple studies in surgical patients, including cardiac surgery.[10,11]

In addition, parenteral iron is substantially less expensive than allogeneic blood transfusion. One gram of either ferric gluconate or iron sucrose costs approximately $688 while 1 unit of blood (which contains approximately 250 mg of iron) costs $761.[12]

Protocol for preoperative use of intravenous iron

The current protocols for iron supplementation are based on the physiologic understanding of the iron content of hemoglobin (1 g of hemoglobin contains 3.3 mg of elemental iron) and the Ganzoni formula; however, for practical reasons iron deficit is not usually calculated, because further intraoperative blood loss will increase preoperative iron deficit.[13] An intravenous iron dose of 1 g will raise the hemoglobin by approximately 2.0 g/dL; use of intravenous iron has reported benefits in successfully treating anemia, and decreasing transfusion rates.[10,13]

The Network for Advancement of Transfusion Alternatives (NATA), recommends that preoperative intravenous iron be administered to patients with ferritin level of less than 100 ng/mL, transferrin saturation less than 20%, or expected blood loss greater than 1500 mL. The cutoff limit to avoid further intravenous iron administration is when ferritin levels are higher than 300 ng/mL and transferrin saturation is greater than 50%, or when there is acute infection.[14] Iron should be administered within sufficient time (3–4 weeks preoperatively) to maximize effective erythropoiesis.[13]

Controversies regarding parenteral iron use

The most feared reaction associated with intravenous iron was anaphylaxis, which happened with increased frequency in combination with high molecular weight dextran.[15]

The Food and Drug Administration (FDA) reported an analysis from 2001 to 2003 on the safety of intravenous iron preparations including iron gluconate, iron sucrose, and high and low molecular weight dextran. Among a total of 30 million doses, the reported incidence of effects was 2.2 per million doses and a mortality of 0.4 per million doses; allogeneic blood transfusion was associated with 10 adverse effects per million units and 4 deaths per million units, which was substantially higher than parenteral iron. The incidence of adverse effects according to iron preparation was: iron sucrose, 0.6 per million doses; ferric gluconate, 0.9 per million doses; low molecular weight dextran, 3.3 per million doses; high molecular weight dextran, 11.3 per million doses. Iron sucrose and iron gluconate were not associated with anaphylaxis. Ferric gluconate has been linked to anaphylactoid reactions in 0.46 per million doses of 100 mg. The preservative benzyl alcohol has been identified as the main culprit, secondary to increased vasoactive reactivity and capillary leak symptoms (tachycardia, hypotension, diarrhea, edema, dyspnea, and chest or abdominal pain). The risk of adverse effects is minimized by decreasing the dose.[16] In addition, patients with reactions to ferric gluconate had no increase in tryptase, which is a marker of mast-cell degranulation and is expected to be elevated in true anaphylaxis.[17]

Preoperative Use of Erythropoiesis-Stimulating Agents

Routine preoperative use of erythropoiesis-stimulating agents (ESAs), occurs mainly in orthopedic surgery (hip and knee replacements) and in cardiac surgery for patients refusing blood transfusions.[18]

Indications of erythropoietin therapy

The degree of erythropoiesis shows a dose-response correlation.[19] In studies in iron-replete nonanemic patients, reticulocytosis reportedly occurs after 3 days of treatment with EPO.[20] Recently it has been shown that EPO increased the reticulocyte life span, especially during the first week after its administration.[21]

Concomitant use of iron when using EPO allows appropriate plasma transferrin saturation to promote optimal erythropoiesis.[19]

Recently, a guideline for perioperative blood conservation in cardiac surgery recommended preoperative epoetin plus parenteral iron for patients undergoing surgery with preoperative anemia, those refusing blood transfusions (Jehovah's witnesses), or those at high risk for postoperative anemia.[22]

Current protocol for preoperative ESA

The use of ESA takes into account the appropriate level of hematinic substrates. A blood-conservation protocol in orthopedic surgery patients using parenteral iron in patients undergoing orthopedic surgery provides concomitant supplementation of vitamin B_{12}, folate, and vitamin C, and a single dose of 40,000 units of EPO. In addition to minimizing intraoperative and postoperative transfusion rate, hemoglobin values were improved at 30 days after surgery. The same group found that patients who received EPO had decreased blood use compared with the group that did not (42% vs 60%, $P = .013$).[23]

In patients undergoing cardiac valvular surgery, a single dose of EPO (500 IU/kg) and iron sucrose (200 mg) on the day before surgery showed a decreased transfusion rate (59% vs 86%, $P = .009$), and a decreased number of units of blood (1.0 vs 3.3 units/patient, $P = .001$) compared with patients receiving placebo.[24]

Regarding the use of multiple preoperative EPO doses, there is significant heterogeneity in practice, which includes different doses, preparations, use of supplemental iron, and so forth.[25]

A decreased rate of postoperative allogeneic blood transfusions in patients receiving preoperative EPO has been shown in a variety of meta-analyses, such as in cardiac surgery (relative risk [RR] 0.53, 95% confidence interval [CI] 0.32–0.88; $P<.01$)[26] and orthopedic surgery (postoperative autologous blood transfusion in up to 27% of patients using EPO compared with up to 71% in patients who did not).[27]

The current recommendation for perioperative use of epoetin alfa (Procrit) as it appears on the package insert is (www.procrit.com/sites/default/files/pdf/ProcritBooklet.pdf):

- 300 units/kg per day subcutaneously for 15 days total: administered daily for 10 days before surgery, 1 dose on the day of surgery, and then for 4 days after surgery, or
- 600 units/kg subcutaneously in 4 doses administered 21, 14, and 7 days before surgery, and on the day of surgery.

The regimen is supported by a study in patients undergoing elective joint replacement surgery, which showed a decreased transfusion rate in patients who received EPO (16%) versus placebo (45%).[28] Another study showing the dose-response effectiveness of preoperative EPO found a transfusion rate of 17% in patients receiving 300 IU/kg, 25% in patients receiving 100 IU/kg, and 54% in the placebo group.[29] The study showed the effectiveness and superiority of weekly versus daily EPO, when comparing patients who receive preoperative EPO 300 units/kg daily for 15 days starting 10 days before, on the day of surgery, and 4 days postoperatively, with a group of patients who received 600 units/kg once weekly beginning 3 weeks before surgery, with a fourth dose on the day of surgery. A decreased postoperative transfusion rate was seen in the patients receiving a weekly (16%) in comparison with a daily (20%) regime; moreover, the weekly regime showed doubling of hemoglobin (1.44 g/dL vs 0.73 g/dL) and a decrease in the total EPO dose (2400 units/kg vs 4500 units/kg) when compared with the daily regime.[30]

The current FDA-approved ESA is epoetin alfa. Indications for its use are total knee or hip replacement surgery, or patients who refuse blood transfusion (Jehovah's witness). The weekly ESA dose provides ease of administration and a decreased total dose, maintaining enhanced hematopoietic response. The recommended dose is 600 units/kg weekly or a total dose of 40,000 units weekly starting 21 days before surgery: 21, 14, and 7 days before surgery, and a fourth dose on the day of surgery. The patient should continue on iron supplementation; the authors favor the administration of concomitant parenteral iron (200 mg iron sucrose or 125 mg ferrous sulfate) along with each dose of epoetin alfa, especially if ferritin levels are less than 100 ng/mL.

Controversies regarding ESA therapy

A prospective study of hemodialysis patients with congestive heart failure or ischemic heart disease who were treated with EPO demonstrated an increased rate of death and nonfatal myocardial infarctions in patients with a "normal" hematocrit target of 42% versus patients with a "low" hematocrit target of 30%.[31] In another study, patients with chronic renal disease receiving EPO therapy had an increased risk of adverse outcomes (composite of death, myocardial infarction, hospitalization for congestive heart failure and stroke) when the hemoglobin level was 13.5 g/dL, compared with patients with a more conservative level of 11.3 g/dL.[32] In addition, in patients with stage IV chronic kidney disease, early EPO therapy showed no significant difference in cardiovascular adverse outcomes in patients with hemoglobin of 13 to 15 g/dL in comparison with those with 10.5 to 11.5 g/dL hemoglobin.[33]

An increased risk of venous thromboembolism (RR 1.57, 95% CI 1.31–1.87) and mortality (hazard ratio 1.10, 95% CI 1.01–1.20) was seen in in 4610 patients with cancer who received ESAs, versus 3562 controls.[34]

In surgical patients undergoing elective spine surgery, risk of deep venous thrombosis (DVT) was higher among patients who received ESAs (4.7%) compared with the patients who did not (2.1%).[35] A meta-analysis by the NATA showed that the risk of DVT increased with the use of recombinant human EPO (Peto odds ratio 1.66, 95% CI 1.10–2.48).[3]

In 2007, the FDA issued a black-box warning to have a conservative approach to anemia management in ESRD patients targeting a hemoglobin level of 11 to 12 g/dL, and recommended the use of EPO in patients with cancer only if they were undergoing active myelosuppressive chemotherapy. The FDA also alerted against the higher risk of mortality, stroke, uncontrolled hypertension, and DVT in patients taking EPO, and recommended prophylactic anticoagulation in perioperative surgical patients treated with epoetin alfa because of the higher risk of DVT. This advice has been incorporated in the Procrit (epoetin alfa) insert. (www.fda.gov/drugs/drugsafety/ postmarketdrugsafetyinformationforpatientsandproviders/ucm126481.htm).

THROMBELASTOGRAPHY

Thrombelastography (TEG) was first described by Hartert in 1948 as a method to assess the global hemostatic function from a single blood sample.[36] TEG demonstrates all phases of hemostasis, from initial fibrin formation, to fibrin-platelet plug construction, through clot lysis (**Fig. 1**). A TEG analysis can also identify imbalances within the hemostatic system, which can help to stratify the risk of bleeding or a thrombotic event. In 2007, Haemonetics (Braintree, MA) acquired the Thrombelastograph, which it continues to market and sell today. The Thrombelastograph analyzes the viscoelastic properties of whole blood samples under low shear conditions, and displays results both graphically and numerically. A whole blood sample of 360 μL is placed into the cuvette and activated with kaolin or heparinase as the activator, depending on the presence of heparin. The Thrombelastograph measures the clot strength by using a stationary cylindrical cuvette that holds the blood sample and oscillates through an angle of 4°45'. Each rotation cycle lasts 10 seconds. A pin is suspended in the blood by a torsion wire and is monitored for motion. The torque of the rotation cuvette is transmitted to the immersed pin only after fibrin-platelet bonding has linked the cuvette and pin together (**Fig. 2**). The strength of these fibrin-platelet bonds affects the magnitude of the pin motion. The output is related to the strength of the formed clot. As the clot lyses, the bonds are broken and the transfer of cuvette motion is decreased. The rotation movement of the pin is converted by a mechanical-electrical transducer to an electrical signal that displays the TEG tracing (**Fig. 3**).[37] The time until initial fibrin formation is the reaction time or r-time. The kinetics of fibrin formation and clot development is the angle. The ultimate strength and stability of the fibrin clot is the maximum amplitude (MA) and clot lysis (fibrinolysis). TEG is a fibrinolysis-sensitive assay, and allows for diagnosis of hyperfibrinolysis in bleeding patients (**Table 1**).

ROTEM

The ROTEM (Rotem Inc, Durham, NC) is a compact and portable device that operates on the principles of thromboelastometry. ROTEM is a viscoelastometric method for analyzing the hemostasis of whole blood and measuring the interactions of coagulation factors, inhibitors, and cellular components during the phases of clotting and lysis over time. ROTEM is most practical for evaluating total hemostatic function in patients.

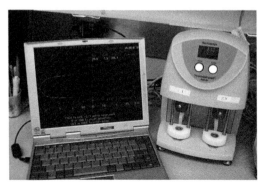

Fig. 1. A thrombelastography (TEG) machine.

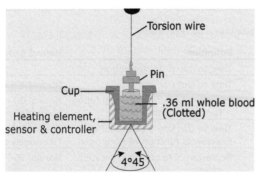

Fig. 2. A pin is suspended in the blood by a torsion wire and is monitored for motion. The torque of the rotation cuvette is transmitted to the immersed pin only after fibrin-platelet bonding has linked the cuvette and pin together.

ROTEM detects hypofunctional and hyperfunctional stages of the clotting process.[38] Whereas standard clotting assays detect the starting time of clotting, ROTEM quickly provides data on the entire process: clotting time, clot formation, clot stability, and lysis, all of which aid in supporting rapid differential diagnosis in bleeding patients. ROTEM helps to differentiate between surgical bleeding and a hemostasis disorder, helps to identify hyperfibrinolysis, the extent of dilutional coagulopathy, and requirement for fibrinogen or platelet substitution, and allows for monitoring of heparin and protamine dosage.[37]

The main descriptive parameters derived by ROTEM are:

CT, corresponding to the time in seconds from the beginning of the reaction to a 2-mm increase in amplitude. CT represents the initiation of clotting, thrombin formation, and the start of clot polymerization.

Clot formation time, the time (seconds) between an increase in amplitude from 2 to 20 mm. This parameter identifies the fibrin polymerization and stabilization of the clot with platelets and factor XIII.

Analytical Software
Graphical Representation

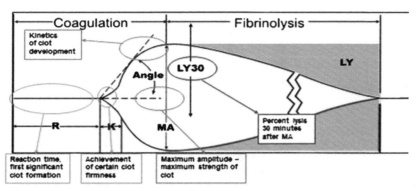

Fig. 3. The characteristics of TEG tracings include R (activation), angle (α), MA (maximal clot strength), and lysis (fibrinolysis). Image: "TEG Tracing Graphic" is used by permission of Haemonetics Corporation. TEG® and Thrombelastograph® are registered trademarks of Haemonetics in the US, other countries or both.

Table 1
Definition and representation of TEG values

		Definition	Normal Range
SP	Split point	Time to initial clot formation	
r	r time	Time to clot size = 2 mm	Normal 4–9 min
R-SP	Delta thrombin	Represents function of coagulation factors up to thrombin	Normal 0.7–1.1 min Factor deficiency if >1.2 min
k	k time	Time to clot size = 20 mm after R Represents function of fibrinogen	Normal 1–3 min Fibrinogen deficiency if >3 min
MA	Maximum amplitude	Represents size of clot at greatest extent	Normal 55–74 mm
G	Clot strength	Calculated from MA Represents strength of clot Calculation done by TEG machine	Normal 5.3–13.2 kd/cm^2 Decreased platelet function if <5.3 kd/cm^2

Maximum clot firmness (MCF), the MA (mm) reached in the tracing, which correlates with platelet count, platelet function, and the concentration of fibrinogen.

Alpha (α) angle, the tangent to the clotting curve through the 2-mm point.

Maximum lysis, the ratio of the lowest amplitude after MCF to the MCF.

Maximum velocity (maxVel), the maximum of the first derivative of the clot curve.

Time to maximum velocity (t-maxVel), the time from the start of the reaction until maxVel is reached.

The area under curve, defined as the area under the velocity curve, that is, the area under the curve ending at a time point that corresponds to MCF (**Fig. 4**).

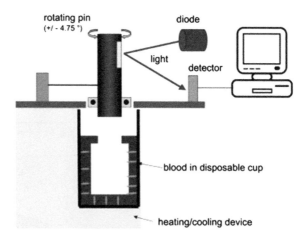

Fig. 4. Test principle of rotational TEG (ROTEM). Citrated whole blood, native whole blood, or plasma (300 μL) and test reagents are pipetted semiautomatically into a single-use plastic cup that is set onto a plastic pin on a rotating vertical axis (±4.75°) guided by ball bearings. The increasing firmness of the clot gradually reduces the movement of the pin. Movement is continuously detected by using a light source, a reflecting mirror on the rotating axis, and a detector chip. The reduction in movement is mathematically transformed into clot firmness (amplitude in millimeters) and plotted against time (in seconds), resulting in a thromboelastometric trace. (*From* Kozek-Langenecker SA. Perioperative coagulation monitoring. Best Pract Res Clin Anaesthesiol 2010;24:27–40; with permission.)

The ROTEM includes 4 tests generally used for monitoring a patient's blood: Hep-TEM, which includes a contact activator plus heparinase for specific detection of heparin; in-TEM, which includes contact activator as an intrinsic pathway assessment of clot formation and fibrin polymerization; ex-TEM, which has tissue factor and provides a view of extrinsic pathway and a quick assessment of clot formation and fibrinolysis; and fib-TEM, which consists of tissue factor and platelet antagonist to provide a qualitative assessment of fibrinogen levels.

The clotting process is detected via a torsion wire that uses a rotating pin, which is fixed on a steel axis stabilized by a ball bearing inserted into a disposable cup. The cup and pin oscillate at about 5°. In conjunction with the optical detection method of ROTEM, this enables it to overcome vibration sensitivities encountered in TEG **(Fig. 5)**.[39]

It is well cited that transfusion decisions vary widely between individuals and institutions with respect to surgery and trauma. Many times products are transfused without laboratory testing. Implementation of rapid point-of-care (POC) testing in surgical applications can help to individualize and direct resuscitation efforts in surgical patients. The ROTEM provides essential data in multiple settings where the potential to measure the clotting process that begins with fibrin formation and continues through the lysis of the clot exists. In trauma studies, ROTEM has been effective in rapidly detecting most coagulation disorders, allowing for the streamlining of massive transfusion protocols in trauma settings.[40] The incorporation and use of ROTEM coupled with transfusion algorithms have been shown in studies to decrease transfusion requirements and postoperative blood loss in patients undergoing cardiac surgery.[41] ROTEM has proved to be popular and effective in managing coagulation when multiple factors are involved. Different to the single factor replacement for hereditary hemorrhagic disorders, the conditions in major perioperative and trauma patients often necessitate the use of multiple components and factor concentrates. Cost savings incurred by using goal-directed coagulation management are significant when considering the shortened surgical times, reduction in frequency of surgical reexploration, shortened length of stay in the intensive care unit (ICU), and less direct and indirect costs of blood products transfused.

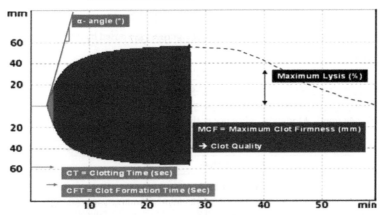

Fig. 5. ROTEM curve and parameters. (*From* Armstrong S, Fernando R, Ashpole K, et al. Assessment of coagulation in the obstetric population using ROTEM(R) thromboelastometry. Int J Obstet Anesth 2011;20(4):293–8; with permission.)

Algorithms

The use of TEG-based algorithms to help guide transfusion practice has been well documented in cardiac surgery, and more recently with trauma patients and rapid TEG (r-TEG). In a study published in 2009 by Ak and colleagues,[42] routine use of a kaolin-activated TEG-guided algorithm reduced the consumption of blood products in patients undergoing elective coronary artery bypass grafting (CABG). The algorithm used focused on the use of fresh frozen plasma, platelets, and antifibrinolytic tranexamic acid (**Table 2**). Utilization of fresh frozen plasma was based on reaction time (r-time) greater than 14 mm, and dose adjusted if greater than 21 mm and greater than 28 mm. Platelet use was based on maximum amplitude (MA) less than 48 mm and dose adjusted if less than 40 mm. The use of tranexamic acid was based on percent clot lysis at 30 minutes (LY30) greater than 7.5%, which indicated fibrinolysis. The results of this study show that the TEG group had significantly lower median units of fresh frozen plasma and platelets in comparison with the other group ($P = .001$). The median number of total allogeneic units transfused (packed cells and blood products) was significantly reduced in the TEG group compared with the other group (median 2, range 1–3 units vs median 3, range 2–4 units, respectively; $P = .001$). The need for tranexamic acid was significantly diminished in the TEG group compared with the other group (10.3% vs 19%, respectively; $P = .007$) (see **Table 2**).

This study shows the promise of the use of a TEG-guided algorithm, but other coagulation profile laboratory tests including bleeding time, prothrombin time (PT), activated partial thromboplastin time (aPTT), fibrinogen, and platelet count are capable of reliably predicting microvascular bleeding after cardiopulmonary bypass, and need to be integrated into the algorithm to accurately treat bleeding.[43] Adopting a type of algorithm that uses different coagulation tests in the care of CABG patients may help improve clinical outcomes, reduce the risk of transfusion-related complications, and decrease the total cost of CABG.[44] In a study performed by Nuttall and colleagues[45] in 2001, the use of a coagulation test–based transfusion algorithm in patients undergoing cardiac surgery with abnormal bleeding after cardiopulmonary bypass reduced nonerythrocyte allogeneic transfusions in the operating room and blood loss in the ICU. The percentage of patients without any transfused nonerythrocyte products in the operating room increased to 30% (**Figs. 6** and **7**).

Table 2
Modified version of the TEG-based transfusion algorithm proposed by Royston and von Kier

TEG Parameter		Treatment
$14 < r < 21$ (mm)	Mild deficiency in coagulation factors[a]	1 unit FFP
$21 \leq r < 28$ (mm)	Moderate deficiency in coagulation factors[a]	2 units FFP
$r \geq 28$ (mm)	Severe deficiency in coagulation factors[a]	4 units FFP
$40 \leq MA < 48$ (mm)	Moderate deficiency in the number/function of platelets	1 unit[b] platelets
$MA < 40$ (mm)	Severe deficiency in the number/function of platelets	2 units platelets
$LY30 > 7.5$ (%)	Exaggerated fibrinolysis	TA

Abbreviations: FFP, fresh frozen plasma; LY30, % lysis at 30 min; TA, tranexamic acid.
[a] If the r time on the h-kTEG was less than one-half of the nonheparinase r time on the kTEG.
[b] Represents single-donor platelets obtained by apheresis, the equivalent of approximately 6 platelet concentrates.
Modified from Royston D, von Kier S. Reduced haemostatic factor transfusion using heparinase-modified thrombelastography during cardiopulmonary bypass. Br J Anaesth 2001;86(4):575–8.

ICU Transfusion Algorithm

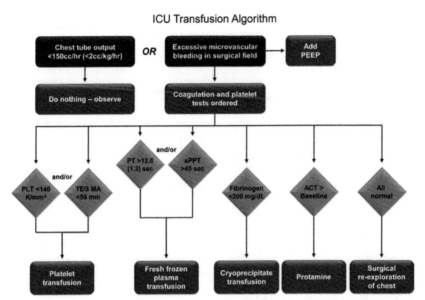

Fig. 6. Operating room transfusion algorithm. ACT, activated clotting time; aPTT, activated partial thromboplastin time; MA, maximum amplitude; PLT, platelet count; PT, prothrombin time. (*Adapted from* Nuttall GA, Oliver WC, Santrach PJ, et al. Efficacy of a simple intraoperative transfusion algorithm for nonerythrocyte component utilization after cardiopulmonary bypass. Anesthesiology 2001;94:780; with permission.)

In 2010, Nuttall and colleagues extended the use of the algorithm to the ICU. After reviewing more than 231 adult patients undergoing cardiac surgery, the cut-points from the operating room algorithm were adjusted to optimize blood use in the ICU. **Fig. 8** shows the updated laboratory values.

Trauma patients can also benefit from the use of TEG, and with the recent addition of r-TEG its clinical implication is more evident. Cotton and colleagues[46] describe r-TEG as being similar to standard TEG while generating several values that describe the clotting cascade. The first value generated is the activated clotting time (ACT), which is the time in seconds between initiation of the test and the initial fibrin

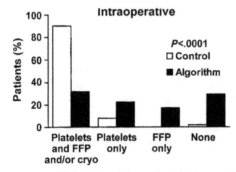

Fig. 7. Percentage of patients transfused intraoperatively before traditional clinical practice and laboratory-guided algorithm. FFP, fresh frozen plasma. (*Adapted from* Nuttall GA, Oliver WC, Santrach PJ, et al. Efficacy of a simple intraoperative transfusion algorithm for nonerythrocyte component utilization after cardiopulmonary bypass. Anesthesiology 2001;94:773–81; with permission.)

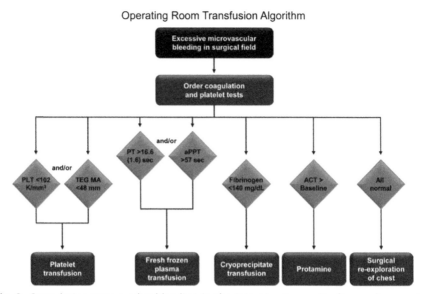

Operating Room Transfusion Algorithm

Fig. 8. Coagulation tests predict bleeding in the intensive care unit after cardiac surgery. ACT, activated clotting time; aPTT, activated partial thromboplastin time; MA, maximum amplitude; PLT, platelet count; PT, Prothrombin time. (*Adapted from* Nuttall GA, Oliver WC, Santrach PJ, et al. Efficacy of a simple intraoperative transfusion algorithm for nonerythrocyte component utilization after cardiopulmonary bypass. Anesthesiology 2001; 94:773–81; with permission.)

formation, increased with factor deficiency or severe hemodilution (normal range, 86–118 seconds). Similar to the ACT, the r-value (also known as the reaction time, 0–1 minutes) expresses the time between the start of the assay and the beginning of clot formation. The k-time (normal range, 1–2 minutes) is the time needed to reach 20-mm clot strength; this is generally increased in states of hypofibrinogenemia. The alpha (α) angle (normal range, 66°–82°) is the slope of the tracing that represents the rate of clot formation. The α-angle is decreased with hypofibrinogenemia or platelet dysfunction. The maximal amplitude (MA; normal range, 54 to the greatest amplitude of the tracing) reflects the platelet contribution to clot strength. Low MA values correspond with states of platelet dysfunction or hypofibrinogenemia. The G-value (normal range, 5300–12,000 dyn/cm^2) is a global measure of absolute clot strength (both enzymatic and platelet contributions) and is decreased in hypocoagulable states. LY30 (normal range, 0.0%–7.5%) is the percent amplitude reduction at 30 minutes after MA and, when elevated, reflects a state of hyperfibrinolysis.[46,47] Holcomb and colleagues[47] published findings on 1974 consecutive trauma patients who were evaluated with r-TEG on admission. In this study the r-TEG data were clinically superior to results from 5 conventional coagulation tests and correlated with the results of the PT, aPTT, international normalized ratio (INR), platelet count, and fibrinogen (**Table 3**).

In addition, r-TEG identified patients with an increased risk of early RBCs, plasma and platelet transfusions, and fibrinolysis. When controlling for age, injury mechanism, weighted Revised Trauma Score, base excess, and hemoglobin, ACT predicted RBC transfusion, and the α-angle predicted massive RBC transfusion better than PT, aPTT, or INR ($P<.001$). The α-angle was a better predictor of fibrinogen with regard to plasma

Table 3
Correlation between TEG parameters and routine coagulation tests

	PT	aPTT	INR	Platelet Count	Fibrinogen
ACT, s	r = 0.35, P<.001	r = 0.47, P<.001	r = 0.52, P<.001	r = −0.15, P<.001	r = −0.17, P<.001
r-value, min	r = 0.24, P<.001	r = 0.32, P<.001	r = 0.37, P<.001	r = −0.14, P<.001	r = −0.17, P<.001
k-time, min	r = 0.21, P<.001	r = 0.44, P<.001	r = 0.34, P<.001	r = −0.25, P<.001	r = −0.32, P<.001
α-angle, degrees	r = −0.23, P<.001	r = −0.41, P<.001	r = −0.33, P<.001	r = 0.34, P<.001	r = 0.53, P<.001
MA, mm	r = −0.22, P<.001	r = −0.35, P<.001	r = −0.27, P<.001	r = 0.42, P<.001	r = 0.63, P<.001
G-value, dynes/cm^2	r = −0.02, P = .445	r = −0.03, P = .325	r = −0.03, P = .411	r = −0.01, P = .872	r = 0.01, P = .902

Abbreviations: ACT, activated clotting time; aPTT, activated partial thromboplastin time; MA, maximum amplitude; PT, prothrombin time; r-value, reaction time.
Data from Holcomb JB, Minei KM, Scerbo ML, et al. Admission rapid thrombelastography can replace conventional coagulation tests in the emergency department: experience with 1974 consecutive trauma patients. Ann Surg 2012; 256(3):476–86.

transfusion (P<.001); MA was a better predictor of platelet count related to platelet transfusion (P<.001); and LY30 (rate of amplitude reduction 30 minutes after the MA is reached) documented fibrinolysis. This method showed improved correlations for patients with transfusion, shock, or head injury (**Table 4**).[47]

These results suggest that conventional coagulation tests could be replaced with r-TEG. The charge for r-TEG ($317) was similar to that of the 5 conventional coagulation tests ($286).[47]

Table 4
Laboratory cut-points for transfusion

Laboratory Values	Blood Product Transfusion
ACT >128 s	Plasma and RBCs
r-value >1.1 min	Plasma and RBCs
k-time >2.5 min	Cryoprecipitate/fibrinogen/plasma
α-angle <56°	Cryoprecipitate/fibrinogen/platelets
MA <55 mm	Platelets/cryoprecipitate/fibrinogen
LY30 >3%	Tranexamic acid
PT >18.0 s	Plasma
aPTT >35 s	Plasma
INR >1.5	Plasma
Platelet count <150 × 10^9/L	Platelets
Fibrinogen <180 g/L	Cryoprecipitate/fibrinogen

Abbreviations: ACT, activated clotting time; aPTT, activated partial thromboplastin time; INR, international normalized ratio; LY30, % lysis at 30 min; MA, maximum amplitude; PT, prothrombin time; RBCs, red blood cells; r-value, reaction time.
Data from Holcomb JB, Minei KM, Scerbo ML, et al. Admission rapid thrombelastography can replace conventional coagulation tests in the emergency department: experience with 1974 consecutive trauma patients. Ann Surg 2012; 256(3):476–86.

Outcomes

Hemorrhage is known to be a major cause of morbidity in trauma and in the surgical setting. Unnecessary transfusions are associated with increased morbidity and increased institutional costs.[48] The benefits of POC testing in surgical patients include rapid turnaround times and specific measurements of hemostatic defects that can help direct therapy as well as provide scientifically based logical treatment guidelines. Clinicians would be able to thus optimize the targeted transfusion therapies with specific coagulation factors instead of empirical administration of components, which carries potentially hazardous consequences.[41] The use of specific tests and algorithms that can be used in the operating room and at the bedside has enabled the incorporation of these tests into transfusion algorithms that more directly address the hemostatic problem and allow treatment using fewer allogeneic blood products, reducing the waste of products and decreasing hospital resources as a whole.[49]

Cell Salvage

The use of intraoperative cell salvage and autologous blood transfusion has become an important incorporated focus and method in blood management strategies. The process involves the suctioning of accumulated blood during a surgical procedure, washing and filtering of the blood, then returning the processed product back to the patient. The main goal of autologous transfusion is to reduce the need for allogeneic blood transfusion and its associated complications. Cell-salvaged blood and allogeneic blood, when compared, have demonstrated an increased mean erythrocyte viability and increased levels of 2,3-disphosphoglycerate and adenosine triphosphate in the salvaged blood. The mean erythrocyte viability has also been reported to be more than 80% with cell salvage.[50] Salvaged RBCs maintain their normal biconcave disc shape, whereas allogeneic blood cells take on a burr cell shape (after 14 days), which is thought to impede the cells' ability to cross the capillary beds. Patients who have had autologous transfusion should have improved oxygen-carrying capacity and tissue oxygen delivery as a result of this process.[50]

The indications for use of cell salvage include:

Anticipated intraoperative blood loss >1 L or 0.20% of blood volume
Preoperative anemia or increased risk factors for bleeding
Patients who have rare blood group types or antibodies
Patients' refusal to receive allogeneic blood transfusion

The American Association of Blood Banks suggests that cell salvage is indicated for surgery when blood would ordinarily be cross-matched or when more than 10% of patients undergoing the procedure require transfusion.

A 2006 Cochrane Collaboration meta-analysis of studies on the use of cell salvage for minimizing allogeneic blood transfusion found that cell salvage was efficacious in reducing the need for allogeneic blood transfusion in adult elective surgery. The use of cell salvage reduced exposure to allogeneic blood transfusion by 39%, with an average saving of 0.67 units per patient, without causing cardiovascular, neurologic, and immunologic adverse clinical outcomes.[51] Cell salvage was found to be most effective in orthopedic surgery, and had no negative impact on morbidity or mortality.

Complications associated with the use of cell salvage are rare, and studies have shown no increase in complications in patients receiving cell salvage. Cell salvage and autologous transfusion are safe and effective at reducing requirements of allogeneic blood transfusion, and are also cost effective in cardiac and orthopedic surgery. Cell salvage should be considered in all cases where significant blood loss is expected

or possible, in patients with preoperative anemia, and in patients who refuse allogeneic blood products.[50]

The investment to incorporate a cell-salvage program is not cheap, but it has been
proved to be cost effective in larger tertiary hospitals. Variation in the case volume and
blood loss in each case, as well as initial capital investment, may vary by institution
and geographic location. In one large center's experience, data from 2328 surgical
patients showed the payback period for such a program as 1.9 months. The capital
that was invested for equipment was $103,551 and the fixed operation costs were
$250,943. The cost of $200 for a unit of allogeneic RBCs was used, and the salvaged
unit of RBC cost was $89.46.[52]

Cell salvage remains a critical component of blood-management efforts for procedures involving high blood loss.

DATA COLLECTION AND EDUCATION

To measure the impact of a comprehensive blood-management program, hospitals
and groups must adopt a transparent data evaluation and distribution system. In
general, the data should include various metrics directed toward providing
evidence-based directional data to help physicians adopt best practice. The success
of a blood-management program should be measured in patient outcomes alongside
financial circumstances. Overall impact on health care system delivery must be
adjusted for the case-mix index, patient-care volume, and cost of blood products.
Blood-waste monitoring should be focused on laboratory waste as well as clinical
waste, which can improve handling procedures such as storage of blood products.
Awareness about patient safety, adverse events, and morbidity associated with the
use of blood products is a key component in changing the culture.

REFERENCES

1. Kumar A, Carson JL. Perioperative anemia in the elderly. Clin Geriatr Med 2008;
   24(4):641–8, viii.
2. Kumar A. Perioperative management of anemia: limits of blood transfusion and
   alternatives to it. Cleve Clin J Med 2009;76(Suppl 4):S112–8.
3. Goodnough LT, Shander A, Spivak JL, et al. Detection, evaluation, and management of anemia in the elective surgical patient. Anesth Analg 2005;101(6):
   1858–61.
4. Auerbach M, Goodnough LT, Picard D, et al. The role of intravenous iron in
   anemia management and transfusion avoidance. Transfusion 2008;48(5):
   988–1000.
5. Macdougall IC. Iron supplementation in the non-dialysis chronic kidney disease
   (ND-CKD) patient: oral or intravenous? Curr Med Res Opin 2010;26(2):473–82.
6. Goddard AF, James MW, McIntyre AS, et al. Guidelines for the management of
   iron deficiency anaemia. Gut 2011;60(10):1309–16.
7. Lachance K, Savoie M, Bernard M, et al. Oral ferrous sulfate does not increase
   preoperative hemoglobin in patients scheduled for hip or knee arthroplasty.
   Ann Pharmacother 2011;45(6):764–70.
8. Kalantar-Zadeh K, Streja E, Miller JE, et al. Intravenous iron versus erythropoiesis-
   stimulating agents: friends or foes in treating chronic kidney disease anemia?
   Adv Chronic Kidney Dis 2009;16(2):143–51.
9. Lee TW, Kolber MR, Fedorak RN, et al. Iron replacement therapy in inflammatory
   bowel disease patients with iron deficiency anemia: a systematic review and
   meta-analysis. J Crohns Colitis 2012;6(3):267–75.

10. Munoz M, Breymann C, Garcia-Erce JA, et al. Efficacy and safety of intravenous iron therapy as an alternative/adjunct to allogeneic blood transfusion. Vox Sang 2008;94(3):172–83.
11. Munoz M, Garcia-Erce JA, Diez-Lobo AI, et al. Usefulness of the administration of intravenous iron sucrose for the correction of preoperative anemia in major surgery patients. Med Clin (Barc) 2009;132(8):303–6 [in Spanish].
12. Shander A, Hofmann A, Ozawa S, et al. Activity-based costs of blood transfusions in surgical patients at four hospitals. Transfusion 2010;50(4):753–65.
13. Munoz M, Garcia-Erce JA, Cuenca J, et al. On the role of iron therapy for reducing allogeneic blood transfusion in orthopaedic surgery. Blood Transfus 2012;10(1):8–22.
14. Beris P, Munoz M, Garcia-Erce JA, et al. Perioperative anaemia management: consensus statement on the role of intravenous iron. Br J Anaesth 2008;100(5):599–604.
15. McCarthy JT, Regnier CE, Loebertmann CL, et al. Adverse events in chronic hemodialysis patients receiving intravenous iron dextran—a comparison of two products. Am J Nephrol 2000;20(6):455–62.
16. Chertow GM, Mason PD, Vaage-Nilsen O, et al. Update on adverse drug events associated with parenteral iron. Nephrol Dial Transplant 2006;21(2):378–82.
17. Coyne DW, Adkinson NF, Nissenson AR, et al. Sodium ferric gluconate complex in hemodialysis patients. II. Adverse reactions in iron dextran-sensitive and dextran-tolerant patients. Kidney Int 2003;63(1):217–24.
18. Testa U. Erythropoietic stimulating agents. Expert Opin Emerg Drugs 2010;15(1):119–38.
19. Goodnough LT. Iron deficiency syndromes and iron-restricted erythropoiesis (CME). Transfusion 2012;52(7):1584–92.
20. Goodnough LT, Brittenham GM. Limitations of the erythropoietic response to serial phlebotomy: implications for autologous blood donor programs. J Lab Clin Med 1990;115(1):28–35.
21. Krzyzanski W, Perez-Ruixo JJ. An assessment of recombinant human erythropoietin effect on reticulocyte production rate and lifespan distribution in healthy subjects. Pharm Res 2007;24(4):758–72.
22. Ferraris VA, Brown JR, Despotis GJ, et al. 2011 update to the Society of Thoracic Surgeons and the Society of Cardiovascular Anesthesiologists blood conservation clinical practice guidelines. Ann Thorac Surg 2011;91(3):944–82.
23. Garcia-Erce JA, Cuenca J, Munoz M, et al. Perioperative stimulation of erythropoiesis with intravenous iron and erythropoietin reduces transfusion requirements in patients with hip fracture. A prospective observational study. Vox Sang 2005;88(4):235–43.
24. Yoo YC, Shim JK, Kim JC, et al. Effect of single recombinant human erythropoietin injection on transfusion requirements in preoperatively anemic patients undergoing valvular heart surgery. Anesthesiology 2011;115(5):929–37.
25. Earnshaw P. Blood conservation in orthopaedic surgery: the role of epoetin alfa. Int Orthop 2001;25(5):273–8.
26. Alghamdi AA, Albanna MJ, Guru V, et al. Does the use of erythropoietin reduce the risk of exposure to allogeneic blood transfusion in cardiac surgery? A systematic review and meta-analysis. J Card Surg 2006;21(3):320–6.
27. Spahn DR. Anemia and patient blood management in hip and knee surgery: a systematic review of the literature. Anesthesiology 2010;113(2):482–95.
28. de Andrade JR, Jove M, Landon G, et al. Baseline hemoglobin as a predictor of risk of transfusion and response to Epoetin alfa in orthopedic surgery patients. Am J Orthop (Belle Mead NJ) 1996;25(8):533–42.

29. Faris PM, Ritter MA, Abels RI. The effects of recombinant human erythropoietin on perioperative transfusion requirements in patients having a major orthopaedic operation. The American Erythropoietin Study Group. J Bone Joint Surg Am 1996;78(1):62–72.

30. Goldberg MA, McCutchen JW, Jove M, et al. A safety and efficacy comparison study of two dosing regimens of epoetin alfa in patients undergoing major orthopedic surgery. Am J Orthop (Belle Mead NJ) 1996;25(8):544–52.

31. Besarab A, Bolton WK, Browne JK, et al. The effects of normal as compared with low hematocrit values in patients with cardiac disease who are receiving hemodialysis and epoetin. N Engl J Med 1998;339(9):584–90.

32. Singh AK, Szczech L, Tang KL, et al. Correction of anemia with epoetin alfa in chronic kidney disease. N Engl J Med 2006;355(20):2085–98.

33. Drueke TB, Locatelli F, Clyne N, et al. Normalization of hemoglobin level in patients with chronic kidney disease and anemia. N Engl J Med 2006;355(20): 2071–84.

34. Bennett CL, Silver SM, Djulbegovic B, et al. Venous thromboembolism and mortality associated with recombinant erythropoietin and darbepoetin administration for the treatment of cancer-associated anemia. JAMA 2008;299(8):914–24.

35. Stowell CP, Jones SC, Enny C, et al. An open-label, randomized, parallel-group study of perioperative epoetin alfa versus standard of care for blood conservation in major elective spinal surgery: safety analysis. Spine (Phila Pa 1976) 2009; 34(23):2479–85.

36. Hartert H. Blutgerninnungstudien mit der thromboelastographic, einen neven untersuchingsver fahren. Klin Wochenschr 1948;26(37–38):577–83 [in German].

37. Ganter MT, Hofer CK. Coagulation monitoring: current techniques and clinical use of viscoelastic point-of-care coagulation devices. Anesth Analg 2008;106(5): 1366–75.

38. Coakley M, Reddy K, Mackie I, et al. Transfusion triggers in orthotopic liver transplantation: a comparison of the thromboelastometry analyzer, the thromboelastogram, and conventional coagulation tests. J Cardiothorac Vasc Anesth 2006; 20(4):548–53.

39. Lindahl TL, Ramstrom S. Methods for evaluation of platelet function. Transfus Apher Sci 2009;41(2):121–5.

40. Davenport R, Khan S. Management of major trauma haemorrhage: treatment priorities and controversies. Br J Haematol 2011;155(5):537–48.

41. Theusinger OM, Spahn DR, Ganter MT. Transfusion in trauma: why and how should we change our current practice? Curr Opin Anaesthesiol 2009;22(2): 305–12.

42. Ak K, Isbir CS, Tetik S, et al. Thromboelastography-based transfusion algorithm reduces blood product use after elective CABG: a prospective randomized study. J Card Surg 2009;24(4):404–10.

43. Nuttall GA, Cook DJ. Transcranial Doppler sonography and cerebral blood flow during cardiopulmonary bypass. Ann Thorac Surg 1997;64(3):891–2.

44. Oliver WC. Coagulation tests predict bleeding in the intensive care unit after cardiac surgery. In: Kroening BJ, editors. Transfusion S. 2010. p. 180A–1.

45. Nuttall GA, Oliver WC, Santrach PJ, et al. Efficacy of a simple intraoperative transfusion algorithm for nonerythrocyte component utilization after cardiopulmonary bypass. Anesthesiology 2001;94(5):773–81.

46. Cotton BA, Minei KM, Radwan ZA, et al. Admission rapid thrombelastography predicts development of pulmonary embolism in trauma patients. J Trauma Acute Care Surg 2012;72(6):1470–5.

47. Holcomb JB, Minei KM, Scerbo ML, et al. Admission rapid thrombelastography can replace conventional coagulation tests in the emergency department: experience with 1974 consecutive trauma patients. Ann Surg 2012;256(3):476–86.

48. Murphy GJ, Reeves BC, Rogers CA, et al. Increased mortality, postoperative morbidity, and cost after red blood cell transfusion in patients having cardiac surgery. Circulation 2007;116(22):2544–52.

49. Enriquez LJ, Shore-Lesserson L. Point-of-care coagulation testing and transfusion algorithms. Br J Anaesth 2009;103(Suppl 1):i14–22.

50. Ashworth A, Klein AA. Cell salvage as part of a blood conservation strategy in anaesthesia. Br J Anaesth 2010;105(4):401–16.

51. Carless PA, Henry DA, Moxey AJ, et al. Cell salvage for minimising perioperative allogeneic blood transfusion. Cochrane Database Syst Rev 2003;(4):CD001888.

52. Waters JR, Meier HH, Waters JH. An economic analysis of costs associated with development of a cell salvage program. Anesth Analg 2007;104(4):869–75.

Thoracic Endovascular Aortic Repair: Update on Indications and Guidelines

Georghios Nicolaou, MB, BCh, FRCPC, Mohamed Ismail, MB, BCh, MSc,
Davy Cheng, MD, MSc, FRCPC, FCAHS*

KEYWORDS

- Endovascular • Thoracic • Aortic • Aneurysm • Hybrid • Rupture • Dissection
- Anesthesia

KEY POINTS

- Thoracic endovascular aortic repair (TEVAR) was initially developed as a treatment for descending thoracic aortic aneurysms in patients deemed unfit for conventional open surgical repair.
- Since then, improvements in endograft design, delivery devices and technical innovations such as hybrid procedures and fenestrated and branched grafts, have allowed endovascular repair to be applied to other thoracic aortic pathologies.
- The dramatic expansion of TEVAR activity has necessitated a better definition for the indications, contraindications, and limitations of this new novel technology.

INTRODUCTION

In 1953, DeBakey and Cooley[1] performed the first successful resection of a fusiform aortic aneurysm with a synthetic graft replacement.[1,2] Since then, open surgical repair of the descending thoracic aorta with resection and graft interposition has become the gold standard in the treatment of descending thoracic aortic aneurysms (DTAAs).[2,3]

Despite significant medical advances, which have allowed operative mortality to decrease to as low as 2.9% in specialized centers, conventional open surgical repair (OSR) is generally associated with substantial morbidity and mortality in a patient population that is often aged and medically debilitated.[2–4] As a result, with the advent of endoluminal technology, thoracic endovascular aortic repair (TEVAR) has emerged as a less invasive treatment modality for patients considered to be unfit for OSR, with a reduction in both morbidity and mortality.

Department of Anesthesia and Perioperative Medicine, London Health Sciences Centre, Schulich School of Medicine & Dentistry, Western University, 339 Windermere Road, Room C3-172, London, Ontario, N6A 5A5, Canada
* Corresponding author.
E-mail address: davy.cheng@lhsc.on.ca

Anesthesiology Clin 31 (2013) 451–478
http://dx.doi.org/10.1016/j.anclin.2013.01.001
anesthesiology.theclinics.com
1932-2275/13/$ – see front matter © 2013 Elsevier Inc. All rights reserved.

AVAILABLE DEVICES

In 2005, the GORE TAG graft (W. L. Gore & Associates Inc, Flagstaff, AZ)[5] was approved by the US Food and Drug Administration (FDA) to treat DTAAs and subsequently, in 2008, the Zenith TX2 TAA Endovascular Graft (Cook Inc, Bloomington, IN)[6] and the Talent Thoracic Stent Graft System (Medtronic Vascular, Santa Rosa, CA)[7] were approved for the treatment of DTAAs and penetrating atherosclerotic aortic ulcers.[3] The Valiant Captivia Thoracic Stent Graft (Medtronic Inc, Minneapolis, MN) and the redesigned Conformable GORE TAG Device (Gore & Associates) have been recently approved (2012) by the FDA for the endovascular repair of isolated lesions (excluding dissections) of the descending segment of the thoracic aorta. This expanded indication includes the treatment of blunt traumatic thoracic aortic injuries. A fifth thoracic device, the Relay stent graft (Bolton Medical Inc, Sunrise, FL) has completed pivotal trial enrollment and awaits regulatory approval.

Hybrid procedures, improvements in endograft design and delivery devices, and fenestrated and branched grafts have allowed TEVAR to be applied to other thoracic aortic pathologies in an off-label manner. Examples include thoracoabdominal aortic aneurysm (TAAA), aortic arch aneurysm, aortic dissection, and ruptured DTAA.[3,8,9]

Fenestrated and branched endografts have been developed as a minimally invasive, totally endovascular alternative for the treatment of complex thoracic aortic aneurysms in high-risk patients. These devices are custom made to fit the specific anatomic requirements of each patient. Fenestrated grafts have openings (fenestrations) within the stent-graft fabric to accommodate visceral arteries. Branched grafts have separate smaller side-arm grafts sutured to the basic stent graft for deployment into an artery to preserve flow into it. Another approach places a self-expanding stent graft through the opening of a fenestrated graft.[8,9]

PREOPERATIVE IMAGING AND EVALUATION

Contrast-enhanced computed tomographic angiography (CTA) or magnetic resonance angiography (MRA) of the chest, abdomen, and pelvis with 3-dimensional (3D) reformatting is performed preoperatively.[3] Imaging can identify patients with aortic anatomy that either precludes the use of stent grafts, requires the use of custom fenestrated or branched stent grafts, or necessitates the use of staged and/or hybrid procedures.[2] Imaging is also used to determine the diameter and length of the endograft(s), and the most appropriate site for vascular access.

The following must be determined: (1) conformation of the aortic arch, (2) location of origins of great vessels relative to the proximal margin of the aneurysm, (3) tortuosity of the descending aorta along its entire length, (4) location of origins of mesenteric vessels relative to the distal margin of the aneurysm, (5) comparative diameters of proximal and distal landing zones, (6) tortuosity and diameter of the iliofemoral arteries, and (7) presence of abdominal aortic graft. In patients who may require coverage of the left subclavian artery, a CTA of the head and neck is obtained to establish the presence of a patent circle of Willis and a nondominant left vertebral artery.[2,3]

SURGICAL CONSIDERATIONS FOR SPECIFIC HYBRID PROCEDURES

A hybrid procedure is a combination of an open surgical approach and an endovascular stenting procedure that uses extra-anatomic bypass techniques to expand the "anatomic" suitability for deployment of stent grafts into zones 0, 1, and 2.[3,8,9] Hybrid procedures can be either staged or done concurrently.[8] Rerouting of supra-aortic branches by transposition or bypass enables endovascular treatment of the aortic arch and proximal descending aorta without the need for aortic cross-clamping, cardiopulmonary bypass (CPB), and/or hypothermic circulatory arrest.[3,8,9] Zones of proximal aortic endograft attachment sites are shown in **Fig. 1**.[3,10]

Left Subclavian Artery Coverage and Revascularization

A proximal landing zone that requires coverage of the left subclavian artery (LSCA) (eg, zones 0, 1, and 2) occurs in 35% to 41% of cases.[11] LSCA revascularization is accomplished by left common carotid artery to LSCA bypass (**Fig. 2**) or LSCA transposition.[12] However, the need for preoperative LSCA revascularization has been the subject of much debate. Some surgeons choose expectant management, with LSCA revascularization for postocclusion symptoms after TEVAR, whereas others advocate routine LSCA revascularization.[2,3,13,14] Others use selective LSCA revascularization before TEVAR, based on patient-specific anatomic considerations, particularly when there is a left dominant vertebral artery, a patent left internal mammary coronary artery bypass graft or an occluded right vertebral artery, and in patients considered at high risk for paraplegia.[2,3,11,13,14]

In an attempt to offer evidence-based guidelines for the management of patients requiring LSCA coverage, a meta-analysis and systematic review of the literature was conducted by the Society for Vascular Surgery (SVS), which discovered that the overall quality of evidence was very low.[13,14] The SVS issued 3 recommendations[14]:

1. In patients who need elective TEVAR whereby achievement of a proximal seal necessitates coverage of the LSCA, routine preoperative revascularization is recommended despite the very low-quality evidence (Grade 2, level of evidence C).

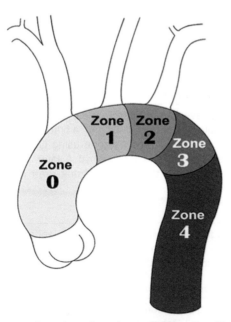

Fig. 1. The zones of proximal aortic endograft attachment sites. (*Adapted from* Criado F, Abul-Khoudoud O, Domer G, et al. Endovascular repair of the thoracic aorta: lessons learned. Ann Thorac Surg 2005;80:857–63; with permission.)

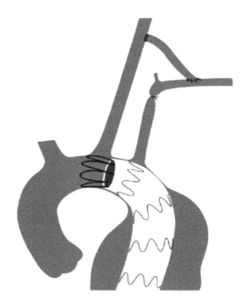

Fig. 2. Left common carotid to left subclavian artery (LSCA) bypass. The proximal LSCA has been ligated to prevent retrograde type II endoleak. (*From* Criado FJ, Barnatan MF, Rizk Y, et al. Technical strategies to expand stent-graft applicability in the aortic arch and proximal descending thoracic aorta. J Endovasc Ther 2002;(9 Suppl 2):II32–8; with permission.)

2. In selected patients who have an anatomy that compromises perfusion to critical organs, routine preoperative LSCA revascularization is strongly recommended despite the very low-quality evidence (Grade 1, level of evidence C).
3. In patients who need very urgent TEVAR for life-threatening acute aortic syndromes whereby achievement of a proximal seal necessitates coverage of the LSCA, revascularization should be individualized and addressed expectantly based on anatomy, urgency, and availability of surgical expertise (Grade 2, level of evidence C).

Hybrid Elephant-Trunk Procedure

In patients who have transverse aortic arch aneurysms with no adequate proximal landing zone but an adequate distal landing zone, a first-stage total arch replacement is performed to create a proximal landing zone using CPB and deep hypothermic circulatory arrest. This procedure is followed at a later setting with the second-stage endovascular repair using the elephant-trunk graft as the proximal landing zone.[8]

Frozen Elephant-Trunk Technique

This technique is a single-stage procedure with conventional surgical repair of the ascending aorta and the aortic arch combined with open antegrade stent grafting of the descending aorta, during circulatory arrest.[9]

Aortic Visceral Debranching Procedures

Aortic visceral debranching procedures allow for endovascular stenting of TAAAs that involve the visceral arteries.[8] Debranching procedures or extra-anatomic bypasses can revascularize the visceral and renal arteries from the iliac arteries in a retrograde fashion or from the descending thoracic aorta above the aneurysm being treated.

Such a procedure is followed by stent grafting of the aneurysm either at the same setting as the debranching procedure or as a first part of a "staged" procedure. A 2-stage procedure is associated with a decreased incidence of spinal cord ischemia (SCI) and renal dysfunction.[15,16] The reason for the decreased incidence of SCI is that a 2-stage procedure avoids extensive segmental artery sacrifice, as occurs in a single-stage procedure.[15]

INDICATIONS AND POTENTIAL USES FOR TEVAR IN THORACIC AORTIC DISEASE
Descending Thoracic Aortic Aneurysms

The incidence of thoracic aortic aneurysms (TAAs) is 10.4 per 100,000 person-years.[2] Aneurysms of the descending thoracic aorta account for approximately 30% to 40% of all TAAs, and their prevalence has tripled over the last 2 decades.[17,18] The disease process is virulent but indolent because it typically grows slowly at an approximate rate of 0.19 cm/y.[18] The annual risk of rupture, dissection, or death is 14.1% in patients with aneurysms larger than 6 cm, compared with 6.5% for aneurysms between 5 and 6 cm.[2] The 5-year survival rate for patients with TAAs treated nonsurgically is 13% to 19.2%, and 60% to 79% for those treated surgically.[17–20]

Open repair
Contemporary results of open repairs of elective DTAAs indicate early mortality rates of 4.8%, paraplegia rates of 3.4%, stroke rates of 2.7%, respiratory failure rates of 9.2%, and renal failure rates of 2.9%. Three-, 5-, and 10-year survival estimates are 72%, 63%, and 38%, respectively.[20]

Endovascular repair
The current guidelines from the Society of Thoracic Surgeons (STS) suggest TEVAR for DTAAs when the aortic diameter is greater than 5.5 cm (Class IIa recommendation, level of evidence B, when the patient has significant comorbidity; Class IIb recommendation, level of evidence C, when the patient has no significant comorbidity).[20] When the aortic diameter is less than 5.5 cm, the STS guidelines advise against TEVAR (Class III recommendation, level of evidence C).[20] The current American College of Cardiology/American Heart Association (ACC/AHA) guidelines suggest TEVAR for DTAAs larger than 5.5 cm, when technically feasible (ACC/AHA Class I recommendation, level of evidence B).[17]

A prospective, nonrandomized, multicenter trial compared 140 patients who underwent endograft exclusion with 94 historical or concurrent patients who underwent open repair. Of the 140 patients, 137 had successful implantation of the endograft. Patients who underwent TEVAR had a significant reduction in perioperative mortality (2.1% vs 11.7%), respiratory failure (4% vs 20%), renal insufficiency (1% vs 13%), SCI (3% vs 14%), mean length of stay in the intensive care unit (2.6 $\pm$ 14.6 vs 5.2 $\pm$ 7.2 days), and overall hospital stay (7.4 $\pm$ 17.7 vs 14.4 $\pm$ 12.8 days). No significant difference was observed in the rate of stroke between the 2 groups (3.6% for the TEVAR group and 4.3% for the open repair group). However, after 2 years of follow-up, there was a 9% incidence of endoleaks and 3 reinterventions associated with TEVAR versus OSR. There was no difference in overall mortality between the 2 groups, at 2 years. At 5 years, the 2 groups differed in their aneurysm-related mortality rates (2.8% for TEVAR and 11.7% for open repair) but not in their rates of all-cause mortality (32% and 33%, respectively).[21,22]

Summary
TEVAR (**Fig. 3**) is less invasive and is associated with a decrease in perioperative morbidity and mortality when compared with OSR. Lifelong surveillance remains

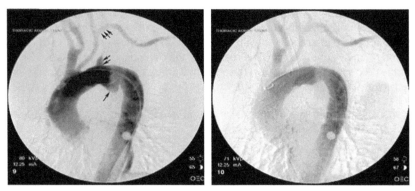

Fig. 3. Aortic angiograms. (*Left*) A prerepair angiogram after LSCA to carotid transfer. Shown are aneurysm (*single arrow*), LSCA stump (*double arrow*), and LSCA to carotid transfer (*triple arrow*). (*Right*) Postrepair angiography. (*From* Gutsche JT, Szeto W, Cheung AI. Endovascular stenting of thoracic aortic aneurysm. Anesthesiol Clin 2008;26:481–99.)

mandatory. However, although OSR is more invasive, it is definitive, with well-defined long-term follow-up in comparison with TEVAR.

Ruptured Descending Thoracic Aneurysms

The incidence of ruptured DTAAs (rDTAAs) is 3.5 per 100,000 person-years, and is the cause of death in 51% of patients with degenerative aneurysms. Mortality from ruptured aneurysms approaches 100% without treatment, with almost 60% of patients dying in the prehospital environment.[2] Recently, TEVAR has been shown to be an alternative to open repair of rDTAAs.

Jonker and colleagues[23] published a meta-analysis comparing the outcomes of TEVAR and open repair in patients with rDTAAs. One hundred forty-three (64%) were treated with TEVAR and 81 (36%) with open repair. Mean age was 70 ± 5.6 years. The 30-day mortality was 19% for patients treated with TEVAR for rDTAAs compared with 33% for patients treated with open repair ($P = .016$). The 30-day occurrence rates of myocardial infarction (11.1% vs 3.5%; $P<.05$), stroke (10.2% vs 4.1%; $P = .117$), and paraplegia (5.5% vs 3.1%; $P = .405$) were increased after open repair in comparison with TEVAR. However, long-term follow-up revealed 5 aneurysm-related deaths in the TEVAR group after 30 days (median follow-up of 17 ± 10 months), whereas no patients died of aneurysm-related causes in the open group after the same period. The estimated aneurysm-related survival at 3 years after TEVAR was 70.6%.[22,23]

Summary

Endovascular repair of rDTAAs is associated with a lower 30-day mortality rate and a lower risk of death, myocardial infarction, stroke, and paraplegia when compared with OSR, and it appears to be the treatment of choice in anatomically suitable patients with a rDTAA.

Blunt Traumatic Thoracic Aortic Injury

Thoracic aortic injury is the second most common cause of death after blunt trauma among patients with major traumatic injuries. It typically occurs with high-speed, deceleration-type injuries, and 80% to 90% of victims die at the scene of the accident. Without surgical intervention, 30% to 50% of initial survivors will die within the first

24 hours. The majority of blunt traumatic thoracic aortic injuries (BTTAIs) occur at the aortic isthmus (80%–90%) just distal to the LSCA.[24]

Traditional open repair has been associated with an average mortality rate of 18% to 28% and a paraplegia rate of 2.3% to 14%.[18] Recently, several meta-analyses have shown improved outcomes with TEVAR when compared with open repair for BTTAI. The aortic injury is classified into 4 grades: grade 1 (intimal injury), grade 2 (intramural hematoma), grade 3 (pseudoaneurysm), and grade 4 (aortic rupture). Intervention is needed for grades 2 to 4, whereas conservative treatment (blood pressure control and follow-up imaging) is reserved for grade 1.[25]

A meta-analysis conducted by Tang and colleagues[26] analyzed 699 procedures (TEVAR 370; open repair 329). These investigators found lower rates of mortality (7.6% vs 15.2%; $P = .0076$), paraplegia (0% vs 5.6%; $P<.0001$), and stroke (0.85% vs 5.3%; $P = .0028$) in patients who underwent TEVAR rather than open repair.[26]

The SVS conducted a meta-analysis and systemic review that included 7768 patients from 139 studies with BTTAIs. Mortality was lower in TEVAR versus open and nonoperative treatments (9%, 19%, and 46%, respectively; $P<.01$). The risk for SCI was higher with open repair compared with TEVAR and nonoperative management (9%, 3%, and 3%, respectively; $P = .01$). The risk for end-stage renal disease (ESRD) was highest in open repair when compared with TEVAR and nonoperative treatment (8%, 5%, and 3%, respectively; $P = .01$). At a median 2-year follow-up, there was a trend toward increased risk of a secondary procedure in endovascular repair versus open repair ($P = .07$).[27]

Summary
Endovascular repair of BTTAI is the preferred treatment of choice in anatomically suitable patients (STS Class I recommendation, level of evidence B).[20] However, as the trauma population tends to be younger, there is a concern for graft migration as aortic remodeling occurs with age and growth. Therefore, adherence to a long-term follow-up protocol is imperative.

Acute Aortic Syndrome

Acute aortic syndrome (AAS) refers to a heterogeneous group of conditions that cause a common set of signs and symptoms, the commonest being aortic pain. AAS includes intramural hematoma (IMH), penetrating atherosclerotic aortic ulcer (PAU), and aortic dissection (AD) (**Fig. 4**).[28]

The Stanford system of classification for AD is applied to IMH and PAU. Stanford type A pathologies involve the ascending aorta and aortic arch, with or without

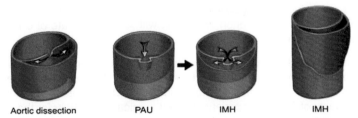

Fig. 4. Aortic dissection (*left*), penetrating atherosclerotic ulcer (PAU) (*middle*), and intramural hematoma (IMH) (*right*), all causing acute aortic syndrome. (*From* Coady MA, Rizzo JA, Elefteriades JA. Pathologic variants of thoracic aortic dissections: penetrating atherosclerotic ulcers and intramural hematomas. Cardiol Clin 1999;17:640.)

descending aortic involvement. Stanford type B pathologies are confined to the descending aorta, distal to the origin of the LSCA.[29]

Regarding initial medical therapy for AAS, the goal is to stabilize the patient, control pain with opiates, lower heart rate (HR) and blood pressure (BP), and reduce the rate of increase or force (dP/dt) of left ventricular ejection.[28] First-line therapy is intravenous β-blockade. A HR of 60 beats/min or lower and a systolic blood pressure of 100 to 120 mm Hg, or the lowest appropriate level for adequate vital-organ perfusion, is recommended (ACC/AHA Class I recommendation, level of evidence C).[17,28,29] In the presence of acute aortic regurgitation, β-blockers should be used with caution because they block compensatory tachycardia (ACC/AHA Class I recommendation, level of evidence C).[17] Labetalol, with both α- and β-blockade, lowers both BP and dP/dt.[28,29] In patients who are β-blocker intolerant, calcium-channel blockers can be used (ACC/AHA Class I recommendation, level of evidence C).[17] If β-blockers alone do not control BP, vasodilators are added (ACC/AHA Class I recommendation, level of evidence C).[17] Vasodilator therapy should not be initiated before HR control, to avoid the associated reflex tachycardia that might aggravate the AD (ACC/AHA Class III recommendation, level of evidence C).[17]

Aortic dissection

The annual incidence of acute aortic dissection (AAD) is 5 to 30 cases per million people,[18] accounting for 80% to 90% of all cases of AAS. The most common risk condition is hypertension (72%).[28]

Type A aortic dissection The mortality rate of untreated acute type A dissection (T_AAD) is 1% to 2% per hour after symptom onset.[28] Without surgery, mortality exceeds 50% at 1 month.[28] At present, urgent surgical repair is the treatment of choice for T_AADs (ACC/AHA Class I recommendation, level of evidence B).[17] Patients with T_AADs in the International Registry of Aortic Dissection (IRAD) database had an overall in-hospital mortality of 27% for patients treated surgically and 56% for those treated medically.[29]

Recently, endovascular techniques have been added as adjuncts to the surgical management of T_AADs. For dissections extending into the descending thoracic aorta, placement of a stent graft into the unrepaired descending aorta can reduce the complications related to the residual dissected vessel. Some surgeons advocate endovascular treatment of T_AADs that extend in a retrograde fashion from a dissection originating in the descending thoracic aorta by covering the tear on the primary entry site. Others propose endovascular treatment of malperfusion states in patients with T_AADs before operative repair of the ascending aorta.[29]

Ye and colleagues[30] reported on a series of 45 patients with Stanford type A dissection, treated with TEVAR. The entry tear was located at the ascending aorta in 10 cases, the aortic arch in 14 cases, and the distal aortic arch or proximal descending aorta in 21 cases where the ascending aorta was also involved by the dissection. The surgical success rate of the cohort was 98%, with a mortality rate of 6.7%. Type I endoleaks occurred in 10 cases.[30]

Uncomplicated type B aortic dissection Uncomplicated type B aortic dissections (T_BADs) are best treated with medical therapy (ACC/AHA Class I recommendation, level of evidence C).[17] Patients with T_BADs in the IRAD database had an overall in-hospital mortality of 29.3% for patients treated surgically and 10% for those treated medically.[29] Medical therapy alone does not stop blood flow to the false lumen and, consequently, 20% to 50% of patients who survive the acute phase develop dilatation of the false lumen at 4 years, requiring intervention.[17,18] As a result, medical therapy alone is associated with a mortality rate of 50% at 5 years.[18]

The INSTEAD (Investigation of Stent Grafts in Aortic Dissection) trial[31] was designed to answer the question of whether TEVAR in patients with chronic uncomplicated T$_B$ADs could reduce late aortic related morbidity and mortality. The investigators examined 140 patients with stable, uncomplicated chronic T$_B$ADs, all of whom were randomized to optimal medical therapy versus optimal medical therapy plus TEVAR of the proximal aortic tear. Patients treated with optimal medical therapy had overall and aortic-related death rates of 4.4% and 2.9%, respectively, whereas the rates in the TEVAR group were 11.1% and 5.6%. At 2 years there was no significant difference in all-cause mortality. Significant aortic remodeling was noted in the TEVAR group, with 91% complete thrombosis at 2 years compared with 19% in the optimal medical therapy group (P<.001).[29,31] This result is significant, as false-lumen thrombosis and true-lumen expansion may prevent late aneurysm formation.[29]

Although TEVAR failed to improve late outcomes compared with medical therapy in uncomplicated chronic T$_B$ADs, results may differ in acute uncomplicated T$_B$ADs. Stent grafting might be more effective in the acute setting before septal fibrosis of the dissecting membrane occurs, which can limit aortic remodeling.[29] More definitive data on the role of TEVAR for acute uncomplicated T$_B$ADs will be forthcoming as results from the ADSORB (European Study of Medical Management vs TAG Device and Medical Management for Acute Uncomplicated Type B Dissection) trial become available.[29,32]

Summary Medical therapy remains the gold standard in uncomplicated T$_B$ADs. However, a recent study showed that patients with uncomplicated T$_B$ADs with false-lumen diameters of greater than 22 mm had a significantly higher risk for aneurysmal formation; this may represent a subset of patients with uncomplicated T$_B$ADs for whom early endovascular management may be appropriate.[29]

Complicated type B aortic dissection Approximately 30% of acute T$_B$ADs are complicated at initial presentation, and 1 in 5 of uncomplicated T$_B$ADs will become complicated, requiring open surgical repair (ACC/AHA Class I recommendation, level of evidence B)[17] or endovascular repair.[33] The goal of intervention is to obliterate the entry tear and achieve end-organ perfusion. Patients presenting with rupture or impending rupture, end-organ malperfusion, limb ischemia, unrelenting pain, and uncontrollable hypertension are designated as having a complicated T$_B$AD.[28,29] The recent IRAD database demonstrated that surgical repair for acute T$_B$AD is associated with a significant risk of cerebrovascular accident (9.0%), paraplegia (4.5%), visceral ischemia/infarction (6.8%), and acute renal failure (18.3%), all of which correlated with postoperative death.[34] The overall in-hospital mortality was 29.3%, and for patients whose procedures were within 48 hours the in-hospital mortality was 39.2%.[34] For patients presenting with malperfusion and rupture, the in-hospital mortality was 27.8% and 62.5%, respectively.[34] The following endovascular techniques are used to repair complicated T$_B$ADs:

Aortic fenestration The goal of endovascular aortic fenestration is to treat malperfusion syndromes by equalization of pressures between the true and false lumens, relieving the dynamic aortic component of obstruction caused by the dissection. Branch-vessel stenting is then used to treat the static obstruction of branch vessels caused by the dissection. However, by preserving flow through the false lumen, aortic fenestration does not address complications such as aneurysm formation and late rupture. Analysis of complicated T$_B$ADs from the IRAD database reveals that malperfusion states were relieved in 9 of 18 patients treated with endovascular fenestration and in 16 of 17 patients treated with stent grafts.[29] Therefore, endograft therapy should be used if a suitable entry tear is present, and fenestration should be reserved for cases whereby malperfusion is present and there is no entry tear amenable to endograft treatment.[29]

Endovascular repair (STS Class I recommendation, level of evidence A) The rationale behind endovascular therapy (**Fig. 5**)[3] is that covering the area of the primary intimal tear with a stent graft promotes false-lumen thrombosis and subsequent aortic remodeling by eliminating antegrade (or occasionally retrograde) flow into the false lumen.[20] In general, stent grafts deployed for the treatment of ADs should extend 20 to 40 mm beyond the primary intimal tear site in both the proximal and distal directions.[29]

In a systematic review, Parker and Golledge[35] reported the findings of multiple centers, over 10 years, of 942 patients who underwent TEVAR for acute T$_B$AD with complications. Procedural success was achieved in 95% of all cases, with emergency conversion being required in 0.6% of patients. Overall in-hospital mortality was 9.1%, with an early complication rate of 8.1% (stroke 3.1%; paraplegia 1.9%; conversion to type A dissection 2%; bowel infarction 0.9%; and major amputation 0.2%). After an average follow-up of 20 months, reintervention was required in 10.4% of patients, with aortic rupture in 0.8% of the cases. Average overall survival was 88% at 20 months.[22,35] Results from IRAD comparing stent grafting with open surgery for treating complicated acute T$_B$ADs showed a decrease in in-hospital mortality (33.9% vs 10.6%) and neurologic/ischemic composite morbidity (20.8% vs 40.0%).[29,33]

A recent review of the Nationwide Inpatient Sample identified 5000 patients who underwent repair of T$_B$ADs (3619 open vs 1381 TEVAR) and found that the TEVAR group had a lower 30-day mortality (10.6% vs 19% for open repair).[36] However, a recent IRAD review demonstrated no difference in 3-year survival in patients with

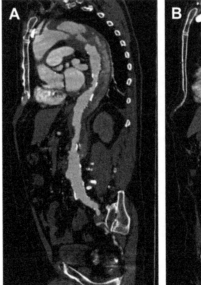
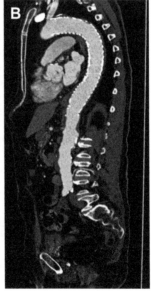

Fig. 5. (*A*) Multiplanar reconstruction of a patient with acute type B aortic dissection. (*B*) Multiplanar reconstruction of the same patient 6 months after successful endovascular repair. (*From* Adams JD, Garcia LM, Kern JA. Endovascular repair of the thoracic aorta. Surg Clin North Am 2009;89:895–912.)

acute T_BADs managed medically (77.6%), surgically (82.8%), or with endovascular therapy (76.2%).[37] These data emphasize the importance of follow-up regardless of the mode of therapy.

Summary Endovascular repair of acute complicated T_BAD is associated with low morbidity and mortality, and has emerged as the treatment modality of choice.

Intramural hematoma

IMH, a precursor of AD, is caused by primary rupture of the vasa vasorum in the aortic medial wall, leading to a concentric hematoma within the media. It has no intimal flap or false lumen. IMH is associated with hypertension, and 70.6% of cases are located in the descending thoracic aorta.[18] On diagnostic imaging IMH appears as a smooth, crescentic, or circular thickening greater than 5 to 7 mm in size. Acute IMH accounts for 5% to 20% of all cases of AAS, with regression in 10%, progression to classic AD in 28% to 47%, and a risk of rupture in 20% to 45%. Long-term surveillance is therefore necessary.[28,29]

A meta-analysis of 143 patients found that patients with lesions of the ascending aorta had a lower mortality with surgery than with medical treatment (14% vs 36%). Patients with lesions of the descending aorta had a similar mortality with medical or surgical therapy (14% vs 20%).[28] As a result, IMH is treated similarly to AD in the corresponding segment of the aorta (ACC/AHA Class IIa recommendation, level of evidence C).[17] The following is recommended[28,29]:

- For patients with type A IMH, open surgery is recommended.
- For patients with uncomplicated type B IMH, best medical treatment and close surveillance is recommended.
- For patients with complicated type B IMH (aneurysmal degeneration of the aorta, aortic diameter greater than 50 mm, persistent pain or hypertension, organ/limb ischemia, hematoma thickness greater than 11 mm, or pleural/pericardial fluid), best medical therapy and TEVAR is recommended (STS Class IIa recommendation, level of evidence C).[20]

Penetrating atherosclerotic aortic ulcer

PAUs are present in 2.3% to 11% of patients with AAS, and two-thirds of cases occur in the descending thoracic aorta. PAU is a condition whereby an atherosclerotic aortic plaque penetrates the internal elastic lamina into the aortic media. It is associated with a type B IMH in 80% of cases. Patients with PAUs are typically older and hypertensive with multiple medical comorbidities. PAU may lead to pseudoaneurysm formation, AD, and aortic rupture.[28,29]

At present, there is no generally accepted therapeutic regimen for PAUs. In general, patients with type A PAUs are treated with surgical resection. Stable patients with type B PAUs may be managed medically, with strict follow-up and serial imaging. Criteria for endograft placement in the acute setting include pain and rupture; in chronic cases, indications include recurrent pain, aortic diameter greater than 55 mm, and increase in size greater than 10 mm per year[29,38] (STS Class IIa recommendation, level of evidence C).[20] Most PAUs are isolated and localized in a relatively normal-sized aorta, which makes them ideal targets for endovascular exclusion. However, patients with PAUs have severe, diffuse atherosclerotic disease, which puts them at an increased risk of atheroembolic complications. Therefore, minimal manipulation of the guide wire and delivery system in the thoracic aorta is imperative.[28]

In 2009, Eggebrecht and colleagues[39] summarized data regarding the success of endografting in the treatment of PAU, reporting high overall technical success rates

(98%) and low rates of in-hospital mortality (7%), neurologic complications (4%), and secondary (5%) and subsequent (2%) aorta-related mortality.

Thoracoabdominal Aortic Aneurysms

Approximately 10% of TAAs occur in the thoracoabdominal aorta. The 5-year survival rate of patients with TAAAs treated nonsurgically is 19% and for those treated surgically, 73.5%.[40] Therefore, an interventional treatment option is mandatory for these patients.

Open surgical repair

Coselli and colleagues[41] reported their experience with OSR of 2286 TAAAs. The 30-day survival rate was 95.0%. Renal failure requiring hemodialysis occurred in 129 patients (5.6%), paraplegia or paraparesis developed in 87 patients (3.8%), pulmonary complications occurred in 734 patients (32.1%), and cardiac events occurred in 181 patients (7.9%). Bleeding requiring a return to the operating room occurred after 57 TAAA repairs (2.5%). Patients who underwent replacement of the entire thoracoabdominal aorta (extent II) had the highest rates of death (6.0%), spinal cord deficit (6.3%), and renal failure (8.3%). Current management strategies enable patients to undergo conventional open TAAA repair with excellent early survival and acceptable morbidity.[41]

Hybrid procedure

Moulakakis and colleagues[42] performed a meta-analysis to assess the safety and efficacy of a hybrid technique in 507 patients with TAAAs or other aortic abnormalities. The pooled estimates for primary technical success and visceral graft patency were 96.2% and 96.5%, respectively. A pooled rate of 7.5% for overall SCI symptoms was observed, whereas for irreversible paraplegia the pooled rate was 4.5%. The pooled estimate for renal failure was 8.8%. The pooled 30-day in-hospital mortality rate was 12.8%. During the mean follow-up period of 34.5 months, a total of 119 endoleaks were identified in 111 patients (22.7%).[42]

The complications typical of TAAA open surgery have not been eliminated by TAAA hybrid repair. Morbidity and mortality rates remain substantial, and TAAA hybrid repair should only be considered in patients who are unsuited for conventional OSR.

Endovascular repair of TAAA

Endovascular repair of TAAA (STS Class IIb recommendation, level of evidence C) is considered when the patient has significant comorbidity.[20] A retrospective review by Bakoyiannis and colleagues[43] reported on outcomes of 155 patients who underwent fenestrated and branched endograft insertion for TAAAs. Technical success was achieved in 94.2% of patients. Twenty-three (18.4%) primary endoleaks were reported. All 26 secondary interventions were elective, most occurring within the first month. The 30-day mortality was 7.1% while the 1-year survival rate was 82.6%. Three (1.9%) patients developed permanent paraplegia and 2 (1.3%) developed permanent paraparesis; renal failure was reported in 9 (5.8%). Overall follow-up mortality was 16.1%.[43]

Fig. 6[44] illustrates a reinforced fenestration, and the implantation of a stent graft with branches to the visceral arteries is shown in **Fig. 7**.[45]

Endovascular repair of TAAAs is technically feasible and shows great promise in patients considered at high risk for open surgery. However, mortality and SCI is still considerable with this technique.

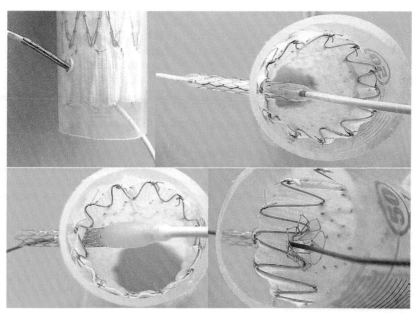

Fig. 6. A fenestration placed in the distal end of a thoracic device. There upper left photo shows a balloon-expandable stent placed through the fenestration, inflated to a diameter matching the target vessel (*upper right*). A larger balloon is then placed into the aortic portion of the stent and used to flare the stent against the aortic graft wall (*lower panels*). (*From* Greenberg R, Eagleton M, Mastracci T. Branched endografts for thoracoabdominal aneurysms. J Thorac Cardiovasc Surg 2010;140(Suppl 6):S171–8; with permission.)

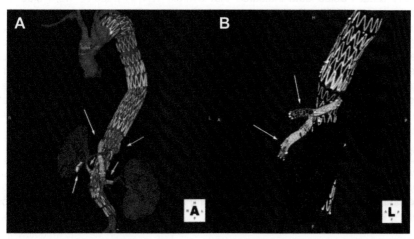

Fig. 7. (*A, B*) Anterior and lateral views of a 3-dimensional reconstruction of a type II thoracoabdominal aortic aneurysm treated with a branched endovascular graft. The celiac and superior mesenteric branches (*white arrows*) are attached to the aortic graft as a side arm and oriented in the direction of the mesenteric vessel. The patient had 2 right renal arteries. The lowest was embolized with coils (*yellow arrow*). The upper right and left renal arteries were incorporated into the repair with reinforced fenestrations (*green arrows*) mated with stent grafts. (*From* Greenberg RK, Lu Q, Roselli EE, et al. Contemporary analysis of descending thoracic and thoracoabdominal aneurysm repair: a comparison of endovascular and open techniques. Circulation 2008;118:808–17; with permission.)

Aortic Arch Aneurysms

OSR of aortic arch aneurysms is associated with a 5% to 7% risk of death and a 2% to 5% risk of stroke.[46] Recently, hybrid procedures have been used to treat complex aortic arch aneurysms in high-risk patients who are not suitable for open surgical repair. In patients with aortic arch aneurysms with severe comorbidities, recent guidelines support an endovascular repair technique (STS Class IIb recommendation, level of evidence C),[20] and for patients who have reasonable surgical risk, the recent guidelines advise against an endovascular repair technique (STS Class III recommendation; level of evidence A).[20]

A systematic review of arch hybrid outcomes in 195 patients showed pooled perioperative mortality and morbidity rates of 9% and 21%, respectively. The most common perioperative complication was stroke (7%). The overall technical success rate was 86%, and the most common reason for technical failure was endoleak (9%). Four aneurysm-related deaths were reported during follow-up (2%).[47]

Summary

Aortic arch hybrid repair is a feasible alternative treatment in patients who are unfit for OSR. Patients with extensive atheromatous involvement of the aortic arch have a high risk of atheroembolization caused by wire and device manipulation, and are not suitable for this technique. Long-term follow-up is necessary to evaluate the efficacy and safety of these new devices.[47]

Summary of Indications and Outcomes for TEVAR in Thoracic Aortic Disease

The most recent large meta-analysis, by Cheng and colleagues,[48] examined TEVAR versus open repair for descending thoracic aortic disease. This analysis included 5888 patients from 42 articles, 38 of which were comparative studies and 4 from registry data. Pooled data indicated that overall, TEVAR patients were older and had more comorbidities than the open surgical patients. There was a significant reduction for TEVAR in comparison with open repair for all-cause mortality at 30 days, paraplegia or paraparesis, transfusions, reoperation for bleeding, renal dysfunction, pneumonia, and cardiac, neurologic, respiratory, and overall complications. There was a decrease in length of hospital stay (−7 days), length of stay in the intensive care unit (−4 days), and procedure time (−142 min) for TEVAR versus open repair. This meta-analysis is consistent with current literature and serves to further validate the aforementioned data. The findings of this study and the indications for TEVAR are summarized in **Tables 1** and **2**.

Contraindications for TEVAR

TEVAR is not recommended in patients with connective tissue disease except as a bail-out procedure or bridge to definitive open surgical therapy, or as a procedure following prior aortic repair when both landing zones lie within previously sited prosthetic grafts.[9]

ANESTHETIC MANAGEMENT
Preanesthetic Evaluation and Preparation

Patients presenting for TEVAR are typically elderly with significant medical comorbidities that can influence operative risk. Published data indicate a high incidence of hypertension (59.1%), coronary artery disease (27.0%), pulmonary disease (20.9%), renal disease (13.6%), and congestive heart failure (11.2%).[2,49] Preoperative evaluation of these comorbidities will identify patients at high risk for complications and allow alterations in perioperative management. Although TEVAR is associated with fewer

Table 1
Outcomes of TEVAR versus open surgical repair for descending thoracic aortic disease

	TEVAR (%)	Open Surgery (%)	I^2, %	OR (95% CI)	P Value
Death, 30-d	5.8	13.9	0	0.44 (0.33–0.59)	<.00001
Death, 1-y	16.0	21.9	0	0.73 (0.53–1.02)	.07
Death, 2- to 3-y	23.0	24.8	0	0.92 (0.63–1.33)	.65
Permanent paraplegia	1.4	4.9	0	0.30 (0.14–0.62)	.001
Stroke	5.0	6.2	23	0.75 (0.50–1.13)	.17
Acute myocardial infarction	2.3	6.3	20	0.81 (0.43–1.53)	.51
Renal dysfunction	5.9	15.7	0	0.40 (0.25–0.63)	<.001
Reoperation for bleeding	0.01	6.5	0	0.26 (0.11–0.62)	.002
Transfused patients	3.9	83.7	23	0.01(0.002–0.04)	<.0001
Reintervention	8.1	9.1	0%	1.01 (0.64–1.60)	.95
Pneumonia	15.9	28.7	44	0.14 (0.23–0.71)	.002
Vascular complications	13.0	21.9	83	0.58 (0.19–1.76)	.34
Overall complications	41.4	69.3	63	0.19 (0.10–0.36)	<.0001

I^2 = percent heterogeneity across trials that cannot be explained by chance variation alone. I^2 >50% indicates high heterogeneity.
Abbreviations: CI, confidence interval; OR, odds ratio.
Data from Cheng D, Martin J, Shennib H, et al. Endovascular aortic repair versus open surgical repair for descending thoracic aortic disease a systematic review and meta-analysis of comparative studies. J Am Coll Cardiol 2010;55:986–1001.

fluid shifts, absence of aortic cross-clamping, and a smaller surgical incision, it is still considered high-risk surgery, based on a perioperative risk of major adverse cardiac events of greater than 5%. At present there is no TEVAR-specific risk stratification tool available. Patients should undergo functional testing, when indicated, based on the ACC/AHA guidelines, for preoperative evaluation of patients undergoing noncardiac surgery.[8,9,50]

Specific Anesthetic Considerations Related to TEVAR

Potential for open conversion
Operative procedures involving endovascular repair of the thoracic aorta have the potential for catastrophic bleeding and cardiovascular collapse.[19,51]

Peripheral vascular disease
Patients who have peripheral vascular disease are at risk for access-site complications such as vascular injury and bleeding. The caliber, degree of atherosclerotic disease, and tortuosity should be preoperatively assessed using CTA or MRA. After TEVAR they should also be assessed for vascular insufficiency.[3,19,51]

Adjunctive procedures
Debranching procedures and retroperitoneal dissections to create surgical conduits (iliac artery or aortic) for vascular access are associated with greater blood loss, longer procedure times, and a longer length of stay in hospital than TEVAR with standard femoral access.[51]

Acute kidney injury following TEVAR
Acute kidney injury (AKI) following TEVAR is multifactorial and can occur as a result of (1) hypoperfusion, (2) mechanical encroachment of the stent graft on the renal vessels,

Table 2
Society of Thoracic Surgeons summary of recommendation classifications and level of evidence for TEVAR

Entity/Subgroup	Classification	Level of Evidence
Penetrating Ulcer/Intramural Hematoma		
Asymptomatic	III	C
Symptomatic	IIa	C
Chronic traumatic	IIa	C
Acute Traumatic Aortic Transection	I	B
Acute Type B Dissection		
Ischemia	I	A
No ischemia	IIb	C
Subacute Dissection	IIb	B
Chronic Dissection	IIb	B
Degenerative descending		
>5.5 cm, comorbidity	IIa	B
>5.5 cm, no comorbidity	IIb	C
<5.5 cm	III	C
Arch		
Reasonable open risk	III	A
Severe comorbidity	IIb	C
Thoracoabdominal/Severe comorbidity	IIb	C

Data from Svensson LG, Kouchoukos NT, Miller DC, et al. Expert consensus document on the treatment of descending thoracic aortic disease using endovascular stent-grafts. Ann Thorac Surg 2008;85(Suppl 1):S1–41.

(3) emboli to the renal arteries, and (4) radiographic contrast-induced nephropathy (CIN). Preexisting renal insufficiency is the most important and predictive risk factor for developing CIN.[8,52]

Strategies to reduce the incidence of AKI following TEVAR
- Maintain a normal cardiac index, a normal mean arterial blood pressure (MAP), and normovolemia.[8,52]
- Use iso-osmolar, nonionic contrast dye and limit contrast dye exposure: a ratio of contrast medium volume to CrCl (creatinine clearance) of greater than 3.7 is associated with increased risk of CIN.
- Substitute intravascular ultrasonography for angiography or use CO_2 angiography.
- Avoid nephrotoxins; stop metformin 48 hours before contrast dye administration, as it can cause lactic acidosis.
- Intravenous bicarbonate: Administer a 3 mL/kg bolus of isotonic bicarbonate, a minimum of 1 hour before the procedure, and continue at a rate of 1 mL/kg per hour for 6 hours after the procedure.
- Acetylcysteine: Administer 1200 mg orally twice daily on the day before, the day of, and the day after the procedure.

Stroke
The incidence of stroke after TEVAR is between 2% and 8%.[11,53] Patients who have had a prior transient ischemic attack (TIA) or stroke are at a higher risk for perioperative

stroke, and should have a computed tomography (CT) or transesophageal echocardiography (TEE) evaluation to grade the severity and mobility of the aortic atheroma.[19] Strokes are related to the severity, mobility, and instrumentation of the vulnerable atherosclerotic plaque within the aorta.[3] In a retrospective study of 530 patients, Ullery and colleagues[53] assessed the vascular distribution of stroke after TEVAR and its relationship to perioperative death and neurologic outcome. Stroke complicated 3.8% of the TEVAR procedures, with 60% involving the posterior circulation and 40% the anterior circulation. Patients who sustained a perioperative stroke had increased in-hospital mortality when compared with those patients whom did not suffer a stroke (20% vs 5.7%).[53] Risk factors for stroke include: (1) history of prior stroke or TIA, (2) chronic renal failure, (3) CT grade IV atheroma (>5 mm) in the aortic arch or proximal descending aorta, (4) wire or catheter instrumentation within the aortic arch or proximal descending aorta in patients who have vulnerable atheroma, (5) coverage of zones 0 to 2, and (6) PAU.[19,53]

Spinal cord ischemia

The most devastating complication of TEVAR is SCI leading to infarction.

Neurologic deficits secondary to TEVAR tend to involve the lower trunk and lower extremities, may lateralize, and range from paraparesis to paraplegia.[2] SCI may be temporary, permanent, immediate, or delayed, and is associated with increased morbidity and mortality.[54] In a recent study, Conrad and colleagues[55] showed that the 5-year survival for patients with SCI was lower than that in patients with no SCI (25% vs 51%, $P<.001$).

In functional terms postoperative SCI may be defined as any neurologic dysfunction, motor or sensory, that occurs in a patient, which did not exist before the thoracic repair and is not attributable to intracranial disorder (ie, stroke or intracranial hemorrhage).[54] The injury seen after SCI (anterior spinal artery [ASA] syndrome) is manifested by a loss of motor function, pinprick sensation, and preservation of vibratory and position sense; this can cause autonomic dysfunction, leading to hypotension or neurogenic shock that can further compromise spinal cord perfusion.[8,19]

The overall incidence of paraplegia or paraparesis after TEVAR, based on clinical series reported in the literature, is 3.9%.[56] It is a multifactorial event, with the following contributing risk factors[8,57,58]:

- Compromised pelvic and hypogastric/iliolumbar circulation supplying the ASA
  - Previous or concomitant abdominal aortic aneurysm (AAA) repair
  - Injury to the external iliac artery
  - Occlusion of the hypogastric artery
- Exclusion of critical intercostal arteries supplying the ASA
  - Coverage of thoracic aortic segment of more than 20 cm or distal coverage within 2 cm of the celiac artery
  - Exclusion of T8 to L2 region of the distal thoracic aorta
  - LSCA coverage in patients without a patent circle of Willis
- Perioperative hypotension
  - Spinal cord perfusion pressure (SCPP) less than 70 mm Hg; risk factor for immediate and delayed SCI
- Severe atherosclerosis of the thoracic aorta
  - Increased risk of emboli to the ASA and athermanous occlusion of the intercostal arteries
- Renal failure
  - Compromised collateral blood supply to the spinal cord

Strategies to reduce the incidence of SCI following TEVAR

- Optimize oxygen delivery. Maintain a normal cardiac index and hemoglobin.[8,57–60]
- Increase the SCPP (ACC/AHA Class IIa recommendation, level of evidence B).[17]
- Maintain MAP above 80 mm Hg, cerebrospinal fluid (CSF) pressure less than 10 mm Hg, and central venous pressure (CVP) less than 10 mm Hg, and preserve LSCA blood flow.
- Pharmacologic protection (ACC/AHA Class IIa recommendation, level of evidence B)[17]:
  - Reduce excitotoxicity. Infuse naloxone at 1 μg/kg/h.[59]
  - Increase blood flow in the spinal cord. Intrathecal papaverine (60 mg) causes vasodilatation, and increases spinal cord blood flow and SCPP.[60]

Hemodynamic manipulation during aortic endograft deployment

The ascending aorta, aortic arch, and proximal descending thoracic aorta represent a hostile environment for endografts, with tortuous anatomy and forceful hemodynamic forces that make accurate positioning difficult. As a result, adjunctive measures to reduce cardiac output (CO) induce asystole, or decrease HR and MAP are required to assist accurate endograft deployment.[61] Adjunctive measures include pharmacologic and nonpharmacologic methods.[61]

Pharmacologic agents should be titratable, short acting, and have a rapid onset of action. Adenosine administered as a bolus at a dose of 0.5 to 1.5 mg/kg produces asystole for 20 to 30 seconds. A target HR of 50 to 60 beats/min can be achieved by using esmolol and dexmedetomidine, and a target MAP of 50 to 60 mm Hg can be achieved by using nitroglycerin, clevidipine, propofol, remifentanil, and volatile anesthetics.[8,61]

Nonpharmacologic measures include rapid transvenous right ventricular pacing (RVP) and right atrial inflow occlusion. RVP results in the loss of atrioventricular synchrony and a reduction in ventricular filling time, causing a decrease in left ventricular preload, stroke volume, and CO. RVP at a rate of 130 to 180 beats/min can lower the systolic blood pressure (SBP) to 50 to 60 mm Hg, and pacing at 160 to 200 beats/min can reduce the SBP to 20 to 30 mm Hg. RVP is associated with more precise placement at the designated location than with any pharmacologic intervention. Accurate proximal endograft deployment can also be facilitated by temporarily occluding the inferior vena cava, leading to preload reduction and hypotension.[61]

The authors pharmacologically induce hypotension with a β-blocker and a vasodilator for deployments in zones 2, 3, and 4, and use RVP for deployments in zones 0 and 1.[61]

Based on these considerations, the following is recommended in conjunction with standard monitoring[19,51]:

- Blood products to be made immediately available
- Large-bore peripheral intravenous access combined with a rapid fluid warmer transfuser, for the administration of blood products and fluids
- Monitoring of urine output; fluid management is directed primarily at maintaining normovolemia
- A right radial arterial line, which will permit monitoring of BP during repair of the proximal thoracic aorta or distal aortic arch if the LSCA has to be covered. Also, a catheter may be placed percutaneously in the left brachial artery for aortic angiography and/or endograft placement
- Central venous access for monitoring the right atrial pressure and for the administration of vasoactive drugs to control the circulation

- Insertion of a spinal drain for CSF drainage (CSFD), and CSF pressure monitoring for spinal cord protection

Anesthetic Technique

TEVAR has been successfully performed under both general anesthesia (GA) and regional anesthesia (RA).

Regional anesthesia

The advantage of spinal or epidural anesthesia is that it allows the patient to remain awake, avoid tracheal intubation, and provide postoperative pain relief. Disadvantages of RA for TEVAR include patient movement, sympathectomy, and no allowance for TEE and neurophysiologic monitoring.[19]

General anesthesia

TEVAR is usually performed under GA.[8,19] Advantages include the ability to control ventilation and limit patient movement. Disadvantages of GA include the potential for airway complications and postoperative central nervous system depression from residual anesthetic drugs.[19] Factors favoring GA include[8]: (1) TEVAR with planned fenestrated or branched endografts, owing to the expected long duration; (2) a need for debranching procedures or for aortic/iliac artery access (through a retroperitoneal incision); (3) planned use of TEE and/or neurophysiologic monitoring; (4) planned hemodynamic manipulations to create a motionless field during stent deployment; and (5) planned central-line placement and/or left brachial artery cannulation.

Regardless of the mode of anesthesia, the intraoperative anesthetic goals during TEVAR are to provide hemodynamic stability while preserving vital organ perfusion and function, and maintaining intravascular volume, adequate oxygenation, and body temperature. These goals are more important to overall outcome than the choice of anesthetic technique.[2,8,19,51]

Specialized Perioperative Monitoring

Transesophageal echocardiography (ACC/AHA Class IIa recommendation, level of evidence B)

Intraoperative TEE can provide the following[8,17,19]: (1) assessment of ventricular function and volume status; (2) diagnosis and confirmation of aortic abnormality; (3) guidance for guide wire, delivery device, and endograft placement within the aorta; (4) classification and detection of endoleaks; (5) verification of aneurysm exclusion by showing static contrast within the aneurysmal sac; and (6) help in identifying proximal and distal stent-graft landing zones, entry and exit points, and true and false lumens of dissections.

Monitoring of spinal cord function

The ideal spinal cord monitor should (1) be noninvasive, (2) be simple enough to use that no additional personnel are required, (3) be highly sensitive and specific to changes in the anterior spinal cord, (4) allow standard anesthesia delivery, (5) exhibit no delay in ischemia detection, and (6) be usable in conscious postoperative patients.[62]

Neurophysiologic monitoring (ACC/AHA Class IIb recommendation, level of evidence B)

Sensory evoked potential monitoring Somatosensory evoked potentials (SSEPs) are cerebral cortical electrical potentials recorded with scalp electrodes during electrical stimulation of the posterior tibial or peroneal nerves of the lower extremities,[17] conducted via the lateral and posterior columns of the spinal cord.[17] There are 4 general problems with SSEP monitoring.[51,63] First, sensory monitoring is more likely to detect lateral and posterior sensory column ischemia and is a poor monitor of the anterior motor column. Second, inhaled anesthetics and hypothermia can interfere with SSEP signals. Third, ischemia affects peripheral nerves, and ischemia in the lower extremities delays conduction from the usual stimulation sites.[51] Fourth, although SSEPs can reliably exclude SCI with a negative predictive value of 99.2%, their sensitivity for its detection is only 62.5%, with no clinically useful predictive value for delayed-onset paraplegia.[63]

Transcranial motor-evoked potential monitoring Transcranial motor-evoked potential (MEP) monitoring is performed by applying paired stimuli to the scalp overlying the motor cortex. The evoked potentials elicited from this stimulation travel from the motor cortex, through cortical spinal tracts, anterior horn cell, peripheral nerve, and finally to the anterior tibialis muscle, where it is recorded.[51] Only electromyogenic responses are specific for the status of the motor neurons in the anterior horn gray matter.[51] An interruption in this pathway will result in the loss or reduction of amplitude in the MEPs. The major problem with MEPs is that it requires experienced personnel for interpretation.

Effects of anesthesia on SSEPs and MEPs Central neuraxial anesthesia is contraindicated if SSEP or MEP monitoring is planned.[17] When conducting SSEP monitoring, volatile anesthetic concentrations should be maintained at half the minimum anesthetic concentration (MAC) because high volatile anesthetic concentrations attenuate cortical signals.[58] The amplitude of MEPs are sensitive to neuromuscular blocking agents and inhalational anesthetics. General anesthetic regimens using intravenous infusions of remifentanil, ketamine, propofol, or etomidate without neuromuscular blockade have been shown to maintain satisfactory MEP signals during operation.[19,51,58]

Supporting evidence for SSEP and MEP monitoring A recent study by Keyhani and colleagues[64] compared both MEPs and SSEPs for spinal cord monitoring in extensive descending thoracic and TAAA repairs (N = 233). Both monitoring modalities had a nearly 90% correlation for spinal cord infarction (correlation statistic = 0.896; $P<.0001$), as well as a 98% negative predictive value for immediate-onset paraplegia. Furthermore, reversible changes in MEPs and SSEPs had no correlation with permanent paraplegia. As such, despite its theoretical advantages, MEP monitoring failed to demonstrate any significant change in clinical management compared with the use of SSEP monitoring alone.[64] In another study, Jacobs and colleagues[65] reported preventing neurologic deficits in 98% of patients undergoing TAAA repair by using MEP monitoring. Because of a lack of general consensus on the effectiveness and type of monitoring that should be used, current thoracic aortic disease guidelines recommend the use of either SSEP or MEP monitoring as valid strategies for the detection of intraoperative SCI.[17,66]

Transcutaneous near-infrared spectroscopy

Transcutaneous near-infrared spectroscopy (NIRS) is currently used for cerebral oximetry in cardiovascular surgery. NIRS assesses the oxyhemoglobin fraction within a focal area of underlying tissue by measuring the differential absorption of 2 wavelengths of near-infrared light (730 and 810 nm) that reflect deoxyhemoglobin and total hemoglobin concentration.[62]

Supporting evidence for NIRS LeMaire and colleagues[62] successfully used NIRS in a pig model to detect induced regional SCI, and Moerman and colleagues[67] used

NIRS to detect SCI during a staged hybrid TAAA repair. Nicolaou and colleagues[68] were the first to use NIRS to accurately detect and treat SCI in humans during TEVAR. One probe was placed over the cervical spine as the control, and one was placed over the lower thoracic spine as the area of interest. In the graph shown in **Fig. 8**, as the MAP was decreased to facilitate stent deployment, the lower cord NIRS saturation decreased. Subsequent CSF drainage improved NIRS. The investigators interpreted this as an improvement in spinal cord perfusion. This patient awoke without a neuro-logic deficit.[68] In summary, NIRS has the potential to satisfy all the criteria for ideal spinal cord monitoring and to provide continuous, real-time information about spinal cord perfusion and oxygenation.

Lumbar CSF pressure monitoring and drainage (ACC/AHA Class I recommendation, level of evidence B)

The physiologic basis for lumbar CSFD is based on the principle that[17]: SCPP = MAP − (CSFP or CVP [whichever is greater]), where SCPP is spinal cord perfusion pressure, MAP the mean aortic pressure, CSFP the cerebrospinal fluid pressure, and CVP the central venous pressure.[17,57,58] Hypoperfusion and ischemia/reperfusion injury may cause spinal cord edema and mediate negative neurotropic substances. CSFD increases SCPP and may restore spinal cord blood flow by decompressing the spinal compartment syndrome caused by spinal cord edema and by removing negative neurotropic substances from the CSF.[69]

Indications for CSFD include[56]: (1) anticipated endograft coverage of T9 to T12 (ASA), (2) thoracic aortic coverage of greater than 20 cm, (3) compromised collateral pathways, (4) symptomatic SCI in a patient who did not have a drain placed preoperatively, and (5) extensive aneurysmal disease (type I and II Crawford classification).

Percutaneous CSFD is performed by inserting a multiorificed, silastic catheter 5 to 10 cm into the subarachnoid space through a 14-gauge Touhy needle, at the L3-L4 or L4-L5 intervertebral interspace. The open end of the catheter is attached to a sterile closed-circuit reservoir, and the lumbar CSFP is measured with a pressure transducer zero-referenced to the midline of the brain. The system should not be attached to

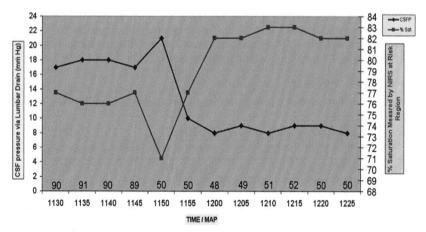

Fig. 8. Relationship between mean arterial pressure, cerebrospinal fluid pressure (CSFP), and the near-infrared spectroscopy (NIRS) saturation over the spinal cord region at risk. (*From* Nicolaou G, Murkin J, Forbes T, et al. Use of spinal near-infrared spectroscopy for monitoring spinal cord perfusion in endovascular repair of thoracoabdominal aneurysm [abstract]. In: outcomes 2009, The Key West Meeting. Barbados, May 27–30, 2009.)

a pressurized flush system, and no heparin should be in the fluid priming the transducer system.[57,66] Lumbar CSF can be drained continuously or intermittently in the operating room to achieve a target CSF pressure of less than 10 mm Hg. There is no consensus on the optimal duration of CSF drain management. The authors' practice is to drain CSF for the first 24 hours after the procedure, to maintain a CSFP of less than 10 mm Hg. If there is no evidence of SCI, the drain is clamped for another 48 hours with continued monitoring of the CSFP and serial neurologic assessments. If the patient remains asymptomatic the drain is then removed 72 hours from the time of insertion.[54,57,58,66]

Contraindications to spinal drain insertion include patient refusal, coagulopathy, and sepsis. Complications of CSFD occur in approximately 1% of patients with spinal drains, with a reported mortality of 0.6%.[57,66] Complications of, and best practices for, CSFD are summarized in **Tables 3** and **4**.

Supporting evidence for CSFD Coselli and colleagues[70] randomized 145 patients undergoing TAAA repair with or without CSFD. Nine patients (13.0%) in the control group developed paraplegia or paraparesis. By contrast, only 2 patients in the CSFD group (2.6%) had deficits develop ($P = .03$). No patients with CSFD had immediate paraplegia.[70] Two independent meta-analyses by Khan and Stansby[71] and by Cina and colleagues[72] concluded that CSFD was advantageous in reducing the risk of SCI in open TAA repairs. In recent years, lumbar CSFD has been shown to be beneficial for the prevention and treatment of SCI after TEVAR.[8,57,58,66] In a prospective observational study using historical controls, Hnath and colleagues[73] showed a significant decrease in the incidence of postoperative spinal cord injury with TEVAR when CSFD was used.

Biochemical markers for the detection of SCI
The protein S100β, which is present in high concentrations in glial and Schwann cells, is released during acute neuronal injury and has been shown to correlate with a decrease in transcranial MEPs.[54] Kunihara and colleagues[69] observed that after TAAA repair, levels of neurotoxic excitatory amino acids, proinflammatory cytokines, and S-100β were found to be higher in the CSF of patients with postoperative SCI than in patients without SCI. Another marker, glial fibrillary acidic protein, was found to be higher in the CSF of patients with SCI. This marker was detectable before the development of clinical symptoms.[54] A limitation of biochemical markers remains the lack of specificity for spinal cord injury versus an intracerebral event.

Postoperative Management

Neurologic examination should be performed immediately on emergence from GA. Any neurologic deficit detected should be considered to be SCI until proven otherwise, and a neurologist should examine the patient.

Table 3
Complications of CSF drainage

Lumbar Puncture	Catheter Presence	CSF Drainage
Nerve root/spinal cord injury	Nerve root irritation	Intracranial hypotension/ bleeding (subdural or intracerebellar hematoma)
Bleeding/neuraxial hematoma	Infection: local/meningitis/ epidural abscess	Headache
Persistent CSF leak	Catheter fracture	Abducens nerve palsy

Data from Refs.[57,58,66]

Table 4
CSF drainage recommendations

	Recommendation
Preoperative	
Coagulation	No LMWH for 24 h (high dose), 12 h (low dose); no clopidogrel × 7 d; no ticlopidine × 10 d; no abciximab × 24–48 h; no eptifibatide or tirofiban × 4–8 h; platelets >100 × $10^3/\mu L^3$; INR <1.3; normal aPTT
Intracranial pressure	Avoid placement of spinal drain if patient has evidence of increased intracranial pressure
Intraoperative	
Insertion of spinal catheter	Sterile technique; must be placed by trained individuals familiar with the risks, contraindications, and anatomy pertinent to the catheterization of the spinal canal; avoid placing in area of localized infection
Awake vs asleep	Awake allows for patient feedback (ie, pain/paresthesia)
Traumatic/bloody tap	Discuss with surgeon; consider delaying surgery for 24 h; delay anticoagulation for 60 min
Hemodynamics	MAP to maintain SCPP >70 mm Hg; CVP <10 mm Hg
Zero transducer	Phlebostatic axis to ensure accurate calculation of SCPP
CSF drainage	CSFP <10 mm Hg to maintain SCPP >70 mm Hg, CSFD ≤20 mL/h, intermittent CSFD with continuous monitoring avoids large volumes of CSFD, which may decrease the risk of intracranial hypotension
Subarachnoid opiates	Avoid, as may exacerbate spinal cord ischemia
Postoperative	
Hemodynamics	Avoid hypotension
New-onset neurologic deficit	Worsening SCI vs neuraxial hematoma; increase SCPP; MRI of spinal cord
Coagulation for drain removal	Platelet count >100 × $10^3/\mu L^3$; INR <1.3; normal aPTT; delay removal 2–4 h after last heparin dose; hold heparin 1 h after catheter removal

Abbreviations: aPTT, activated partial thromboplastic time; CSFD, cerebrospinal fluid drainage; CSFP, cerebrospinal fluid pressure; CVP, central venous pressure; ICH, intracranial hemorrhage; INR, international normalized ratio; LMWH, low molecular weight heparin; MAP, mean arterial blood pressure; MRI, magnetic resonance imaging; SCPP, spinal cord perfusion pressure.

Data from Feezor RJ, Lee WA. Strategies for detection and prevention of spinal cord ischemia during TEVAR. Semin Vasc Surg 2009;22:187–92; and Fedorow CA, Moon MC, Mutch WA, et al. Lumbar cerebrospinal fluid drainage for thoracoabdominal aortic surgery: rationale and practical considerations for management. Anesth Analg 2010;111:46–58.

Management of SCI following TEVAR[8,19,57–59,66]

1. Optimize oxygen delivery
   a. Optimize the cardiac index
   b. Hematocrit 30% or greater
2. Maximize SCPP
   a. Maintain a perioperative MAP above 90 to 110 mm Hg through volume expansion and by using an α-agonist (eg, norepinephrine, phenylephrine, vasopressin)
   b. Therapeutic CSFD to maintain CSFP below 10 mm Hg
   c. CVP less than 10 mm Hg
3. Reduce neurotoxic excitatory neurotransmitters[61]
   a. Naloxone infusion at 1 μg/kg/h, continue for 48 hours postoperatively

4. Serial neurologic examination
    a. To assess for improvement or worsening of the neurologic deficit
5. Magnetic resonance imaging
    a. To exclude a spinal hematoma or any other spinal cord abnormality

SUMMARY

TEVAR has revolutionized thoracic aortic surgery and has increased the options available to the aortic specialist in treating thoracic aortic disease. Although current devices do not allow perfusion of intercostal arteries, TEVAR is less invasive and is associated with a decrease in perioperative morbidity and mortality when compared with OSR. In patients with: (1) traumatic thoracic aortic injury, (2) acute complicated T_BADs, (3) DTAAs larger than 5.5 cm with feasible anatomy, and (4) ruptured DTAAs with suitable anatomy, TEVAR is considered the treatment of choice. Ideally, TEVAR should be performed in specialized aortic centers providing a full range of diagnostic and treatment options, using a multidisciplinary team approach.

However, despite encouraging results from a large number of publications in recent years, the long-term durability of TEVAR still remains largely unknown. Follow-up with serial imaging studies is necessary to detect device failure. As endovascular techniques and technology continue to evolve, TEVAR use will continue to expand at a rapid pace. Randomized controlled trials to examine the long-term efficacy and safety of TEVAR in comparison with open surgery and conservative medical management are necessary to better define patient selection and the role of TEVAR in the treatment of thoracic aortic disease.

ACKNOWLEDGMENTS

The authors wish to acknowledge Ms Brieanne McConnell for her assistance in facilitating literature searches, retrieval, and citation management.

REFERENCES

1. DeBakey ME, Cooley DA. Successful resection of aneurysm of the thoracic aorta and replacement by graft. JAMA 1953;152:673–6.
2. Findeiss LK, Cody ME. Endovascular repair of the thoracic aortic aneurysms. Semin Intervent Radiol 2011;28(1):107–17.
3. Adams JD, Garcia LM, Kern JA. Endovascular repair of the thoracic aorta. Surg Clin North Am 2009;89:895–912.
4. Achneck HE, Rizzo JA, Tranquilli M, et al. Safety of thoracic aortic surgery in the present era. Ann Thorac Surg 2007;84:1180–5.
5. Makaroun MS, Dillavou ED, Kee ST, et al. Endovascular treatment of thoracic aortic aneurysms: results of the phase II multicenter trial of the GORE TAG thoracic endoprosthesis. J Vasc Surg 2005;41:1–9.
6. Matsumura JS, Cambria RP, Dake MD, et al. International controlled clinical trial of thoracic endovascular aneurysm repair with the Zenith TX2 endovascular graft: 1-year results. J Vasc Surg 2008;47:247–57.
7. Fairman RM, Criado F, Farber M, et al. Pivotal results of the Medtronic vascular talent thoracic stent graft system: the VALOR trial. J Vasc Surg 2008;48:546–54.
8. Argalious M. Endovascular aortic repair in the descending thoracoabdominal aorta [abstract 322]. In: Programs and abstracts of the American Society of Anesthesiologists' Annual Meeting. Chicago, IL, October 15–17, 2011. p. 1–9.

9. Grabenwoger M, Alfonso F, Bachet J, et al. Thoracic endovascular aortic repair (TEVAR) for the treatment of aortic diseases: a position statement from the European Association for Cardio-Thoracic Surgery (EACTS) and the European Society of Cardiology (ESC), in collaboration with the European Association of Percutaneous Cardiovascular Interventions (EAPCI). Eur Heart J 2012;33(13):1558–63.
10. Criado F, Abul-Khoudoud O, Domer G, et al. Endovascular repair of the thoracic aorta: lessons learned. Ann Thorac Surg 2005;80:857–63.
11. Feezor RJ, Martin TD, Hess PJ, et al. Risk factors for perioperative stroke during thoracic endovascular aortic repairs (TEVAR). J Endovasc Ther 2007;14(4):568–73.
12. Criado FJ, Barnatan MF, Rizk Y, et al. Technical strategies to expand stent-graft applicability in the aortic arch and proximal descending thoracic aorta. J Endovasc Ther 2002;(9 Suppl 2):II32–8.
13. Rizvi AZ, Murad MH, Fairman RM, et al. The effect of left subclavian artery coverage on morbidity and mortality in patients undergoing endovascular thoracic aortic interventions: a systematic review and meta-analysis. J Vasc Surg 2009;50(5):1159–69.
14. Matsumura JS, Lee WA, Mitchell RS, et al. The Society for Vascular Surgery Practice Guidelines: management of the left subclavian artery with thoracic endovascular aortic repair. J Vasc Surg 2009;50(5):1155–8.
15. Bischoff MS, Di Luozzo G, Griepp EB, et al. Spinal cord preservation in thoracoabdominal aneurysm repair. Perspect Vasc Surg Endovasc Ther 2011;23(3):214–22.
16. Lin PH, Kougias P, Bechara CF, et al. Clinical outcome of staged versus combined treatment approach of hybrid repair of thoracoabdominal aortic aneurysm with visceral vessel debranching and aortic endograft exclusion. Perspect Vasc Surg Endovasc Ther 2012;24(1):5–13.
17. Hiratzka LF, Bakris GL, Beckman JA, et al. 2010 ACCF/AHA/AATS/ACR/ASA/SCA/SCAI/SIR/STS/SVM guidelines for the diagnosis and management of patients with Thoracic Aortic Disease: a report of the American College of Cardiology Foundation/American Heart Association Task Force on Practice Guidelines, American Association for Thoracic Surgery, American College of Radiology, American Stroke Association, Society of Cardiovascular Anesthesiologists, Society for Cardiovascular Angiography and Interventions, Society of Interventional Radiology, Society of Thoracic Surgeons, and Society for Vascular Medicine. Circulation 2010;121(13):e266–369.
18. Coady MA, Ikonomidis JS, Cheung AT, et al. Surgical management of descending thoracic aortic disease: open and endovascular approaches: a scientific statement from the American Heart Association. Circulation 2010;121:2780–804.
19. Gutsche JT, Szeto W, Cheung AT. Endovascular stenting of thoracic aortic aneurysm. Anesthesiol Clin 2008;26:481–99.
20. Svensson LG, Kouchoukos NT, Miller DC, et al. Expert consensus document on the treatment of descending thoracic aortic disease using endovascular stent-grafts. Ann Thorac Surg 2008;85(Suppl 1):S1–41.
21. Bavaria JE, Appoo JJ, Makaroun MS, et al, Gore TAG Investigators. Endovascular stent grafting versus open surgical repair of descending thoracic aortic aneurysms in low-risk patients: a multicenter comparative trial. J Thorac Cardiovasc Surg 2007;133:369–77.
22. Cao CQ, Bannon PG, Shee R, et al. Thoracic endovascular aortic repair-indications and evidence. Ann Thorac Cardiovasc Surg 2011;17:1–6.

23. Jonker FH, Trimarchi S, Verhagen HJ, et al. Meta-analysis of open versus endovascular repair for ruptured descending thoracic aortic aneurysm. J Vasc Surg 2010;51(4):1026–32.
24. Nicolaou G. Endovascular treatment of blunt traumatic thoracic aortic injury. Semin Cardiothorac Vasc Anesth 2009;13(2):106–12.
25. Azizzadeh A, Keyhani K, Miller CC 3rd, et al. Blunt traumatic aortic injury: initial experience with endovascular repair. J Vasc Surg 2009;49:1403–8.
26. Tang GL, Tehrani HY, Usman A, et al. Reduced mortality, paraplegia, and stroke with stent graft repair of blunt aortic transections: a modern meta-analysis. J Vasc Surg 2008;47:671–5.
27. Lee AW, Matsumara JS, Mitchell RS, et al. Endovascular repair of traumatic thoracic aortic injury: clinical practice guidelines of the Society for Vascular Surgery. J Vasc Surg 2011;53:187–92.
28. Tsai TT, Nienaber CA, Eagle KA. Contemporary reviews in cardiovascular medicine: acute aortic syndromes. Circulation 2005;112:3802–13.
29. Patel PJ, Grande W, Hieb RA. Endovascular management of acute aortic syndromes. Semin Intervent Radiol 2011;28(1):10–23.
30. Ye C, Chang G, Li S, et al. Endovascular stent-graft treatment for Stanford type A aortic dissection. Eur J Vasc Endovasc Surg 2011;42:787–94.
31. Nienaber CA, Rousseau H, Eggebrecht H, et al. INSTEAD Trial randomized comparison of strategies for type B aortic dissection: the INvestigation of STEnt Grafts in Aortic Dissection (INSTEAD) trial. Circulation 2009;120(25):2519–28.
32. Gore & Associates. A European study of medical management versus TAG device and medical management for acute uncomplicated type B dissection (ADSORB). Available at: ClinicalTrials.gov. Accessed March 22, 2010.
33. Fattori R, Tsai T, Myrmel T, et al. Complicated acute type B dissection: is surgery still the best option? A report for the International Registry of Acute Aortic Dissection (IRAD). JACC Cardiovasc Interv 2008;1:395–402.
34. Trimarchi S, Nienaber CA, Rampoldi V, et al. Role and results of surgery in acute type B aortic dissection: insights from the International Registry of Acute Aortic Dissection (IRAD). Circulation 2006;114(Suppl 1):1357–64.
35. Parker JD, Golledge J. Outcome of endovascular treatment of acute type B aortic dissection. Ann Thorac Surg 2008;86:1707–12.
36. Sachs T, Pomposelli F, Hagberg R, et al. Open and endovascular repair of type B aortic dissection in the Nationwide Inpatient Sample. J Vasc Surg 2010;52(4):860–6.
37. Tsai TT, Fattori R, Trimarchi S, et al. Long-term survival inpatients presenting with type B acute aortic dissection: insights from the International Registry of Acute Aortic Dissection. Circulation 2006;114:2226–31.
38. Botta L, Buttazzi K, Russo V, et al. Endovascular repair for penetrating atherosclerotic ulcers of the descending thoracic aorta: early and mid-term results. Ann Thorac Surg 2008;85(3):987–92.
39. Eggebrecht H, Plicht B, Kahlert P, et al. Intramural hematoma and penetrating ulcers: indications to endovascular treatment. Eur J Vasc Endovasc Surg 2009;38:659–65.
40. Coselli JS, Conklin LD, LeMaire SA. Thoracoabdominal aortic aneurysm repair: review and update of current strategies. Ann Thorac Surg 2002;74:S1881–4.
41. Coselli JS, Bozinovski J, LeMaire SA. Open surgical repair of 2286 thoracoabdominal aortic aneurysms. Ann Thorac Surg 2007;83(2):S862–4 [discussion: S890–2].
42. Moulakakis KG, Mylonas SN, Avgerinos ED, et al. Hybrid open endovascular technique for aortic thoracoabdominal pathologies. Circulation 2011;124:2670–80.

43. Bakoyiannis CN, Economopoulos KP, Georgopoulos S, et al. Fenestrated and branched endografts for the treatment of thoracoabdominal aortic aneurysms: a systematic review. J Endovasc Ther 2010;17:201–9.
44. Greenberg R, Eagleton M, Mastracci T. Branched endografts for thoracoabdominal aneurysms. J Thorac Cardiovasc Surg 2010;140(Suppl 6):S171–8.
45. Greenberg RK, Lu Q, Roselli EE, et al. Contemporary analysis of descending thoracic and thoracoabdominal aneurysm repair: a comparison of endovascular and open techniques. Circulation 2008;118:808–17.
46. Patel HJ, Deeb GM. Ascending and arch aorta: pathology, natural history, and treatment. Circulation 2008;118:188.
47. Antoniou GA, El Sakka K, Hamady M, et al. Hybrid treatment of complex aortic arch disease with supra-aortic debranching and endovascular stent graft repair. Eur J Vasc Endovasc Surg 2010;39:683–90.
48. Cheng D, Martin J, Shennib H, et al. Endovascular aortic repair versus open surgical repair for descending thoracic aortic disease a systematic review and meta-analysis of comparative studies. J Am Coll Cardiol 2010;55:986–1001.
49. Davies RR, Goldstein LJ, Coady MA, et al. Yearly rupture or dissection rates for thoracic aortic aneurysms: simple prediction based on size. Ann Thorac Surg 2002;73(1):17–27.
50. Fleisher LA, Beckman JA, Brown KA, et al. ACC/AHA 2007 guidelines on perioperative cardiovascular evaluation and care for noncardiac surgery: a report of the American College of Cardiology/American Heart Association Task Force on Practice Guidelines (Writing Committee to Revise the 2002 Guidelines on Perioperative Cardiovascular Evaluation for Noncardiac Surgery) developed in collaboration with the American Society of Echocardiography, American Society of Nuclear Cardiology, Heart Rhythm Society, Society of Cardiovascular Anesthesiologists, Society for Cardiovascular Angiography and Interventions, Society for Vascular Medicine and Biology, and Society for Vascular Surgery. J Am Coll Cardiol 2007;50(17):e159–241.
51. Miller R. Anesthesia for vascular surgery. In: Miller R, Erikkson L, Fleisher L, editors. Miller's anesthesia: expert consult. 7th edition. Philadelphia: Churchill Livingstone Elsevier; 2009. p. 2015–8.
52. Goldfarb S, McCullough PA, McDermott J, et al. Contrast-induced acute kidney injury: specialty-specific protocols for interventional radiology, diagnostic computed tomography radiology, and interventional cardiology. Mayo Clin Proc 2009;84(2):170–9.
53. Ullery BW, McGarvey M, Cheung AT, et al. Vascular distribution of stroke and its relationship to perioperative mortality and neurologic outcome after thoracic endovascular repair. J Vasc Surg 2012;56(6):1510–7.
54. Feezor RJ, Lee WA. Strategies for detection and prevention of spinal cord ischemia during TEVAR. Semin Vasc Surg 2009;22:187–92.
55. Conrad MF, Ye JY, Chung TK, et al. Spinal cord complications after thoracic aortic surgery: long-term survival and functional status varies with deficit severity. J Vasc Surg 2008;48(1):47–53.
56. Rizvi AZ, Sullivan TM. Incidence, prevention, and management in spinal cord protection during TEVAR. J Vasc Surg 2010;52(Suppl 4):86S–90S.
57. Fedorow CA, Moon MC, Mutch WA, et al. Lumbar cerebrospinal fluid drainage for thoracoabdominal aortic surgery: rationale and practical considerations for management. Anesth Analg 2010;111:46–58.
58. Sinha AC, Cheung AT. Spinal cord protection and thoracic aortic surgery. Curr Opin Anaesthesiol 2010;23:95–102.

59. Acher C. It is not just assisted circulation, hypothermic arrest, or clamp and sew. J Thorac Cardiovasc Surg 2010;140(6):S136–41.

60. Lima B, Nowicki ER, Blackstone EH, et al. Spinal cord protective strategies during descending and thoracoabdominal aortic aneurysm repair in the modern era: the role of intrathecal papaverine. J Thorac Cardiovasc Surg 2012;143(4): 945–952.e1.

61. Nicolaou G, Forbes TL. Strategies for accurate endograft placement in the proximal thoracic aorta. Semin Cardiothorac Vasc Anesth 2010;14(3):196–200.

62. LeMaire SA, Ochoa LN, Conklin LD, et al. Transcutaneous near-infrared spectroscopy for detection of regional spinal ischemia during intercostal artery ligation: preliminary experimental results. J Thorac Cardiovasc Surg 2006;132:1150–5.

63. Achouh PE, Estrera AL, Miller CC III, et al. Role of somatosensory evoked potentials during thoracic and thoracoabdominal aneurysm repair. Ann Thorac Surg 2007;84:782.

64. Keyhani K, Miller CC III, Estrera AL, et al. Analysis of motor and somatosensory evoked potentials during thoracic and thoracoabdominal aortic aneurysm repair. J Vasc Surg 2009;49:36–41.

65. Jacobs MJ, Mess WH, Mochtar B, et al. The value of motor evoked potentials in reducing paraplegia during thoracoabdominal aneurysm repair. J Vasc Surg 2006;43(2):239–46.

66. Ullery BW, Wang GJ, Low D, et al. Neurological complications of thoracic endovascular aortic repair. Semin Cardiothorac Vasc Anesth 2011;15(4):123–40.

67. Moerman A, Van Herzeele I, Vanpeteghem C, et al. Near-infrared spectroscopy for monitoring spinal cord ischemia during hybrid thoracoabdominal aortic aneurysm repair. J Endovasc Ther 2011;18:91–5.

68. Nicolaou G, Murkin J, Forbes T, et al. Use of spinal near-infrared spectroscopy for monitoring spinal cord perfusion in endovascular repair of thoracoabdominal aneurysm [abstract]. In: Outcomes 2009, The Key West Meeting. Barbados, May 27–30, 2009.

69. Kunihara T, Kubota S, Wakasa S. Prevention of spinal cord injury after thoracoabdominal aortic aneurysm repair. In: Grundmann R, editor. Diagnosis and treatment of abdominal and thoracic aortic aneurysms including ascending aorta and the aortic arch. New York, USA: InTech; 2011. p. 187–208.

70. Coselli J, LeMaire S, Koksoy C, et al. Cerebrospinal fluid drainage reduces paraplegia after thoracoabdominal aortic aneurysm repair: results of a randomized clinical trial. J Vasc Surg 2002;35:631–9.

71. Khan SN, Stansby G. Cerebrospinal fluid drainage for thoracic and thoracoabdominal aortic aneurysm surgery. Cochrane Database Syst Rev 2004;(1):CD003635.

72. Cina CS, Abouzahr L, Arena GO, et al. Cerebrospinal fluid drainage to prevent paraplegia during thoracic and thoracoabdominal aortic aneurysm surgery: a systematic review and meta-analysis. J Vasc Surg 2004;40:36–44.

73. Hnath JC, Mehta M, Taggert JB, et al. Strategies to improve spinal cord ischemia in endovascular thoracic aortic repair: outcomes of a prospective cerebrospinal fluid drainage protocol. J Vasc Surg 2008;48:836–40.

Anesthetic Considerations for Electrophysiologic Procedures

Ryan Anderson, MD, PhD, Izumi Harukuni, MD*,
Valerie Sera, MD, DDS

KEYWORDS

- Anesthesia • Electrophysiology • Cardiology • Pacemaker • Defibrillator
- Catheter ablation

KEY POINTS

- Anesthesiologist involvement with procedures in the electrophysiology laboratory has significantly increased in recent years because of the complexity of procedures and patient comorbidity.
- The electrophysiology laboratory can present challenges to providing a safe anesthetic because of physical barriers between patient and anesthesia provider, unfamiliar equipment, remote location, and working with staff unfamiliar with anesthesia provider's needs.
- Although most procedures in the electrophysiology laboratory can be performed using conscious sedation, patient and procedural factors will often warrant a general anesthetic.
- Commonly used medications can affect the sinoatrial or atrioventricular node activities and cardiac conduction.
- Monitoring during anesthesia care in the electrophysiology laboratory should reference the American Society of Anesthesiologists standards for monitoring.
- The electrophysiology laboratory uses a high amount of ionizing radiation for imaging; hence anesthesia providers should exercise the ALARA (as low as reasonably achieved) principle for minimizing exposure.

INTRODUCTION

The array of diagnostic and therapeutic procedures performed in the cardiology electrophysiology laboratory has undergone rapid expansion in recent years. An increasing number of facilities and cardiologists are performing these procedures, and the number of patients for whom these procedures are indicated is growing. In the authors' institution, demand for assistance from anesthesiologists in the electrophysiology laboratory has grown by a factor of 10 in the past 5 years.

Division of Adult Cardiothoracic Anesthesia, Department of Anesthesiology and Perioperative Medicine, Oregon Health and Science University, 3181 Southwest Sam Jackson Park Road, UHS-2, Portland, OR 97239, USA
* Corresponding author.
E-mail address: harukuni@ohsu.edu

Anesthesiology Clin 31 (2013) 479–489
http://dx.doi.org/10.1016/j.anclin.2013.01.005
1932-2275/13/$ – see front matter

In 2011, a survey of cardiologists set out to analyze the sedation practice in academic electrophysiology laboratories in the United States.[1] Although the respondent size was small, important findings from the survey included that some patients were transitioned into deep sedation or general anesthesia often with no supervision from an anesthesiologist, and among the respondents who believed anesthesiologists should be present for more than 50% of the cases, the explanation for the absence of an anesthesiologist was lack of availability, difficulty in scheduling, and long turnover times.

Because of the complexity of the procedures and associated patient comorbidity, anesthesia providers will become more involved in providing care in the electrophysiology laboratory. Anesthesia providers must be prepared to handle a broad range of case complexity, from the stable patient undergoing light sedation to the critically ill patient undergoing a general anesthetic for a lengthy and complex procedure. This article addresses the implications of providing anesthesia safely and effectively in the electrophysiology laboratory.

ENVIRONMENT AND EQUIPMENT
Remote Location

Like most "out of operating room" locations, the environment can present challenges to providing a safe anesthetic. Existing electrophysiology laboratories were not designed with the anesthesia provider in mind. Consequently, limited space is available for anesthesia equipment and providers, and the space that exists is often some distance from the patient. Imaging equipment creates a physical barrier, and the patient tables do not have the same adjustment capabilities that operating room tables have. Monitors that display vital signs are often difficult to see from the anesthesia provider's area. These factors make monitoring cumbersome and cause adjustments in care, such as starting additional intravenous lines or managing the airway, to be difficult or impossible once the procedure in underway. Movement of the fluoroscopy table is controlled by the cardiologist performing the procedure and may occur without warning to the anesthesia provider. Extra attention should be given to securing the airway circuit, intravenous lines, and monitoring cables. Modern technology for ablation uses magnetic resonance imaging (MRI) to guide catheters in the atrium for mapping, which mandates the use of MRI-compatible equipment and trained personnel.

Because of the remote location, a lengthy delay can occur from the initial request until the arrival of additional anesthesia providers, technicians, equipment, or drugs, if they should be needed unexpectedly. As a result, anticipating the need for help and having a low threshold for requesting it is of paramount importance.

Room Setup

Room setup and planning must take into account the complicating factors that the electrophysiology laboratory introduces into providing anesthesia. Large pieces of equipment that are specifically required in electrophysiology procedures include a fluoroscopy machine, a large back table, an MRI system, defibrillators, and a radiocontrast infusion system (**Fig. 1**). Imaging equipment will often rotate around the patient and can dislodge the breathing circuit, intravenous tubing, and monitoring cables. This possibility is important to anticipate, and these items should be adequately secured and given adequate length by adding extensions when necessary.

The physical barriers between the patient and anesthesia provider complicate both monitoring and delivery of care, such as placing additional lines or managing the

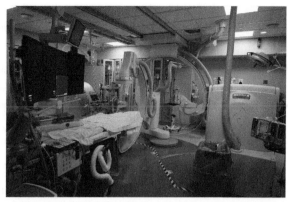

Fig. 1. Large pieces of equipment specifically required in electrophysiology procedures include a fluoroscopy machine, a large back table, an MRI system, defibrillators, and a radio-contrast infusion system.

airway. Therefore, it is advisable to make conservative management decisions (eg, additional intravenous access, secured airway) early in the case so as to avoid the need for rescue interventions during the procedure, when these become increasingly difficult or impossible to perform. Converting sedation into a general anesthetic in a patient who is unstable while the procedure is already underway is a dangerous endeavor with a narrow margin for error.

Drugs Frequently Used in the Electrophysiology Laboratory

The intracardiac catheters used during electrophysiology laboratory procedures are prothrombotic, and therefore heparin is used to reduce the risk of thrombus formation. Anticoagulation is monitored by the activated clotting time (ACT), which is maintained at greater than 300 seconds by intermittent boluses or infusion. Isoproterenol is a direct-acting, relatively selective β_1- and β_2-adrenergic agonist that is used to induce tachyarrhythmias during mapping. Its β_1 effect increases the sinoatrial node rate and atrioventricular conduction velocity while it decreases the refractory period. The β_2 effects can cause vasodilatation and hypotension. Isoproterenol is a strong central nervous system stimulant, and an infusion has been reported to increase the level of consciousness measured by bispectral index monitoring.[2]

Monitors

Monitors during anesthesia should reference the American Society of Anesthesiologists standard monitoring guidelines. End-tidal carbon dioxide (ETCO$_2$) monitoring is not mandatory for light sedation, but once the imaging equipment is in place and the patient draped, it may be the only means of confirming respirations. ETCO$_2$ is recommended for moderate to deep sedation[3] or patients at high risk for obstruction or respiratory difficulties. Esophageal temperature monitoring has been shown to reduce the risk of thermal esophageal injury during atrial fibrillation ablation.[4] Placement of an arterial line may be indicated if the patient is particularly prone to cardiac arrhythmias, consequent hypotension, and compromised cardiac output.

INDICATIONS

Detailed indications for each electrophysiology laboratory procedure are outlined in **Table 1**, including

Table 1
Indications for electrophysiology laboratory procedures and device implantation

Device/Procedure	Indications
Permanent pacemaker	High-degree atrioventricular block (second-degree Mobitz, third-degree) Symptomatic bradycardia/sinus pauses Sick sinus syndrome Symptomatic bi-/trifascicular block Pause-dependent VT Recurrent syncope from carotid stimulation Heart failure Hypertrophic obstructive cardiomyopathy Idiopathic dilated cardiomyopathy Heart transplantation with bradycardia

Implantable cardioverter-defibrillator	Primary prevention
	  Impaired left ventricular function (EF <30%)
	  Hypertrophic cardiomyopathy
	  Long QT syndrome with syncope
	  Brugada syndrome with syncope
	  Arrhythmogenic right ventricular dysplasia
	  Cardiac sarcoidosis
	Secondary prevention
	  Cardiac arrest
	  Sustained ventricular tachycardia

Cardiac resynchronization therapy	Must meet all of the following criteria: EF ≤35%, QRS >120 ms, sinus rhythm, NYHA class III or IV symptoms on optimal medical therapy
Cardioversion	Supraventricular tachycardia Reentrant tachyarrhythmias (atrial fibrillation/flutter, AVNRT, VT)

Ablation	Curative for:
	  Atrial fibrillation/flutter
	  AVNRT
	  Ectopic and reentrant atrial tachycardia
	  Wolff-Parkinson-White syndrome
	  Idiopathic monomorphic VT
	  Bundle branch reentry tachycardia
	  Automatic junctional tachycardia
	Palliative for:
	  Sustained VT in patients with CAD or nonischemic cardiomyopathy
	  Atrial fibrillation and multifocal atrial tachycardia when performed on the atrioventricular node

Abbreviations: AVNRT, atrioventricular nodal reentrant tachycardia; CAD, coronary artery disease; EF, ejection fraction; NYHA, New York Heart Association; VT, ventricular tachycardia.

- Radiofrequency ablation for tachyarrhythmias, such as atrial fibrillation, atrial flutter, supraventricular tachycardia, and ventricular tachycardia
- Permanent pacemaker (PPM) placement for high-grade heart block and symptomatic bradycardia[5]
- Cardiac resynchronization therapy for symptomatic heart failure with impaired left ventricular (LV) function and widened QRS complex[6]
- Implantable cardiac defibrillator (ICD) placement for primary and secondary prevention of sudden cardiac death in patients with severely impaired LV function

(ejection fraction <30%), history of ventricular tachyarrhythmia, long QT syndrome, hypertrophic cardiomyopathy, arrhythmogenic right ventricular dysplasia, and Brugada syndrome[5,7]

- Lead extractions for infected, broken, or recalled PPM/ICD leads

CONTRAINDICATIONS

Electrophysiology studies/procedures are contraindicated for

- Patients with acute myocardial infarction, because rapid pacing may increase its extent,
- Patients unable to lie flat because of respiratory failure or heart failure, in which case consultation for general anesthesia is warranted,
- Patients with contraindications to anticoagulation (eg, intracranial bleeding), and
- Patients who are pregnant, because of exposure to high radiation levels.

ANESTHESIA CONSULTATIONS

Several patient factors warrant an anesthesia consultation, such as the possibility of a difficult airway, obesity, obstructive sleep apnea, pulmonary disease, congestive heart failure, hemodynamic instability, psychiatric or neuromuscular disorders, and medication/substance use that complicates the administration of sedative agents (ie, chronic opioid or benzodiazepine use, alcohol abuse). Procedural factors that warrant an anesthesia consultation include patients presenting for arrhythmia ablation, complicated lead extraction (laser lead extraction), biventricular pacemaker placement, and a procedure and/or a patient requiring a general anesthetic.

PATIENT PREPARATION

Patients are commonly scheduled as outpatients and are admitted to a preprocedure holding area on the day of the procedure. A complete history and physical examination should be performed. Patients undergoing electrophysiology procedures are likely to be on several medications for their cardiac disorder and to have comorbidities that often accompany cardiac disease. These medications include anticoagulants and antiplatelet medications, diuretics, antihypertensive agents, and antiarrhythmic medications. Particular attention should be given to the possibility of allergy to iodine contrast, possibility of pregnancy, presence of devices, and history of previous heart surgery, particularly the placement of artificial heart valves.

Preprocedure testing may include a 12-lead electrocardiogram and laboratory tests including a complete blood cell count and chemistry/metabolic and coagulation panels. Many patients present for electrophysiology procedures after failed ablation, recent myocardial infarction resulting in complete heart block requiring permanent pacemaker placement, or chronic heart failure with severely impaired LV function requiring an ICD and/or biventricular pacemaker placement. A recent echocardiogram is valuable in assessing ventricular function and valvular abnormalities. Interrogation of an existing device should be performed before the scheduled procedures are initiated.

TECHNIQUES AND BEST PRACTICE
Sedation Versus General Anesthesia

Factors that influence the type of anesthetic required for a case in the electrophysiology laboratory are the type of procedure, patient factors, cardiologist preference, and patient preference. Most procedures are minimally invasive and therefore would not require a general anesthetic. Pain that accompanies vascular access and incisions can usually be managed with liberal infiltration of local anesthetic. Light sedation can be given in the form of titrated doses of opioid and benzodiazepine or infusion of propofol. One procedure that may warrant a deeper level of sedation or general anesthetic is the complex ablation of atrial fibrillation, which necessitates a motionless patient and can take several hours. The disadvantages of a general anesthetic are the increased risk associated with intubation and the delay in recognition of and intervention for thromboembolism. However, general anesthesia has been reported to be associated with higher success rates for certain procedures, such as pulmonary vein isolation.[8]

ICD placement is the other procedural indication for deep sedation or a general anesthetic. Placement of the device is similar to that of a PPM; however, after the ICD is placed, it is typically tested to ensure proper functioning of the antitachycardia therapy through inducing ventricular tachyarrhythmia with an externally placed defibrillator, which then should trigger the device to deliver a shock that terminates the arrhythmia. This process is brief but moderately painful, although the pain can be preempted by a propofol bolus or the procedure can be performed entirely under general anesthesia. Alternatively, the electrophysiologist may elect not to test the device. The anesthesia provider should be aware of the cardiologist's plan before the case is underway.

Commonly Used Medications

During placement of a biventricular pacemaker, the use of long-acting neuromuscular blocking agents should be avoided because they have the potential to mask diaphragmatic stimulation by the coronary sinus lead because of the proximity of this lead to the phrenic nerve. The effect of volatile anesthetics on cardiac conduction is conflicting. In vitro sevoflurane has been shown to prolong the action potential duration and accessory pathway effective refractory period and was clinically shown to prolong QTc, which may affect the induction of tachyarrhythmia and electrophysiologic measurements.[9] Isoflurane prolongs the atrial refractory period and delays ventricular repolarization. Desflurane at 2 minimum alveolar concentration shortens the atrial action potential duration and effective atrial refractory period.[10] The clinical significance of this is minimal or nonexistent.

Fentanyl is the most commonly used opioid during sedation or general anesthesia for electrophysiology procedures and has been shown to enhance vagal tone and cause bradycardia. Electrophysiology study has shown that fentanyl prolongs sinus node recovery time but not sinoatrial conduction time in pediatric patients.[11] The use of remifentanil and/or dexmedetomidine is controversial or contraindicated in electrophysiology procedures because it significantly depresses sinus and atrioventricular nodal function, which causes undesired and misleading measurements of cardiac conduction and can be a problem in inducing tachyarrhythmia.[12–14]

Specific Considerations

PPM implantation Patients may have normal ventricular function or severely impaired ventricular function with or without congenital heart abnormalities. Implantation of PPMs can usually be performed under sedation, with local anesthetic to cover the stimulation of vascular access and incision of the pocket for the device. Most PPMs have a right atrial and right ventricular lead, which are inserted through the subclavian, cephalic, or axillary veins. Leads are connected to the body of the device, which is then sewn into the subcutaneous pocket in the prepectoral space. Devices are preferentially placed on the side of the nondominant hand so as to minimize effects of its placement. In some instances, such as subpectoral placement or device planned, deeper sedation or general anesthesia is indicated. Prophylactic antibiotics are administered in device implantation.

ICD and biventricular pacemaker implantation As described in the "Indications" section for these devices, patients may have a significant history of ventricular arrhythmias, ischemic cardiomyopathies, and/or severely reduced ventricular function. The basic procedure is similar to the implantation of PPMs except a biventricular pacemaker has a third, "coronary sinus" lead. Placement of this lead can be difficult, thus increasing the length of the procedure. If general anesthesia is chosen, long-acting muscle relaxants should be avoided as mentioned earlier. The ICD is tested at the end of procedure by inducing ventricular tachyarrhythmia with "R on T" through a ventricular lead. Additional (2 sets) external defibrillator pads should be applied before the procedure as a backup in the event of device failure. During testing, sedation may be deepened with small intravenous boluses of propofol.

Catheter ablations Most catheter ablations are performed with moderate sedation and standard monitoring; however, they can be lengthy (many hours), and maintaining patient comfort and minimizing movement can be difficult. Excessive patient movement and exaggerated respiratory movement may result in poor catheter stability and unsuccessful ablation.[15] High-frequency jet ventilation has been successfully used under general anesthesia to improve the catheter stability and reduce the procedure time.[16] A temperature probe is placed to monitor the esophageal temperature to reduce the risk of injury to the esophagus. Heparin bolus followed by continuous infusion is used to maintain the ACT at greater than 300 to prevent thrombosis during left atrial instrumentation. Using the nasal airway to rescue the airway obstruction should be avoided to prevent excessive nasal bleeding.

During intracardiac mapping for ectopic foci, drugs that affect the sympathetic nervous system should be avoided if possible. During tachyarrhythmia induction, inotropic or vasoactive agents may become necessary to maintain hemodynamic stability.

Lead and/or device extractions Indications for lead and/or device extractions are infection, malfunctions, and device recalls. Device extractions should be performed in a traditional or hybrid operating room. The anesthesia provider should be familiar with various methods and potential complications, including vascular injury resulting in excessive bleeding, hemothorax, and/or cardiac tamponade. The capability of emergent cardiac surgery with cardiopulmonary bypass should be readily available.[5]

Electrical (direct-current) cardioversion With atrial fibrillation/flutter lasting longer than 48 hours, a transesophageal echocardiogram should be performed to confirm the absence of intracardiac thrombi before cardioversion; anticoagulation is required for at least 3 weeks before and 4 weeks after cardioversion.

POSTPROCEDURE CARE

Most electrophysiology procedures are performed on an outpatient basis, and the discharge criteria are no different from those for any other procedure involving sedation or general anesthesia. Short procedural time coupled with minimally invasive technique leads to lower required amounts of anesthetic medication, resulting in fewer anesthesia-related complications and a shorter recovery time. Still, patients with significant comorbidities warrant a more conservative approach to their care to reduce the risk of complications. The post-electrophysiology procedural care unit should have the same level of equipment as the post-anesthesia care unit. Patients should be monitored for rhythm, hemodynamics, and signs and symptoms of potential complications through the following:

- Vital signs (cardiac perforation/tamponade commonly manifest as hemodynamic instability)
- Airway patency
- Bilateral breath sound and chest radiograph (after subclavian access, for pneumothorax and/or hemothorax)
- Neurologic examination (for potential stroke or nerve injury)
- Access-site check (for bleeding, hematoma)
- Distal perfusion, pulse check
- Device pocket check (for bleeding, hematoma)
- Twelve-lead electrocardiogram (to evaluate rhythm, PPM function)
- Confirm device (PPM/ICD) function

AVOIDING COMPLICATIONS

The key to avoiding problems in the electrophysiology laboratory is understanding the underlying condition, procedures performed, and potential complications for each case. The remote location and unfamiliarity with the facility, equipment, and staff will aggravate the challenges to the anesthesia providers. Communication with the cardiologist and other staff in the electrophysiology laboratory is paramount.

Vascular access–related complications are frequently encountered (3%–4%).[17] The access site should be assessed immediately after the procedure, and evidence of hematoma, continued bleeding, impaired perfusion distal to the site, and neurologic injury requires immediate attention. The anesthesia provider should be informed of details regarding the closure technique and specific care instructions for the site, such as the duration of lying flat or pressure to be held, and communicate these to the post-anesthesia care unit nurse. If access was obtained in the chest or neck, the anesthesia provider should pay particular attention to evidence of pneumothorax or hemothorax. Oversedation, loss of airway, necessity of airway intervention, or conversion to general anesthesia is reported to occur in 40% of non–general anesthesia electrophysiology procedures.[18]

Specific Considerations

PPM and ICD placement

Most complications are related to vascular access (eg, bleeding, infection, hematoma, vascular injury, pneumothorax, and hemothorax) and the device pocket (eg, hematoma, infection, dehiscence). Rare complications include cardiac injury from perforation with tamponade, valvular damage, and lead dislodgement.

Biventricular pacemaker placement

Complications are similar to those of PPM/ICD placement. Because of the anatomy of the coronary sinus (CS), there is a risk for its dissection or perforation, which may result in significant hemodynamic instability. Careful attention should be given to volume status because patients undergoing this procedure have heart failure and a very limited ability to tolerate excessive volume load.

Catheter ablation

During the procedure, hemodynamically unstable arrhythmias or complete heart block requiring immediate therapy could be observed. In addition to the standard resuscitation drugs, various antiarrhythmic drugs should be readily available. Defibrillation/transcutaneous pacing pads should be applied before the procedure.

The most significant complications are thermal injury to the esophagus and the occurrence of an atrioesophageal fistula (0.01%–0.2%).[17,19] The use of an esophageal temperature probe is recommended to reduce the risk. Koruth and colleagues[20] described a case series involving the use of mechanical esophageal displacement guided by esophagogram to prevent the esophageal injury. This technique requires general anesthesia.

Cardiac perforation and tamponade occurs in less than 1% to 2% of cases.[17,19] Intracardiac echocardiography is useful to confirm the diagnosis. Immediate termination of the procedure, removal of the instruments from cardiac chambers followed by reversal of anticoagulation (eg, using protamine or factor VII and/or XI), and percutaneous pericardial drainage should be performed. Observation through transthoracic echocardiography should be performed to determine the necessity of open surgical repair.

The incidence of thromboembolism and stroke is rare but will increase with left heart instrumentation. ACT is targeted at greater than 300 seconds to decrease the risk. Valvular damage, endocarditis, pulmonary vein stenosis, and phrenic nerve injury are other major complications.

External cardioversion

External cardioversion can precipitate ventricular arrhythmias through delivering the shock on the ST segment or T wave. Transient myocardial depression, recurrent arrhythmia, thermal injury, and thromboembolisms are other potential complications. Providers should observe safety measures to prevent current passage to themselves.

RADIATION SAFETY

Radiation exposure to anesthesiologists doubled after electrophysiology laboratories were introduced.[21] Each anesthesia provider should have knowledge of the effect of ionized radiation and the concept of "as low as reasonably achieved" (ALARA),[22] which is attained by the following;

- Increased distance from the source
- Decreased exposure time
- Protection with maximum barriers with front and back coverage via a lead apron, a thyroid shield, and leaded glasses; stationary barriers, such as leaded glass between the radiation source and anesthesia provider, add additional protection.
- Requiring anesthesia providers who are frequently in the EP laboratory to wear a personal dosimeter.

SUMMARY

EP laboratory can present challenge to providing a safe anesthesia care because of physical barriers between patients and anesthesia provider, unfamiliar environment, remote location, and working with staff unfamiliar with anesthesia provider's needs. Although most procedure in EP laboratory can be performed with conscious sedation, patients and procedural factors will often warrant general anesthesia and anesthesiologists involvement. Importance of familiarizing to environment, equipment as well as understanding patient's condition, and procedures, and radiation safety should be emphasized.

REFERENCES

1. Gaitan BD, Trentman TL, Fassett SL, et al. Sedation and analgesia in the cardiac electrophysiology laboratory: a national survey of electrophysiologists investigating the who, how, and why? J Cardiothorac Vasc Anesth 2011;25:647–59.
2. O'Neill DK, Aizer A, Linton P, et al. Isoproterenol infusion increases level of consciousness during catheter ablation of atrial fibrillation. J Interv Card Electrophysiol 2012;34:137–42.
3. Standards for Basic Anesthetic Monitoring (Effective July 1, 2011). American Society of Anesthesiologists Web site. Available at: http://www.Asahq.org/For-Members/Standards-Guidelines-andStatements.aspx. Accessed November 30, 2012.
4. Perzanowski C, Teplitsky L, Hranitzky P, et al. Real-time monitoring of luminal esophageal temperature during left atrial radiofrequency catheter ablation at the pulmonary fibrillation: observations about esophageal heating during ablation at the pulmonary vein ostia and posterior left atrium. J Cardiovasc Electrophysiol 2006;17:166–70.
5. Elsik M, Fynn S. Permanent pacemakers and implantable defibrillators. In: Mackay JH, Arrowsmith JE, editors. Core topics in cardiac anesthesia. 2nd edition. Cambridge (England): Cambridge University Press; 2012. p. 241–8.
6. Saxon LA, DeMarco T. Cardiac resynchronization therapy in heart failure: indications. UpToDate Web site. Available at: http://www.uptodate.com/contents/cardiac-resynchronization-therapy-in-heart-failure-indications?source=search_result&search=Cardiac+resynchronization+therapy+in+heart+failure&selected Title=1%7E150. Accessed October 23, 2012.
7. Epstein AE, DiMarco JP, Ellenbogen KA, et al. ACC/AHA/HRS 2008 guidelines for device-based therapy of cardiac rhythm abnormalities: a report on the American College of Cardiology/American Heart Association Task Force on Practice Guidelines. Circulation 2008;117:e350–408.
8. Di Biase L, Conti S, Mohanty P, et al. General anesthesia reduces the prevalence of pulmonary vein reconnection during repeat ablation when compared with conscious sedation: results from a randomized study. Heart Rhythm 2011;8:368–72.
9. Caldwell JC, Fong C, Muhyaldeen SA. Should sevoflurane be used in the electrophysiology assessment of accessory pathways? Europace 2010;12:1332–5.
10. Richardson AJ, Pierce JM. Anesthesia and electrophysiological disorders. In: Mackay JH, Arrowsmith JE, editors. Core topics in cardiac anesthesia. 2nd edition. Cambridge (England): Cambridge University Press; 2012. p. 249–56.
11. Fujii K, Iranami H, Nakamura Y, et al. Fentanyl added to propofol anesthesia elongates node recovery time in pediatric patients with paroxysmal supraventricular tachycardia. Anesth Analg 2009;108:456–60.
12. Niksch A, Liberman L, Clapcich A, et al. Effects of remifentanil anesthesia on cardiac electrophysiologic properties in children undergoing catheter ablation of supraventricular tachycardia. Pediatr Cardiol 2010;31:1079–82.
13. Hammer GB, Drover DR, Cao H, et al. The effect of dexmedetomidine on cardiac electrophysiology in children. Anesth Analg 2008;106:79–83.
14. Shook DC, Savage RM. Anesthesia in the cardiac catheterization laboratory and electrophysiology laboratory. Anesthesiol Clin 2009;27:47–56.
15. Kumar S, Morton JB, Halloran K, et al. Effect of respiration on catheter-tissue contact force during ablation of atrial arrhythmias. Heart Rhythm 2012;9:1041–7.

16. Elkassabany N, Garcia F, Tschabrunn C, et al. Anesthetic management of patients undergoing pulmonary vein isolation for treatment of atrial fibrillation using high-frequency jet ventilation. J Cardiothorac Vasc Anesth 2012;26:433–8.
17. Patel KD, Crowley R, Mahajan A. Cardiac electrophysiology procedures in clinical practice. Int Anesthesiol Clin 2012;50:90–110.
18. Trentman TL, Fassett SL, Mueller JT, et al. Airway intervention in the cardiac electrophysiology laboratory: a retrospective review. J Cardiothorac Vasc Anesth 2009;23:841–5.
19. Dagres N, Hindricks G, Bode K, et al. Complications of atrial fibrillation ablation in a high-volume center in 1,000 procedures: still cause for concern? J Cardiovasc Electrophysiol 2009;20:1014–9.
20. Koruth JS, Reddy VY, Miller MA, et al. Mechanical esophageal displacement during catheter ablation for atrial fibrillation. J Cardiovasc Electrophysiol 2012;23:147–54.
21. Katz JD. Radiation exposure to anesthesia personnel: the impact of an electrophysiology laboratory. Anesth Analg 2005;101:1725–6.
22. Phillips G, Monaghan WP. Radiation safety for anesthesia providers. AANA J 2011;79:257–67.

Index

Note: Page numbers of article titles are in **boldface** type.

A

Anesthesiology Clin 31 (2013) 491–503
http://dx.doi.org/10.1016/S1932-2275(13)00024-4
1932-2275/13/$ – see front matter © 2013 Elsevier Inc. All rights reserved.

Moving?

Make sure your subscription moves with you!

To notify us of your new address, find your **Clinics Account Number** (located on your mailing label above your name), and contact customer service at:

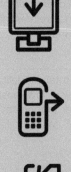

Email: journalscustomerservice-usa@elsevier.com

800-654-2452 (subscribers in the U.S. & Canada)
314-447-8871 (subscribers outside of the U.S. & Canada)

Fax number: 314-447-8029

Elsevier Health Sciences Division
Subscription Customer Service
3251 Riverport Lane
Maryland Heights, MO 63043

*To ensure uninterrupted delivery of your subscription, please notify us at least 4 weeks in advance of move.

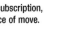

Printed and bound by CPI Group (UK) Ltd, Croydon, CR0 4YY

03/10/2024

01040442-0010